RELIGION AND CULTURE IN THE MIDDLE AGES

Soul-Health

Series Editors
Denis Renevey (Université de Lausanne)
Diane Watt (University of Surrey)

Editorial Board
Miri Rubin (Queen Mary University of London)
Jean-Claude Schmitt (École des Hautes Études en Sciences Sociales, Paris)
Fiona Somerset (Duke University)
Christiania Whitehead (University of Warwick)

RELIGION AND CULTURE IN THE MIDDLE AGES

Soul-Health

THERAPEUTIC READING IN LATER MEDIEVAL ENGLAND

DANIEL McCANN

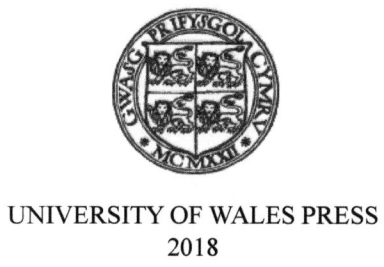

UNIVERSITY OF WALES PRESS
2018

© Daniel McCann, 2018

All rights reserved. No part of this book may be reproduced in any material form (including photocopying or storing it in any medium by electronic means and whether or not transiently or incidentally to some other use of this publication) without the written permission of the copyright owner except in accordance with the provisions of the Copyright, Designs and Patents Act. Applications for the copyright owner's written permission to reproduce any part of this publication should be addressed to University of Wales Press, University Registry, King Edward VII Avenue, Cardiff CF10 3NS.

www.uwp.co.uk

British Library Cataloguing-in-Publication Data
A catalogue record for this book is available from the British Library.

ISBN   978-1-78683-331-0
e-ISBN   978-1-78683-332-7

The right of Daniel McCann to be identified as author of this work has been asserted in accordance with sections 77 and 79 of the Copyright, Designs and Patents Act 1988.

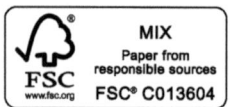

Typeset by Eira Fenn Gaunt, Pentyrch, Cardiff
Printed by CPI Antony Rowe, Melksham, Wiltshire

Contents

Series Editors' Preface   vii
Acknowledgements   ix
Abbreviations   xi
Note on Editions and Translations   xiii

Introduction: *Cura Animarum*   1

1   Apprehensive Medicine   27

2   Lyrical Treatment   51

3   Compassionate Healing   81

4   Longing for Health   111

5   Dangerous Reading   133

Conclusion: Sowle-hele   153

Notes   159
Select Bibliography   179
Index   189

Series Editors' Preface

Religion and Culture in the Middle Ages aims to explore the interface between medieval religion and culture, with as broad an understanding of those terms as possible. It puts to the forefront studies which engage with works that significantly contributed to the shaping of medieval culture. However, it also gives attention to studies dealing with works that reflect and highlight aspects of medieval culture that have been neglected in the past by scholars of the medieval disciplines. For example, devotional works and the practice they infer illuminate our understanding of the medieval subject and its culture in remarkable ways, while studies of the material space designed and inhabited by medieval subjects yield new evidence on the period and the people who shaped it and lived in it. In the larger field of religion and culture, we also want to explore further the roles played by women as authors, readers and owners of books, thereby defining them more precisely as actors in the cultural field. The series as a whole investigates the European Middle Ages, from *c.*500 to *c.*1500. Our aim is to explore medieval religion and culture with the tools belonging to such disciplines as, among others, art history, philosophy, theology, history, musicology, the history of medicine, and literature. In particular, we would like to promote interdisciplinary studies, as we believe strongly that our modern understanding of the term applies fascinatingly well to a cultural period marked by a less tight confinement and categorization of its disciplines than the modern period. However, our only criterion is academic excellence, with the belief that the use of a large diversity of critical tools and theoretical approaches enables a deeper understanding of medieval culture. We want the series to reflect this diversity, as we believe that, as a collection of outstanding contributions, it offers a more subtle representation of a period that is marked by paradoxes and contradictions and which necessarily reflects diversity and difference, however difficult it may sometimes have proved for medieval culture to accept these notions.

Acknowledgements

This book is the result of my postdoctoral research fellowship, generously funded by the Leverhulme Trust. I thank them for their crucial assistance; without it this book and my chance of an academic career would not have been possible. Since 2012, the University of Oxford has been a home for me, and this book has benefited enormously from that institution and the vast resources and expertise it holds. In that respect it is a book born out of many interactions and conversations, and so I owe thanks to my colleagues and friends here. Such support came to me in the form of Freya Johnston at St Anne's College, Edward Wilson from Worcester College, and Timothy Michael from Lincoln College: thank you all for your patient support and advice. I owe particular thanks to a number of the medievalists I met here: Mishtooni Bose, Kantik Ghosh, Laura Ashe, Marion Turner, Annie Sutherland, Philip Knox, Anya Adair, Kylie Murray, John C. Hirsh and Andy Orchard. Each has provided me with stimulating discussion, raucous wit and unique professional examples. Time is a more precious resource than anything else and my colleagues here have been extremely generous with theirs. For that I am truly grateful.

I owe especial thanks to a number of other medievalists. Mary Carruthers and Peregrine Horden have been two constant sources of support and encouragement, and I am very grateful for the time and attention each has given me since I came to Oxford and before that time. Also, Giuseppe Pezzini deserves a special commendation for spending his time (and patience) in teaching me Latin. Denis Renevey also deserves particular thanks, and he has been extremely generous with his time, expertise and advice. John Thompson and Malcolm Andrew also deserve thanks as my early mentors, as they encouraged me to develop into a medievalist, and made the majority of time at Queen's University Belfast stimulating and enjoyable. Sr Maggie Ross has been a constant source of spiritual and intellectual advice, and I always enjoy our coffees together. The greatest debt of gratitude, however, is to Vincent Gillespie. I first met him in the form of my external examiner, and after a robust viva he has become both my mentor and my friend. His depth of knowledge is matched only by his generosity and scholarly humility, and he has always offered me his time, attention and advice. This book is, in many ways, the result of our conversations and the comments he made on early drafts. I am, and will always be, extremely grateful to him and the example he has given me.

Finally, I owe my dear wife Kathrin and my darling daughter Eloise a great deal of thanks. They have proved infinitely patient and kind with the grumpy man writing makes of me. Kathrin has been a constant source of support, encouragement, wisdom and love; and Eloise has been an inexhaustible source of joy. I dedicate this book to them, though no words can ever express the profound gratitude I feel for them and their love. Danke meine Lieben!

Abbreviations

EETS Early English Text Society (1864–)
 O. S. Original Series (1864–)
 E. S. Extra Series (1867–1920s)
 S. Supplementary Series (1970–)

MED *Middle English Dictionary*, ed. Hans Kurath and S. M. Kuhn (Ann Arbor: University of Michigan Press; London: Oxford University Press, 1952–) Online Version (Michigan, December 2001): *http://quod.lib.umich.edu/m/med/*

PL *Patrologia cursus completus series Latina*, ed. J. P. Migne, 221 vols (Paris: Garnier Frères, 1844–1905).

PG *Patrologia cursus completus series Graeca*, ed. J. P. Migne, 161 vols (Paris: Garnier Frères, 1857–1905).

Note on Editions and Translations

Due to considerations of space, frequently cited editions of Middle English texts are given full references here on a per-chapter basis, with the specified short forms used for the rest of the book. All quotations are taken from the following editions:

I: The Speculum Vitae and The Prick of Conscience
Ralph Hanna (ed.), *Speculum Vitae: A Reading Edition*, EETS O. S. 331 (Oxford: Oxford University Press, 2008). Hereafter: *SV.*

Ralph Hanna and Sarah Wood (eds), *Richard Morris's Prick of Conscience: A Corrected and Amplified Reading Text*, EETS O. S. 342 (Oxford: Oxford University Press, 2013). Hereafter: *PoC.*

II: The Penitential Psalms
Valerie Edden (ed.), *Richard Maidstone's Penitential Psalms: Edited from Bodleian MS Rawlinson A.389* (Heidelberg: Carl Winter, 1990). Hereafter: *MPP.*

III: The Prickynge of Love
Harold Kane (ed.) *The Prickynge of Love*, 2 vols (Salzburg: Institut für Anglistik und Amerikanistik der Universität Salzburg, 1983). Hereafter: *Prickynge*. Punctuation has been modernised.

IV: A Talking of the Love of God
Salvina Westra (ed.), *A Talking of the Love of God* (The Hague: Martinus Nijhoff, 1950). Hereafter: *Talking*. Punctuation has been modernised.

V: The Chastising of God's Children
Joyce Bazire and Eric Colledge (eds), *The Chastising of God's Children, and The Treatise of Perfection of The Sons of God* (Oxford: Basil Blackwell, 1957). Hereafter: *Chastising*.

VI: Works of Walter Hilton, the Cloud-author, and Julian of Norwich
Thomas H. Bestul (ed.), *The Scale of Perfection* (Kalamazoo, Michigan: Medieval Institute Publications, 2000). Hereafter: *Scale*.

Fumio Kuriyagawa (ed.), *Walter Hilton's Eight Chapters on Perfection* (Tokyo: Keio University, 1967). Hereafter: *Eight Chapters on Perfection*.

Carl Horstmann (ed.), *Of Angels Song*, in *Yorkshire Writers: Richard Rolle of Hampole, an English Father of the Church, and His Followers*, 2 vols (London: Swan Sonnenschein, 1895–96), vol. 1, pp. 175–82. Hereafter: *Angels Song*.

Carl Horstmann (ed.), *Epistle on the Mixed Life*, in *Yorkshire Writers: Richard Rolle of Hampole, an English Father of the Church, and His Followers*, 2 vols (London: Swan Sonnenschein, 1895–96), vol. 1, pp. 264–92. Hereafter: *Mixed Life*.

Phyllis Hodgson (ed.), *The Cloud of Unknowing and The Book of Privy Counselling*, EETS, O. S. 218 (London: Oxford University Press, 1944). Hereafter: *Cloud*.

A Tretyse of þe Stodye of Wysdome þat Men Clepen Beniamyn; *A Pistle of Preier*; *A Pistle of Discrecioun of Stirings*; and *A Treatise of Discrescyon of Spirites* are all in Phyllis Hodgson (ed.), *Deonise hid Divinite and Other Treatises on Contemplative Prayer related to The Cloud of Unknowing*, EETS O. S. 231 (London: Oxford University Press, 1955). Hereafter: *Stodye*; *Pistle*; *Discrecioun of Stirings*; *Discrescyon of Spirites*.

Julian of Norwich: A Revelation of Love, ed. Marion Glasscoe (Exeter: University of Exeter Press, 1976). Hereafter: *Revelation*.

Translations
Translations from the Latin, unless otherwise noted, have been prepared with the kind expertise of Dr Giuseppe Pezzini. Any errors remain my own.

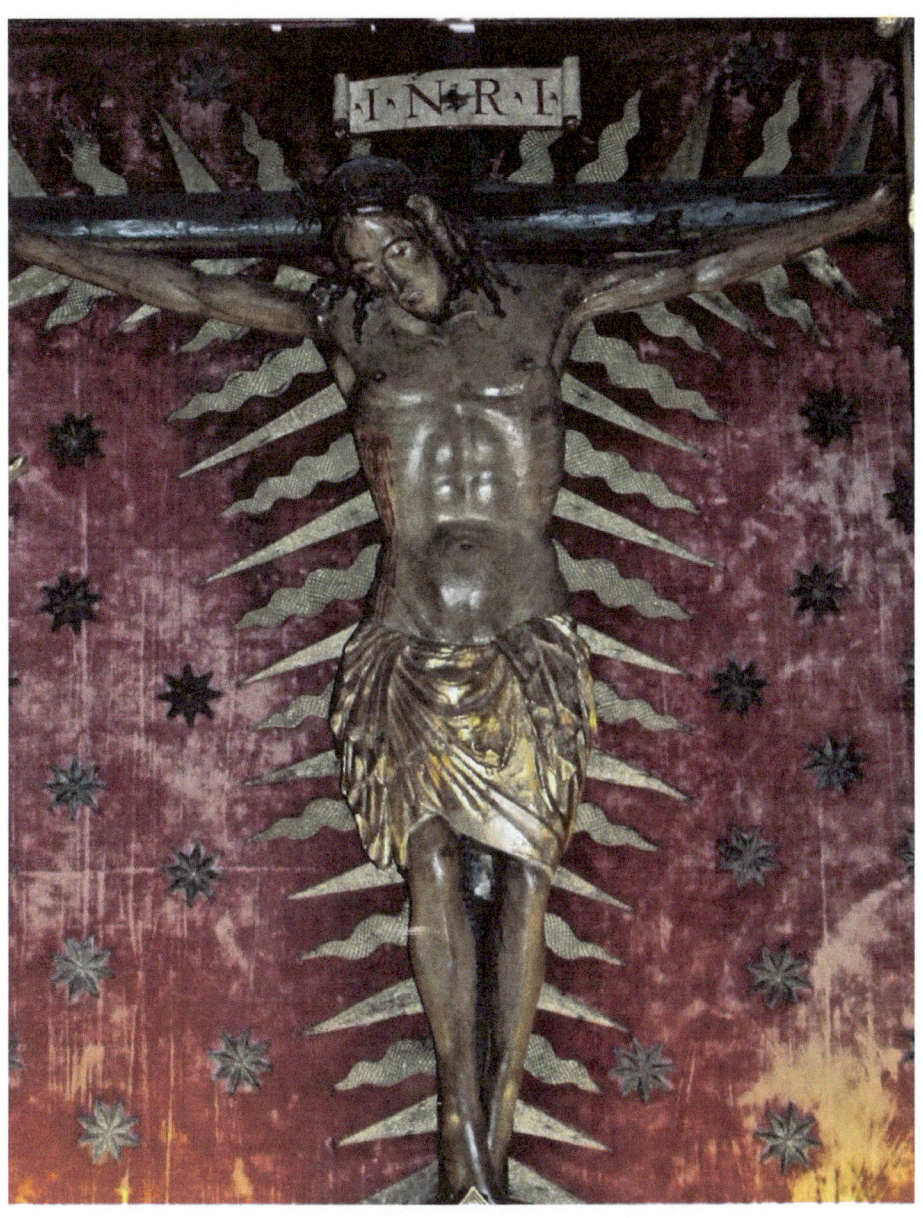

Figure 1 Christ on the Cross – San Marcello al Corso (*c*.1440s). The photograph is by Mr Edoardo Fanfani, who has kindly given permission to use it.

Introduction: *Cura Animarum*

The wooden and gold-dusted crucifix that hangs in the Italian Church of San Marcello al Corso has a fascinating history that combines passion with plague as much as health with harm (Figure 1). A product of the fourteenth-century Sienese school of art, this crucifix is the miraculous survivor of a fire which destroyed the whole Church in 1519. Such durability soon proved providential. In 1522 the inhabitants of Rome faced that most perennial of medieval threats: an outbreak of the pestilence or plague. It was a fairly widespread occurrence in Italy, and captivated the contemporary imagination so much so that many held the current Pope, Adrian VI, responsible for it. While many fled the city, many did not. Those who remained decided to take action rather than wait to succumb to the ravages of the plague. They took the bold move of holding a penitential procession through the city with the miraculous Cross of San Marcello. The result was yet further proof of the crucifix's power, as the plague was lifted from the city and eventually Italy. This crucifix, held to be the most realistic depiction of Christ's agony in all of Italy at the time, evoked penance and compassion within the crowds – emotions which proved powerful enough to dispel the plague. Yet, as with all intense emotions evoked by religious artefacts, there are darker tones and hues to the history of this crucifix and its healing potential.[1]

A disturbing rumour wreathes its origins. It was believed that the sculptor of the crucifix, in order to achieve the most authentic depiction of Christ's agony as possible, abducted a peasant charcoal burner and slowly killed him. The man's final sufferings were supposedly sketched in detail by the sculptor, and used as the visual template for the figure on the crucifix itself. While most likely a legend designed to enhance the fame of the artefact, it is nevertheless part of its social history: passion and plague, health and harm, devotion and death all come together here in the story of this crucifix. It works, therefore, to illustrate not only the complex interconnection between religious emotions and premodern ideas of healing, but also the often disturbing intensity of religious emotions themselves. As such, it serves as an excellent introductory anecdote for the central concern of this book: that the health of the soul can be obtained by reading texts which evoke only the most difficult and dangerous of passions. Thus, this is a book about reading, about the psychology of literary response, and about precisely how texts can evoke and manipulate emotions to create the state termed *salus animae* – the health of the soul. It is also a book about later medieval religious cultures, specifically those in medieval England which placed emphasis upon the medical treatment of the soul, its need for urgent healing and reformation, and the literary means of affecting it.

In terms of medical and theological knowledge, medieval England does not exist in splendid isolation. The more advanced university medicine from Italy and France does make its way to England, often through continental physicians receiving noble patronage and/or ecclesiastical benefices in the fourteenth century.[2] Moreover, medical and religious discourses continued to overlap and interconnect in the vernacular, so that the idea of spiritual health 'becomes a potent metaphor for both religious and the laity'.[3] What is distinctly English, however, is the focus on practicalities and pastoral care.[4] From the twelfth to the fifteenth centuries, theology in England 'continued to be seen as a practical science, which could be applied and diffused through sermons' and other means in the vernacular.[5] This can be seen most clearly in the Middle English texts which offer spiritual medicine/therapeutics: they are distillations of earlier theological knowledge on the emotional treatment of the soul designed for practical application in the work of pastoral care.

This book seeks to understand how texts of religious instruction and guidance offered their readers – both clerical and lay – modes of emotional stimulation to enable the health of the soul. While the book will focus on late medieval England and its rich treasure trove of beautiful and intense religious texts in the vernacular, its range will be far broader than that. Medieval medicine, medieval psychology, the arts of rhetoric and grammar, and of course the cultural impacts of medieval theology, will all be marshalled to explore this most fascinating aspect of the *cura animarum* – the treatment of the soul through a 'medicyne of words', through texts of passion.[6] As a result of this focus, the book contributes to a series of ongoing scholarly debates. First and foremost, it engages with the burgeoning field of medical humanities, which has received a great deal of recent interest and expansion.[7] A movement away from simple medical history to a more interdisciplinary and nuanced engagement with the cultural and social diffusion of medical knowledge continues to gather momentum. This book, as part of that field, seeks to explore the connection between literature, medicine and theology in the medieval period. In this way it is distinct from the important work of Glending Olson, whose *Literature as Recreation* explored the therapeutic aspects of reading in the Middle Ages. That book focused on the hygienic justification of literature in the period, and on the therapeutic potential of specific genres.[8] While an inspirational and interdisciplinary book, it did not address medieval religious texts in detail, nor texts which evoke 'depressive' emotional states – joy and laughter were its focus, not pain, penance or suffering. Later, Brian Stock offered something of a remedy to this, and addressed in a series of articles the medical significance of meditation in the history of reading.[9] Though his work noted the potential dangers of meditation in the *lectio divina*, it focused on it in a general sense, not specifically on medieval English vernacular religious texts that were read in similar ways.

The present book will explore these aspects directly, and aims to further our understanding of the therapeutic aspects of religious texts. In so doing it will also engage with the connection between literature and emotion, and the so-called 'affective turn' in medieval studies. The literature on these topics is vast, but the central issue is one of definition. Affect, emotion and passion are all terms that have been used in different ways and contexts.[10] Each term carries different nuances and disciplinary resonances, be they medical, neurological, psychopathological, or socio-cultural. The most dominant in recent years has been the term 'affect'. Its popularity in the social sciences hardly needs any summary, but what does need clarification is the epistemological assumption of that term. Affect in this context often incorporates the perspectives of the natural sciences, specifically neuroscience, and as such it signifies an essentialist and biological model of the emotions.[11] While this is of course interesting, there are consequences: affect in this sense posits something that is inherent in human beings and, to an extent, not subject to historical or cultural change.

This is not the case in the medieval period: while medieval thinkers of course saw emotion as biological, or more accurately as inherent, their engagements with the emotional aspects of humanity were constantly revised, adapted, and re-modelled in accordance with (or reaction to) Christian, medical and philosophical discourses. In theory and in practice, emotions were understood in the medieval period through a complex network of interconnected and embedded 'explanatory models of reality'.[12] As such, the concept of the emotions was inherently interdisciplinary, and so inherently subject to discursive framing, and thus discursive change: frameworks mediate the passions, and frameworks change in time. This key factor has been acknowledged in recent work on the subject of the emotions.[13] As always, the devil is in the detail: the frameworks applied to the passions are contextual, and changing, and at the same time there is a sense that the passions are not simply socially constructed, but rather that they are both innate and changing.[14]

Complicating matters is the complexity of context: the medieval terms for emotions are varied, and include terms such as *motus animae, perturbatio, affectus, passio, inclinatio, accidentia animae*. Each term can have precise meanings relative to the overarching theological, philosophical or medical works in which each occurs; and some of them can be used as more general terms for a range of bio-psycho-socio phenomena. As a result, using passions is also problematic, as it can lack a certain terminological precision and – as Knuutila notes – is all too easily conflated with the modern usage of passion, meaning intense emotion.[15] While intense feeling is key to this book, a term is needed that can delineate various aspects of intense feelings in relation to texts while still being sufficiently flexible to incorporate specific medical or theological meanings. Emotion is the term it shall use. Despite its anachronistic nature, it is, as others note, a sufficiently capacious term that permits both a greater depth of analysis, and more comparative engagements across genres and texts. It is also more psychologically rich, and 'refers to a phenomenon that is both cognitive and affective – an idea that has always been present in medieval reflections on affectivity'.[16] It is the emotions that religious texts seek to evoke in order to treat the soul, and this book will speak of them in that way. As such, this book is concerned not with the social construction of the emotions, nor of their individual expression *per se*, but rather with how medieval texts were understood to evoke passionate states within the souls of their readers.

In this way, the book is part of the ongoing interest in psychological issues in medieval literary studies. Here too, as elsewhere, the popularity of the 'affective turn' is evident, and is most strongly developed in relation to Middle English religious, devotional, and mystical texts. The work on medieval religious texts and subjectivity by Vincent Gillespie, Alistair Minnis and William Pollard generated new perspectives and influential critical terminologies, while making the case for the importance of the psychological in matters of literary response and its affective impact.[17] Denis Renevey and Nicholas Watson's monographs on Richard Rolle highlighted the complexity of the '*affectus*' in what can loosely be termed 'mystical writing', and the ways in which Middle English authors engaged – and transformed – antecedent Latin material on the powers and passions of the soul.[18]

In recent years the work of Jennifer Bryan on medieval selfhood and its relation to religious writing, and Michelle Karnes's work on the role of imagination in meditative texts, have offered new insights into the connections between literary texts and premodern psychologies.[19] Focusing specifically on affect and reading, Mark Amsler offers an account of the constitutive relationship between text and reader. His idea of 'affective literacy' argues that reading texts constitutes a psychologically formative process that engages the senses as well as the psychology of the reader.[20] In a similar way, Ayoush Lazikani notes that twelfth-century religious texts offer moments of 'co-feeling' – that they aim to stir emotion, to 'introduce new modes of feeling' but that they are ultimately 'dependent on the affective capacities of readers and audiences'.[21] Her work responds to Sarah McNamer and the whole concept of 'affective scripts'.[22] For McNamer, texts designed to evoke affect are 'intimate scripts' that the reader essentially performs. Her work relies to some extent on William Reddy's conception of 'emotives' – first-person utterances that are often performative – and the performance theory of Judith Butler. Her overall thesis posits that certain lyrical texts can evoke affect and enable a composite affect/identity performance. In a later publication she revisits aspects of this model, adding some additional detail and expanding its applicability to a wider range of literary texts.[23] Her central contention is that medieval studies ought to embrace 'a broad understanding of emotion as practice, as performance, as process – always in some sense in the making and open to inflection by culture'.[24] Citing Boyd's work on the role of literature in psychological development, she asserts that such 'affective scripts' can offer models of behavioural, cognitive and affective possibility that a reader can develop, augment or resist in the hermeneutic engagement with a text.[25]

It is an important contribution to the field; however, the theoretical model lacks sufficient capacity: many texts from the period are evocative of the emotions without having a first-person narrator, or a clear sense of their performative character. Rarely do medieval texts concern themselves with a single emotion; rather, many of them are involved in evoking a more complex and layered state of emotional response: joy with fear, horror with hope, and love with hate. Performance theory does not offer sufficient purchase on texts that are designed to evoke not only contrasting states of emotional response, but also of perspective and identity. Many of the texts this book will explore seek to encourage not so much a subjectivity, but an intersubjective modality of self-awareness – one predicated upon strong feelings. Many penitential or Passion lyrics are not concerned with just one emotion, nor one perspective: the reader is encouraged, almost simultaneously, to view a scene of agony and suffering from the narrator's perspective, from Christ's, from His Mother's – from a position that is concerned with the interrelationship between people and emotions.[26] While the term 'affective script' is useful, one weakness is that it can contain a certain element of the philosophy of suspicion – a sense that there is something inauthentic, unreal or disingenuously dramatic, about emotional response elicited through reading. Texts which aim to make their readers feel a certain way are no more cynical than those very readers, and are concerned not so much with 'scripting' emotional response as with providing models of possibility – with possible feelings, possible moments and possible selves, all blended together. Emotion is as much a part of the ontological emergence and development of the person as any other, and texts which aim to evoke emotions are thus also engaged in altering and shaping selfhood in other, more nuanced, ways.

Ultimately, McNamer's model seeks to attend to 'the illumination of the *hows* of affective history'– with how texts 'script' emotional response.[27] Such a goal is admirable, but it is not achievable through this particular method. As Carruthers notes, 'works of art do not just simulate or represent human feelings but *produce* them in those who are experiencing the work'.[28] Production is the key word here, and the texts this book will explore are concerned with producing specific emotions – a goal that is intimately connected to the formal lineaments of their composition. The term affective scripts, by its very nature, generalises formal and compositional aspects, homogenising the distinctive forms, genres and structures of medieval texts into an undifferentiated mass. It ignores the medieval period's own fascinating ideas of precisely *how* texts work to evoke emotion – ideas which can greatly enhance literary analysis. This book will, therefore, approach texts that extoll their medicinal potential not as 'scripts', but as *compositions* which work to *compose* a psychological state within their readers – as carefully crafted assemblages of rhetorical form, vivid imagery and grammatical structure designed to evoke emotions intense enough to enable *salus animae*, or the health of the soul. To that end, it will focus on the pre-eminent example of a 'medicyne of words', the Vernon manuscript. This enormous manuscript, roughly datable to the 1390s, contains a vast number of distinct religious texts in both Middle English and Anglo-Norman. It covers an impressive range of devotional and spiritual writings popular throughout the period: items such as the *South English Legendary* (altered here to be more suited to private reading) and *Ancrene Wisse*, sit alongside Richard Rolle's *Ego Dormio*, Walter Hilton's *Scale of Perfection*, even the more traditionally pastoral A-text of *Piers Plowman*, and a selection of religious lyrics. Such diversity in material suggests that the manuscript was intended for the 'encouragement of inward devotion in persons of various needs and capacities who could at least read the texts'.[29] Significantly, it has an 'index' appended to it later, which aids the reader in navigating its expansive contents – essentially reconfiguring it for more casual consultation. Despite the range of material it contains, the index and the incipit of the manuscript nevertheless suggest an overall function: to evoke *salus animae*. Indeed, from its opening, the manuscript states a single and fascinating therapeutic purpose: to provide, through the emotive power of its contents, 'in latyn tonge Salus anime and in englyhs tonge Sowle-hele'.[30]

Medicine of Words

The phrase 'medicyne of words' was coined by Richard Rolle, a fourteenth-century English hermit who, it can be said with some certainty, was not a medical doctor. Yet, this fact often results in a form of critical misapprehension which views Rolle's use of medical language as simply rhetorical ornament or flourish. As this book will show, when Rolle asserts that his Psalter commentary is a 'medicyne of words', he is not being arch or superficially clever. Rather, he is drawing upon widespread cultural understandings regarding the very definition of health, and the medicinal potential of the act of reading itself. Therapy comes in many forms, and is here figured by Rolle as a textually mediated treatment of emotional extremes: to read the Psalter will cause the reader to oscillate between emotional states, 'to forthink synne with teres, now hyghtand ioy'.[31] It is, of course, an understanding of reading common to the entire historical period and to medieval England in particular. As Vernon's incipit makes clear, it is concerned with *salus animae*, with the connection between the health of the soul and its own textual contents. The concept of health is, therefore, one of far greater complexity throughout the Middle Ages, and is not distinct from religious connotations.[32] This is clear lexically, as the Latin word for health – *salus* – can also mean salvation. The word's interesting semantic range unites what modern culture would consider the conceptually distinct domains of religion and medicine. So too the word therapy, coming from the Greek *therapeutes*, means 'active worshipper' as well as treatment.[33]

As a cultural concept, 'treatment' is more broadly conceived in premodern cultures and includes biological, psychological and social factors that go above and beyond modern understandings of biomedical efficacy.[34] The idea of 'sowle-hele', therefore, bears witness to this interconnection and complexity, and is a valid concept ultimately derived from Ancient and Classical philosophy. Plato's *Timaeus* considers who provides superior treatment – those who provide for the health of the body (physicians) or those who provide for the health of the soul (philosophers).[35] Thus, when Rolle asserts the efficacy of his medicine of words, or when Vernon makes the claim that its contents can promote the health of the soul, both make a deliberate and culturally normative connection between reading and healing. Throughout the literature of the period, this connection that can be found time and again. As medieval medicine attests, reading can heal. Initially, its benefits were confined to the physical aspects of the body and its digestive processes. In the *De Medicina* of Aurelius Cornelius Celsus (*c*.AD 50), the act of reading – *lectio* – could be used to treat a range of bodily conditions. It can do so because it constitutes a form of physical exercise:

> Now the chief means of preserving [health] is exercise, which ought always to precede a meal, more severe with him who has been studying less hard, and whose concoction is perfect; gentle with him who is exhausted, and who has concocted but in part. Reading aloud, martial weapons, the ball, running and walking, are means of exercise convenient enough.[36]

To read is to exert oneself, as the activity makes specifically physiological demands upon the body. This is possible because reading is understood here as a vocal rather than sub-vocal activity: *lectio* is here the *clara lectio* – or reading aloud. Such an activity naturally requires exertion of breadth and body, making the lungs work harder, and necessitating that the body adopts a firm posture. In this way it is seen as the therapeutic equivalent of a range of more conventionally familiar exercises such as running and walking. Given the physical requirements of *clara lectio*, it will impact the body directly. Here the main benefit is aiding digestion. The word 'concoction' has a specific medical meaning and refers to 'the action of the innate heat of the body in "cooking" food or morbific matter, permitting its digestion'.[37] Reading aloud, along with the other forms of physical exercise mentioned here, aids digestive processes in persons with optimal or less than optimal natural heat. As a form of exercise, reading can thus engage with the natural heat in the body and augment it for maximum digestive benefit. Celsus later notes the wider therapeutic impact of reading upon digestion: 'he whose stomach is infirm, ought to read aloud and walk' after eating a meal.³⁸ Conversely, he also notes that persons who suffer from 'gravedoes' – head colds or nasal catarrh – should avoid 'reading after food' due to its ability to manipulate the body's natural heat.³⁹ Thus, reading aloud constitutes a regimental treatment that one practises as a part of daily life before eating.

Later, Galenic medicine would augment the very idea of regimen itself, situating it within the more expansive theoretical medical framework offered by the *res non-naturales* – or non-natural things.⁴⁰ This framework is transmitted by Johannitius's *Isagoge ad Techne Galieni* – the Latin translation of an Arabic synopsis of various passages of Galen and Hippocrates. It had an enduring appeal throughout the period, and was translated many times. The framework itself consists of six 'things' which refer not to the body and its organs, but rather to broadly conceived personal and environmental factors. When regulated with precision and care, these factors help ensure that the humours of the body are kept in balance or *eucrasia*. This state promotes good and lasting health for as long as the regimen is maintained. Taken together, these factors deal with a wide range of human activities, concerning the air and the environment, eating and drinking, exercise and rest, sleeping and waking, evacuation and repletion, and the passions of the soul.⁴¹ In this schema reading aloud falls under the second non-natural as one of many forms of physical exercise. This understanding of the medical potential of *lectio* continued through Antiquity and into the Middle Ages, and was very common in monastic circles.⁴²

Beyond exercise, reading aloud possesses an extended therapeutic potential by being able to promote health through manipulating the sixth non-natural: the passions of the soul – the emotions. Such an understanding is a persistent medieval one, and is witnessed in the widespread and influential Middle English translations of the *Regimen sanitatis salernitanum*. This text, called the *Secretum Secretorum*, notes that reading 'delectabil bookis' is an excellent form of therapy, as it is 'bettir for helth and digestion if þe man haue ioy and gladnes'.⁴³ Reading for pleasure thus has health benefits, as it can restore balance to the passions of the soul and by extension promote harmony within the body.⁴⁴ Medieval medicine was clear on the psychosomatic impacts of emotion:

> Some incidental states of the soul have an effect on the body, such as those which bring the natural heat from the interior of the body to the surface of the skin. Sometimes this happens suddenly, as with anger; sometimes gradually and agreeably, as with sensations of delight. Some affections, again, contract and suppress the natural heat – either suddenly, as with fear and terror, or gradually, as with anguish. There are some which disturb the natural energy both in the interior of the body and on the exterior, for instance, sorrow.⁴⁵

Emotional disturbances are also physical disturbances. Certain passions of the soul can cause profound changes in the body's internal balance of heat and fluids, and so by extension can change its overall humoral balance, thereby increasing the likelihood of disease. Fear, sorrow and terror are seen here as generating less desirable physiological impacts. If experienced frequently, these emotions and their physiological impacts can become habituated within the body, and potentially permanent.

Over time the emotions are incorporated within a more detailed classificatory schema. In his influential *Liber de anima seu sextus de naturalibus*, Avicenna (*d*.1037) connects the main emotions to specific motive powers within the soul. They are two in number – the concupiscible and irascible powers.⁴⁶ He notes that 'fear, pain, and distress belong to the accidents of the irascible power through the communion of the apprehensive powers, for when they are moved as a consequence of an intelligible or imaginable form, there will be fear'.[47] Leaving aside for the moment the role imagination plays in evoking them, it is clear that the emotions of the irascible power exert a potentially very dangerous influence on health. Better by far is the physiological influence of moderate joy, or *gaudium*, as it will not cause rapid changes but instead a more moderate and gradual diffusion of heat and vital spirit. Monastic culture has long recognised this therapeutic potential. The idea of *recreatio* covers not simply the modern sense of play, but also that of re-creation or restoration.[48] It is given more direct articulation through the concept of *hilaritas*, which demonstrates 'the healing and persuasive benefits of witty mirth against melancholy and over-seriousness'.[49] Such comments cover reading material that is directly comic or witty, and which promotes a state of moderate joy among the emotions – the state most conducive to good health. Yet not all reading material provokes laughter or is conducive to moderate joy, and specifically monastic understandings of reading and reading practices reimagine and expand the therapeutic potential of *lectio* enormously, allowing it to engage with multiple non-naturals at once.[50]

The monastic *lectio divina*, or divine reading, is a key motivator in this expansion. It is supplemented, and furthered in specific ways, by the interconnected reading practice known as *lectio spiritualis*.[51] Taken together, both reading processes were vastly influential during the Middle Ages. The first and most important, the *lectio divina*, is comprised of four interconnected stages that increase in psychological and cognitive intensity, and are termed *lectio*, *meditatio*, *oratio* and *contemplatio*.[52] *Meditatio*, the second stage of the *lectio divina*, is rich in complex and subtle meanings that derive from secular as well as religious sources, and carries the idea of meditation itself as well as the idea of physical exercise. At this stage *clara lectio* and *lectio divina* have complementary therapeutic significance. Yet, beyond physical exercise lies another non-natural: diet.

The first two stages of the *lectio divina* are often given their own term – *ruminatio*, or rumination. It is similarly rich in meaning, covering not simply 'considered thought' but also the physical act of chewing. It is used essentially as a figure for the monastic reader's activity: slowly and deliberately reading and softly reciting a text. The term, therefore, covers not just processes of mastication and ingestion, but also digestion as well. As Carruthers notes, *ruminatio* is an 'image of regurgitation, quite literally intended; the memory is the stomach, the stored texts are the sweet-smelling cud originally drawn from the gardens of books (or lecture), they are chewed on the palate'.[53] This is more than metaphor, as the monastic practice of reading deliberately includes the idea of 'spiritual nutrition' through the mouth of the heart (*ore cordis*), and so by extension includes an appreciation of reading's dietary significance.[54] As diet is one of the non-naturals, there is a medical resonance embedded within the *lectio divina* at a fundamental level. This is reinforced by a companion idea to eating the text: belching its contents forth from memory.[55] Ingestion, digestion and eructation are all part of the monastic reading process and are vividly realised functional analogies regarding its impact upon those who practise it. In Augustine, this dietary significance is given a much more forceful medical articulation:

> Deus et dominus noster curans et sanans omnem animae languorem, multa medicamenta protulit de Scripturis sanctis, velut de quibusdam armariis suis, cum lectiones divinæ legerentur . . . Multa lecta sunt, et magna, et necessaria; quanquam ita sint omnia: sed tamen alia secretius in

Scripturis absconduntur, ut quærentes exerceant; alia vero in promptu et in manfestatione ponuntur, ut desiderantes curent.[56]

(Our Lord and God takes care of and heals every ailment of the soul, and so he produced many medicines from the holy Scriptures (which you could call the shelves of his pharmacy or drugstore) when the divine readings were being read . . . There have been many things read, both important and necessary. They are all like that, of course, and yet some things are hidden more thoroughly in the Scriptures in order to stretch and test the students, while others are set there openly and ready to hand for the immediate treatment of patients.)

Reading is a process that essentially consists of ingesting pharmaceuticals. The text, here the Scriptures, is no longer a collection of words but rather a concoction of medicines uniquely adapted to the individual constitution of the reader. Such reading is a universal medicine capable of entering patients in the most direct and physical of ways – through the mouth. It is administered by Christ – the ultimate doctor who cures through the ultimate medicine: the *verbi medicina*, or medicine of the word (Ps 93:7). This is a complex allusion to both Christ as the Word, and to the Scriptures themselves, and is an integral part of Augustine's broader conception of Christ the physician – the *Christus Medicus* topos.[57] It is subject to further elaboration in Augustine's idea of the poultice of words, or *fomenta verborum*:

Conscientia tua saniem collegerat, apostema tumuerat, cruciabat te, requiescere non sinebat: adhibet medicus fomenta verborum, et aliquando secat; adhibet medicinale ferrum in correptione tribulationis: tu agnosce medici manum; confitere, exeat in confessione et defluat omnis sanies.[58]

(Your conscience had gathered up evil humours, with boils it had swollen, it was torturing you, it suffered you not to rest: the Physician applies the fomentations of words, and sometimes He lances it, He applies the surgeon's knife by the chastisement of tribulation: do thou acknowledge the Physician's hand, confess thou, let every evil humour go forth and flow away in confession.)

Words are a form of medicine, one that works to remove corruption to restore health. It is hardly a pleasant process, and is rendered here a difficult and intensive purgation of conscience. This passage is a deft combination of a range of ideas and practices: it forges connections between confession, self-examination, medical treatment, and the act of reading. To read these medical words is to effect a powerful purgation of the conscience. As a result, the *lectio divina* engages with another non-natural: evacuation and repletion. Initially, it would seem only to point towards internal bodily processes of matter excretion and replenishment. Yet the Latin translation used for evacuation highlights its significance: *purgatio*. This word has a complex and multifaceted range of meanings, and is used in medical, theological and poetic contexts. Throughout both the classical and medieval periods reading is held to affect an internal purgation – an ability seen most clearly in the term *catharsis*. Derived from Plato, this technical philosophical term designates a procedure of emotional cleansing enabled and completed by poetic or rhetorical works of sufficient skill and impact. Crucially, this term is rendered as *purgatio* by Calcidius's widely influential translation of Plato's *Timaeus*. As a result there is a conceptual overlap between medical and poetic theory: a reading practice of sufficient psychological intensity can enable a purgation of the emotions themselves. The *lectio divina*, that most psychologically intense form of reading, involves the reader's memories, passions and sensations. Thus, it too possesses this purgative aspect: it has the ability to effect radical changes within the reader's mental state, and is vividly presented by Augustine as one of Christ's verbal treatments of the conscience.

From here the medical significance and impact of *lectio divina* becomes more psychologically focused, and deals with the final non-natural: the passions of the soul. The connection is unambiguous, as the *lectio divina* requires the presence and evocation of emotional states:

Quis vivit sine affectionibus? Et putatis, fratres, quia qui Deum timent, Deum colunt, Deum diligunt, nullas habent affectiones? Vere, hoc putabis, et putare audebis, quod affectiones habeat tabula, theatrum, venatio, aucupium, piscatus, et non habeant opera Dei et non habeat meditatio Dei interiores affectiones quasdam suas?[59]

(What man does live without affections? And do ye suppose, brethren, that they who fear God, worship God, love God, have not any affections? Will you indeed suppose and dare to suppose, that painting, the theatre, hunting, hawking, fishing, engage the affections, and the meditation on God does not engage certain interior affections of its own?)

Without passion there can be no real reading, and certainly no medicine of words. On a purely functional level the *lectio divina* makes great demands on the memory of the reader, and 'a memory cannot be stored without an emotion'.[60] More importantly, without passion there can be no treatment. In order for the textual medicine of the Scriptures to be accessed, the reader must have emotional reactions to those therapeutic words.

The importance of such reactions is given greater emphasis in an interconnected reading practice: *lectio spiritualis*. This form of reading came to prominence during the twelfth to fourteenth centuries, and while it draws structurally from the *lectio divina* it has its own distinct elements, such as a focus on the act of writing.[61] It is more directly attuned to the interior evocation of emotional states, and 'offers various methods for interior reflection that mainly deal with the reader's own affective response to a text, especially Scripture'.[62] This is due to the self-reflexive elements in the practice, what Stock terms its 'subjective, personal, or autobiographical element', all of which focus more directly upon the interior states and mental processes of the reader.[63] As the practice does not actually require a text, only the memory of a passage or line, it is much more focused upon the cascade of subjective thoughts, images, ideas and emotions that a memorised passage can induce. The difference is one of attention. The *lectio divina* focuses upon the text, upon listening to the *voces paginarum*, and towards a deeper understanding of the Scriptures and the act of prayer. The *lectio spiritualis* focuses upon the emotional reaction to the text, upon its psychological impact – it makes the reader's psychology into a text.[64] It too has a therapeutic aspect centred specifically upon the emotive potential of its 'internal coherence of words, images, narratives, and subjective experiences'.[65]

Both reading practices would appear to function in a similar manner to the non-monastic idea of reading's therapeutic potential, as they both manipulate the emotions. However, there is a very significant difference. While engaging the passions is key in *lectio divina* and *lectio spiritualis*, it is done not to promote balance or moderate joy. As Augustine notes, the Scriptures constitute a 'bitter medicine'.[66] Monastic reading practices have a sharper taste, and offer more demanding pharmaceuticals than other 'delectabil bookis'. Their bitter treatment achieves health not by gently moderating the emotions, but by forcefully evoking them, bringing them to states of intensity that compel the reader closer to God. Their medicinal operation goes beyond *hilaritas* and towards something more powerful – to a therapeutic practice that concerns itself with purging the soul, with reforming it through intense feeling. Such ideas and models of reading have an abiding influence over the Middle Ages. As the Cistercian Itier of Vassy (*c*.1200) notes, 'neither metrics nor verses bring health to the soul. / True restorers are piety, tears, and good works'.[67] While the remark comes from a text on the vanity of versification, it does not itself disprove the idea of therapeutic reading; rather, it makes the case that the health of the soul is dependent upon emotional states that are difficult, unpleasant, and intense. Such sentiments express the emotional expectations of monastic reading, and underpin Rolle's own reading practices as much as they do his 'medicyne of words'. Moreover, they expand the ambit of therapeutic reading to include any material that can evoke the required emotions at the required intensity.

Other vernacular texts of meditative guidance also note the manifold therapeutic potential of reading, and the importance of its ability to engage the emotions. As the early fifteenth-century translation of St Catherine's *Dialogue*, the *Orchard of Syon*, notes,

> In þis orcherd, whanne ȝe wolen be conforted, ȝe mowe walke and se boþe fruyt and herbis. And albeit þat sum fruyt or herbis seeme to summe scharpe, hard or bitter, ȝit to purgynge of þe soule þei ben ful speedful and profitable . . . taste of sich fruyt and herbis resonably aftir ȝoure affeccioun, & what ȝou likeþ best, aftirward chewe it wel & ete þereof for heelþe of ȝoure soule.[68]

Reading is here an aggregate treatment that combines multiple regimental practices through its flexible figurative rendering. To read is to take exercise by walking through an expansive orchard. It also offers a good diet, full of the food of 'fruyt and herbis' that the reader should 'ete thereof'. Yet these very foodstuffs can be bitter, and so function as purgative medicines that remove impurities and which are ingested 'resonably aftir youre affeccioun'. Exercise, diet, purgation and the passions are all combined here in this presentation of reading. Crucially, though, they are all directed towards a single goal – the 'heelþe of ȝoure soule'. Such a medicine of words is in effect the ultimate form of regimen, embracing most of the non-naturals and operating in a multi-layered manner. Yet the medicine is not gentle. While the references to diet and exercise seem neutral, those regarding purgation and the passions do not. These medicinal words can be 'scharpe, hard or bitter' in their purgative function, and can evoke emotions with a speed and intensity that is far from subtle. Soul health is achieved through emotions more forceful and depressive. The fifteenth-century vernacular commentary on the Office for Brigittine Nuns, *Myrour of Our Lady*, makes this connection between religious reading and dangerous emotions unambiguous:

> Other bokes ther be that ar made to quyken & to sturre up the affeccyons of the soule, as som that tel of the sorowes & dredes of dethe, & of dome & of paynes, to sturre vp the affeccyons of

drede & of sorow for synne . . . when ye rede these bokes, ye oughte to laboure in youre self inwardly, to sturre vp your affeccyons accordingly to the matter that ye rede.[69]

Reading operates as a catalyst for the emotions, working to evoke and enhance specific ones within the soul. Its function is one of dynamic augmentation: the words used to describe it, 'sturre' and 'quicken', have a visceral and generative quality that convey reading's ability to enliven and invigorate.[70] Moreover, both words have medical connotations, meaning to recover from illness. Reading is not a passive or casual act, but instead orientated towards the health of the soul through its ability to evoke these powerful emotional states. Yet those very states, despite being extolled as beneficial, are understood by medieval medicine as dangerous or damaging. Medical theory is clear that the passions from the irascible power of the soul have the potential to be very harmful. As Trevisa's vernacular translation of Bartholomeus Anglicus's *De Proprietatibus Rerum* notes, madness and melancholia can be caused 'sometyme of passiouns of þe soule, as of besynes, and grete þouȝtes of sorwe, and of to greet studie, and of drede'.[71] Dread, sorrow, and excessive reading, ought to be avoided as they can cause disease. This begs an important question of monastic reading practices themselves: how can emotions, widely understood to be dangerous, operate therapeutically?

Medicine and theology are deeply interconnected during the period, and medieval monasticism was not medically ignorant: from its earliest stages, and most clearly after the Benedictine reform, monastic culture had a keen interest in maintaining the health of the monks. Moreover, many medical texts – from medical compendia to vernacular herbals – were associated with, produced by, or at least held in monastic libraries.[72] To assert that dangerous emotions generated through reading are therapeutically significant is not, therefore, a mistake born of ignorance; rather, it is a deliberate recommendation that comes from a complex understanding of the state of the soul, the nature of sin, and the potential use of the soul's affective powers.

Both medieval theology and medieval medicine spend considerable time and energy dealing with a shared topic: the soul and its relation to the body. In their own ways, each is concerned with an aspect of health – be it health understood as bodily balance, or health understood as the salvation of the soul. Yet, for medieval theology, there is an added element of complexity: the soul is inherently damaged due to *natura lapsa* – Fallen Nature – and is literally sick with sin. While in part remedied through Christ's sacrifice, sin and its effects nevertheless persist. To heal the soul further requires not simply further action, but also a more precise diagnosis of what sin is. Early monastic theologians such as Clement of Alexandria, Origen, and Augustine explore this in great detail, and understand sin as essentially an emotional disorder. All sinful acts arise from an inability to control emotional urges that are directed towards, or stem from, the wrong things.[73] As Origen notes, sinners are those who 'feel sadness about mundane things, who fear suffering or death, who desire things they do not have, and who irrationally bind their soul to allegedly good things which are not good'.[74] It is the object of the emotions which determines their merits or dangers, not the emotions themselves. Sin is here understood as emotion without reasonable limit and without reasonable cause. Such misguided and misaligned emotions have profound consequences for the health of the soul, not just the body.

During the eleventh and thirteenth centuries, with the dissemination and dominance of the medical theories of Salerno, and of the works of Averroes (*d*.1198) and Avicenna, (*d*.1037) the theological engagement with the soul and its nature undergoes profound changes and takes on a new level of intensity and purpose. This fusion of medical and theological knowledge can be seen in the works of a range of influential theologians. William of St Thierry's (*d*.1148) *De natura corporis et animae*, and Isaac of Stella's (*d*.1169) *Epistola de anima*, repeat the standard division of the soul into irascible and concupiscible powers, but do not ascribe any negative impacts to a specific division and its emotions.[75] The main focus is understanding which division specific passions belong to. For John Blund (*d*.1245) this was quite important. In his *Tractatus de anima*, he keys specific pairs of emotions into either the concupiscible or irascible parts of the soul, and endows them all with a functional agenda. As Boquet and Nagy note, his work 'perfected a scheme coming from the Fathers, according to which the emotions of the concupiscible aspired towards virtue, while the emotions of the irascible kept away the vices'.[76] This becomes all the more important when the number of emotions expand from these central four into more complex sets. As Richard of St Victor (*d*.1173) notes, there are seven main emotions 'hope and fear; joy and grief; hatred, love, and shame. All of these can be ordered at one time and disordered at another'.[77] The passions are not in and of themselves pathological; rather, it is whether they are in order or disorder that is important. Richard's other key text, *De quatuor gradibus violentae caritatis* (*The Four Degrees of Violent Love*), is in many ways a reaction to the popular medical concern with love sickness, and notes how a potent and potentially harmful emotion that operates like a wasting illness can in fact be a virtue when directed towards its proper object: God.[78]

Other texts, such as Hugh of St Victor's (*d*.1141) *De unione corporis et spiritus*, and Alcher of Clairvaux's (*d*.1180) influential *De spiritu et anima*, fuse medical and theological knowledge, and use similar divisions and taxonomies for the purposes of understanding the dual natures of Christ. In each the passions are not seen as explicitly dangerous or beneficial, only that they belong to specific powers and have broad utility in pursuing virtue and fleeing vice. As a result of this, the passions begin to have more of a utility than a danger. In William of Auvergne's (*d*.1249) *De Virtutibus*, the initial passions of the soul can be transformed – through focus on proper or improper objects – into affects. These affects are in essence the foundations of vice or virtue, as when they are repeatedly experienced they form dispositions towards certain modes of behaviour. In this way, virtue becomes 'a passionate habitus or way of being, motivated and morally connoted by emotion. In this conception, affective intensity was no longer regarded as harmful, and it survived in the lasting disposition of virtue'.[79] However, it is the work of John of la Rochelle (*d*.1245) which represents the most significant development in the theological understandings of the emotions and their potential utility.

The *Tractatus de divisione multiplici potentiarum animae* (*c*.1233) and *Summa de anima* (*c*.1235) collectively offer an account of the emotions that has greater classificatory and taxonomical precision than all prior accounts. It proves to be extremely influential.[80] His views of the soul and its emotions not only inform those of his most famous student, St Bonaventure (*d*.1274), but also those of Odo Rigaldi (*d*.1275), Albert the Great (*d*.1280) and Thomas Aquinas (*d*.1274).[81] The result is that his account becomes the dominant perspective on the emotions until the later Middle Ages when Aquinas's summary of it become more popular, and is itself revised through the work of Duns Scotus (*d*.1308), William of Ockham (*d*.1347) and John Buridan (*d*.1358). Over the course of each text he provides a complex and careful engagement with the soul, and draws from medical and theological sources. He not only refers to and employs the *Pantegni*'s widely disseminated model of the passions, but also asserts that 'just as the organ of the apprehensive sensible virtue is primarily the brain, so the organ of the motive virtue is the heart, *as the natural scientists say*'.[82] His understanding of the passions is of particular interest:

> Qui quidem IIII affectus anime omnium sunt vitiorum et virtutum principia ac communis materia. Cum ergo prudenter modeste, fortiter et iuste amor et odium instituuntur, in virtutes insurgunt, prudentiam scilicet, temperantiam, fortitudinem et iustitiam; que quasi origines atque cardines sunt omnium virtutem, quia hec cum affectuose et virtuose in anima instituuntur, per odium mundi et sui perficit in amorem Dei et proximi, per contemptum temporalium et inferiorum crescit in desiderium eternorum et supernorum.[83]

> (These four affections of the soul are the beginnings of all vices and virtues, and the common substance. Therefore whenever love and hate are instituted with wisdom, moderation, strength and justice, they are raised into virtues, i.e. wisdom, temperance, fortitude and justice, which are almost the origins and the cornerstones of all virtues, since when they are instituted in the soul with charity and virtue, through the hate of the world and itself it [i.e. the soul] improves in the Love of God and one's neighbour, and through the contempt for temporal and inferior things it grows in the desire of eternal and supernal things.)

The soul's sickness, like its health, has a shared source: the emotions. There is no specification here of dangerous ones, or the location of them within a specific division of the soul. Instead, all emotions can become dangerous irrespective of whether they come from the irascible or concupiscible powers. What makes the difference is whether the emotion is controlled, subject to proper moderation and guidance, and directed towards the correct object. Sin comes from within, not without: love and hate are simply capacities which can exert either positive or negative influence upon the soul depending on how they are used. While each of these four emotions still has its own unique physiological impacts, each can further the health of the soul if properly governed. The key line here is the specification that these four are 'the beginnings of all vices and virtues': there is another, more advanced, level to the soul's potential salvation or corruption. From here the account becomes taxonomically more complex, as John takes the irascible and concupiscible powers and specifies a series of emotions that reside in each – emotions which are rendered indistinguishable from virtues or vices. The therapeutic treatment of the emotions simply starts with the four basic ones, and is effected more fully through the specific sets of emotions that reside within the irascible and concupiscible powers.

In the concupiscible power there are twelve emotions that are arranged into contrasting sets. The first set 'are desiring, longing, rejoicing, delighting, loving, liking'.[84] The second set are contrary states, and take the form of 'scorning, which is the opposite of desiring, of detesting, which is the opposite of longing, of deploring which is the opposite of rejoicing, of lamenting which is the opposite of delighting, of hating which is the opposite of loving and liking'.[85] He makes a further specification regarding pity and envy, noting that 'since to pity is to share the sadness about others' evils, and to envy is to be sad about others' goods, they are included under sadness'.[86] Initially this does not appear to be very significant, but as John develops his account it becomes clear that some of these emotions are extremely similar to vices or virtues – pity and envy being perhaps the most easily recognisable. In the subdivision of the irascible power this overlap is even more evident. As with the concupiscible power, he divides the irascible into a series of contrary sets. The first set are 'ambition and hope, pride, arrogance, contempt' and 'bravery, anger, and rising/insurrection'.[87] Depending upon their object and level of intensity, many of these emotions could be a virtue or a vice: hope, pride, arrogance and bravery have a wider significance in Christian thought. This is emphatically more the case with their contrasting pairs:

> Paupertas spiritus opponitur ambicioni; que est appetitus fuge honoris et excellencie. Desperacio uero est appetitus resiliens ab arduo obtinendo; et est contraria spei. Humiliacio uero est amor subiectionis fugiens excellenciam; et est contraria superbie uel dominacioni. Reuerencia uero est, ex consideracione excellencie alterius, resilicio in propriam paruitatem, siue ueneracio rei uel persone alicuius propter suam excellenciam; et est contraria comtemptui.[88]

(Poverty of Spirit, which is the desire to flee honour and distinction, is opposed to ambition. Despair is a desire to withdraw from the obtaining of something arduous; and it is contrary to hope. Humiliation is the love of subjugation that flees distinction; and it is contrary to pride and imperiousness. Reverence is withdrawing to one's own smallness in considering the distinction of someone else; and it is contrary to contempt.)

At this level within the soul there is no clear or absolute conceptual boundary between an emotion and a state of virtue or vice. The whole passage has a strong theological resonance to it, and reads much like a catechetical list of vices and virtues. Many of the emotions listed here are held as key virtues inseparable from an advanced Christian life: poverty of spirit is one of the Beatitudes, and reverence must always be cultivated when thinking about God. This is keenly evident shortly after this passage, when the contrary to bravery is specified as being a series of interlinked emotions of 'penitence, impatience and fear'. Of these penitence and fear have considerable theological significance and application. The overall result of this moves beyond mere classificatory and taxonomic work, and articulates the potential utility – and danger – of the emotions.

If the irascible and concupiscible powers contain such states of virtue and vice, then the precise and systematic manipulation of the emotions has the potential to bring the soul either closer to salvation or damnation: to its ultimate *salus* or *infirmitas*. This is nothing short of a revolution in the systematic thinking regarding the treatment or reformation of the soul, and its relevance for the *cura animarum* is fully realised by John. His *Summa De Vitiis* (*c*.1235–6), a popular text which informed the great *Summa theologica* of Alexander of Hales (*d*.1245), combines his analysis of the passions with a complete synthesis of prior accounts and engagements with the vices.[89] Its aim is to 'organise the arguments of the great thinkers, without neglecting the practical requirements for those whose job it was to care for the soul on a daily basis', to combine 'moral discourse with a solid psychological knowledge that exploits the most recent acquisitions in the study of the science of the soul'.[90] Written with practical use in mind, the text contains several schematic tables, one of which connects vices to specific subdivisions within the soul: avarice and wrath emerging from the concupiscible and irascible parts of the soul.[91] Its medical overtones are far from accidental: understanding, classifying, combating and removing the emotional origins of sin really is the treatment of the soul.

An understanding of the importance of emotion is a key development in pastoral care during the inter-conciliar period and the decades after the Fourth Lateran Council. During this time the *cura animarum* underwent an intellectual revolution, with a new emphasis placed upon on the education of the clergy, and the provision of texts and decrees that would facilitate it. The practice of pastoral care began to be understood as something not simply benefiting from a university education, but as being the apex of it – as the *ars artium*. All the arts of the *trivium* and *quadrivium* were in this sense subordinate to the cure of souls, the 'sit ars artium regimen animarum', and so clerics ought to be trained in all those 'things that are known to pertain to the care of souls'.[92] Like medicine today, pastoral care is an applied science that takes a pragmatic approach regarding the utility of all manner of learning. As Jerome notes, 'if we find something useful in them, we apply it to our doctrine'.[93] Contemporary legislative documents support this understanding. As Leonard Boyle has noted, the *Cum ex eo* decree made provision for more clerics to attend university and undertake a liberal arts education; with the requirement that they would then return to their parish with new skills and techniques relevant for the *cura animarum*.[94]

Pastoralia, the vast and variegated literature of pastoral care, demonstrates how theological speculation was distilled into more functionally orientated texts. While the precise origins of this form of writing are hard to pinpoint, they are nevertheless traceable. In the twelfth and thirteenth centuries a number of key theologians working in Paris including John of la Rochelle, Alexander of Hales, Hugh of St Cher (*d*.1263), Peter the Chanter (*d*.1197), and William de Montibus (*d*.1213), composed numerous texts that offered summary information and easily accessible quotations and excerpts for students.[95] While not elaborate or sophisticated, these early texts are nevertheless attempts to systematise – to offer an easier way of training others, and to provide readily available raw materials and quotations for sermons, homilies, confessions, and other aspects of religious life (e.g. *Peniteas Cito*). Later examples of *pastoralia* are more elaborately schematic, using numerical division, tables and other forms of *ordinatio*. All of them, however, are designed to be practical and instructive. They seek to use the insights of theology for the practice of the *regimen animarum*.

An example of this concern with treating the soul is evident in other texts more directly influential in medieval England. Written between 1220 and 1245, Robert Grosseteste's *Templum Dei* is an extremely influential pastoral manual that connects specific sins with specific ailments and infirmities, and notes the medical treatments – *medicina* and *preparatio* – for them.[96] To cast the sickness of sin out of the soul requires the use of *misericors* (pity), *pauper spiritu* (poverty of spirit), *humilitas* (humility) and *penitentia* (penance). These emotions are essentially therapeutic treatments and eventually become ways of being or 'habitus'. This is similar to William of Auvergne's model of passions becoming affects, each affect becoming a habitus, before turning into a virtue. With Grosseteste, the model moves a stage further with the virtues eventually becoming the *Beatitudines*, or Beatitudes. In any case, the emotions function therapeutically, and operate on the soul in a specific manner:

> In hac tabula est tota cura officii pastoralis, ut obstetricante manu per vinum et oleum contra vulnera et infirmitates educatur coluber tortuosus, et preambulis preparationibus detur medicina purgativa inducens sanitatem, et inductam conservet quousque pro infirmitatibus dotes et pro vulneribus beatitudines inducantur.[97]

(In this table there is all the duty of the pastoral office, that the twisting snake is to be taken out by the hand of the obstetrician with wine and oil against wounds and illnesses, and a purgative medicine is to be given during the preliminary preparations, a medicine which induces health, and once induced it conserves it until gifts and blessings are brought about instead of illnesses and wounds.)

The soul requires a medicine that is purgative, and far from gentle. There is a degree of force here, one given potent articulation via the visceral imagery. To treat the soul and its emotions, to promote sowle-hele, requires the experience of emotions that are intensive and operate intensively. Emotional states long understood as dangerous become, through the interconnection between medicine and theology, salutary ones which work to counter the origin of sickness within the soul: sin or vice. This medicinal conception of the emotions underpins the office of pastoral care, Rolle's 'medicyne of words', and the very idea of therapeutic reading that the Vernon manuscript is based upon. The religious texts in that vast compendium are in essence and purpose texts of emotional treatment, and to read them is to evoke states of passionate intensity within the soul – to make it feel strongly, to heal it.

Words of Fire and Fruit

Ex supradictis potest constare, quod tota virtus et omni efficacia orationis vocalis pendet et habet provenire ex toto clamore cordis atque compunctione et devotione et intentione mentis. Unde evidens est illam orationem esse penitus inutilem que fit tantum sono oris et non contritione cordis, mente ab ea recedente et corde fugiente, et aliud quam de ea cogitante.[98]

(From what we have just said it can be evinced that all the virtue and all the efficacy of an oral prayer depends and has to derive from the cry of the heart, the compunction, the devotion and the intention of the mind. Hence it is evident that the prayer that is made only with the sound of the mouth and not with the contrition of the heart, with the mind withdrawing from it and the heart fleeing and thinking about something else, is completely useless.)

Without emotion there can be no real prayer. Its efficacy is dependent upon specific emotions that must accompany the words of prayer at all stages. Only with adequate compunction and devotion will prayer prove effective in purging the soul of sin: as Peter the Chanter here asserts, a lack of these emotions will ensure that prayer 'does not purge'.[99] Words, emotions and purgation all come together here in a manner that stresses their interdependence. In a broader sense, such a statement is equally applicable to the idea of therapeutic reading itself. If a text does not evoke any emotions, or does not evoke them with sufficient strength, then the soul remains as it is – sick. This raises an important methodological question: how exactly do texts evoke emotions?

The answer lies in medieval psychology and the arts of grammar and rhetoric. Texts are, to greater and lesser degrees, arrangements of words – words designed and organised to create specific psychological impacts. If a grouping of words is to achieve a medicinal effect, then they must be selected, arranged and used with the utmost care and consideration by the writer. There is, therefore, a fundamental link between composition and cognition

– a link which finds its origins in medieval psychology. As mentioned earlier in this chapter, Avicenna notes that the emotions can be stimulated 'as a consequence of an intelligible or imaginable form'.[100] When stimulated, the mechanisms of human sense perception, thought and recollection will evoke the emotions: sense data, either mediated directly through the senses, or simulated through the work of imagination, will exert a force on the mind; human psychology cannot behave otherwise. Words, when read, engage the faculties of imagination and memory. Yet, what words generate are more than simply images within the mind. More precisely, reading a text will generate memory phantasms: not images seen by the senses directly but rather verbal simulations recreated imaginatively through the work of memory; literally a re-presentation of composite items stored in the memory.[101] Medieval arts of rhetoric and poetic are deeply concerned with these processes of imaginative recreation/re-presentation, and the psychological impact and importance of vivid images. The category of vividness is given some considerable critical attention, understood via the key terms *ekphrasis* and *enargeia*:

> Literary impact is created by the presentation of a *phantasia*, but can only be adequately generated when presented by those that have a clarity of manifestation (*enargeia/declaratio*) that is peculiar to themselves and which therefore permits *katalepsis* or *comprehensio* on the part of the audience. This imaginative vividness, this gifted imagination, endues the poet with the power of communication that generates strong reactions in the mind of the reader or hearer and allows the audience to become co-creators of the phantasm generated in the imagination.[102]

Every poetic image is in this way a memory phantasm, a composite of both simulated sense data and the immediate affective reaction to that sense data – a 'feeling-toned' combination of sense and intention.[103] Each verbally mediated phantasm will move the soul in the most technical of ways, will stimulate not simply the senses but also the affections through the simulation of sense data: descriptions of delicious food and foul smells are naturally geared towards certain senses via the *enargeia* of their presentations, but they will also evoke passions of desire and aversion by virtue of the mechanisms of human psychological response.

Throughout the later Middle Ages there is a sustained scholarly interest in the psychological impacts of poetic and aesthetic stimuli, and a sharper focus on their pastoral potential.[104] The arts of rhetoric and poetic are understood as important tools in the cure of souls. In Robert Grosseteste's *De Artibus Liberalibus*, the merits of the arts of the *trivium* and *quadrivium* are noted, and the importance of poetic composition in evoking emotional states is stressed. As the fifteenth-century translation makes clear, rhetoric is the art that can 'excite and awake theym that bien slugges and sleepers, to gyve audacite to fereful and tymerous'.[105] Engagement with the works of Averroes, Avicenna and Aristotle in the generation after Grosseteste proved pivotal, as it allowed poetry to become reconfigured as a branch of rhetoric. Its ability to move the soul to 'love the good and flee the bad' via the psychologically intense 'imaginative syllogism' made poetry an important part of moral philosophy.[106] The poetic images in a text will, through their vivid descriptive power, generate emotions. This is the case for all texts, but it is especially the case for those texts which seek to heal the souls of their readers.

An excellent example of this can be found in the devotional compilation the *Pore Catiff* (*c.*1380s) – a text which seeks to treat its readers by bringing them into 'þe ground of helþe'.[107] Its therapeutic ambitions are predicated upon the ability to evoke strong emotions, and to that end it offers 'summe short sentencis excitinge men to heuenli desiir'.[108] Emotion is key to the text, as it asserts that 'loue is perfeccioun of lettris, vertu of prophecies, fruyt of truþe, helpe of sacramentis, stablyng of wittis & kunnyng'.[109] Such words on love come from Richard Rolle's *Form of Living* – a writer whose engagement with love took it to new heights of lyrical and devotional intensity. Their inclusion here, therefore, is a direct statement not only of the text's demanding ambitions, but also of the practical connection between the liberal arts and those therapeutic passions. If texts are supposed to excite their readers, to provide emotions that will heal the soul, then they must employ all the power that poetic writing can command. Over its course, the text displays awareness of the utility of poetic narrative, as it offers exemplary accounts of specific saints in its discussion of the commandments to exhort its readers and hearers. It opts not for a bare furnishing of facts, but instead embellished and adorned narrative moments designed to accentuate and enhance its didactic and affective impact. Its early discussion of penance is one such instance:

> Crist diede in þe cros bodili þat we dure in þe cros of penaunce, aȝenstondinge synne to oure lyues eende. Þe cros of penaunce haþ foure partis. Þe ffirst is sorwe for þe lesyng of þe loue of god, þe secunde is sorwe for þe leesyng of þe ioie of heuene, þe þridde is sorwe for disseruyng of þe peyne of helle, and þe ferþe is sorwe for seruyng to feendis & to synne. Crist was biried þat we hide oure goode dedis fro fauour & preisyng of þe world.[110]

This is a paradigmatic instance of *translatio*, as penance is brought to poetic life via the gruesome death of Christ. Through it penance becomes transformed, and the reader is compelled to think of one of the most frequent manifestations of sacramental life in fresh and evocative ways. It is no longer a ritual act, but a form of personal crucifixion that is itself a participation in Christ's own suffering. The text then moves to enumerate the four parts of penance, keying them into each part of the Cross itself. This central image – the Cross – is itself a universal locus of emotional import and force, and by deploying it the text seeks to use that force to move the reader in specific ways. It generates, via universal mental reflexes, a perception in the mind of the Cross and a feeling associated with it. Yet here, via the poetic presentation of the Cross, this psychological process is extended and drawn out, with the 'feeling-tone' of the central image partitioned into four, each referenced to sorrow and each repeated successively. In practice we get not one 'feeling-tone' but rather four: the image and its emotional import deepen and thicken, drawing the reader in and indeed into more precisely modulated states of emotional response.

The art of poetic composition is central to this, as the passage employs repetition and a form of parallelism that are effective both didactically and in evoking emotions. Each beam of the Cross is essentially the same – sorrow; though in each case sorrow for a different reason. Reiteration and slight variation of detail allow the impact this description has on the passions to be maintained and extended. The reader cannot get bored with the metaphor due to the structured shifts in detail, yet the affective content of each shift is nevertheless the same. Repetition of the clause endings is a subtle but effective stylistic and structural choice. Through this technique the 'sorwe' the text describes is magnified and thematically connected, made both integral and inescapable as it binds the passage together structurally in much the same way that penance is connected to the Cross. Such versified writing amplifies the central point of the passage by taking that image and spreading it out, making it inescapable through the rhythmic parallelism. Rhythm envelops the reader in the emotional embrace of the image through its own ability to manipulate human psychological processes: as a manifestation of music, rhythm offers greater precision in timing and pacing the reader's sequential movement among the various parts of this emotional picture. Through the use of versified writing one unified image is able to generate four unified emotional impacts; all of which are then transposed to the idea of confession itself. The reader learns, in a very general sense, to feel a certain way about a certain topic. By rendering penance as a form of crucifixion, the passage at once endows it with a specific solemnity and connects it with the Passion for emotive import: the metaphor provides gravitas and delimits a specific set of emotional responses. The feelings of pity for Christ's crucifixion and death, and the sense of reverence for that event, are now transposed to another area of Christian life. The reader is also implicated in this, as the sorrows of the Cross and the sorrow of penance are now more emphatically the result of sin – of the behaviour of the reader.

The arts of rhetorical and poetic composition are thus as important as the mechanisms of human psychology for understanding how texts can evoke emotional states. Rhetoric often gets the lion's share of attention here, and rightly so – the idea of the imaginative syllogism is key for understanding the psychological aspects of poetic images. However, equally important and at a much more fundamental level is the art of grammar. While rhetorical and poetic arrangements of words can generate mental images that exert a concerted force on the mind, the raw elements of this force come from the very words themselves. Citing St Bernard, the text notes that just as 'good speche & chaast wordis eechen vertu & grace in þe soulis of spekers & heerers, so foule wordis of lecherie & of oþir synnes defoulen þe soulis boþe of hem þat speken & of hem þat heeren'.[111] Words have a unique potential to impact upon the psychological disposition of the person. They are powerful, and can be dangerous or useful depending on how they are employed and arranged. The entire text is in a way an extended example of this point: while it castigates those who use and listen to such poetically arranged narratives it nevertheless employs similar techniques of poetic composition. The arts of grammar and rhetoric are tremendously powerful, and so their pastoral potential is clear – provided they are applied to the promotion of virtue. Yet, the potential ambiguity regarding their use underscores this central point: it is words themselves which possess great force, one that can only be contained, harnessed and augmented through their formal arrangement. Such an aspect of language is given considerable attention by medieval grammar theory, as it explores the means by which words can evoke passions.

The art of grammar (*ars grammatica*) exerted a particularly strong hold over the intellectual endeavours of the Middle Ages, was a foundational aspect of any education, and was the first subject of the *trivium* and *quadrivium*. Its range was considerable, containing both elementary and highly advanced aspects, and dealing with the activity of interpretation and composition.[112] As a result, it is a rather diffuse discipline which impacts upon a range of different contexts – poetic, logical, scientific, and even theological. Grammar's engagement with the relationship between language and emotion is of considerable interest and influence, evident even in the most elementary grammar texts:

> Interiectio est pars orationis interiecta aliis partibus orationis ad exprimendos animi affectus; aut metuentis, ut ei; aut optantis, ut o; aut dolentis, ut heu; aut laetantic, ut evax.[113]

(The interjection is a part of speech thrown in between the other parts of speech to express the affects of the soul; either of someone who fears, like ei; or of someone who wishes, like o; or of someone in pain, like heu; or of someone merry, like evax.)

Some of the soul's most potent emotions find expression and articulation through the interjection. This particular part of speech has a significant and fascinating connection to emotion, and operates differently from nouns, verbs and the other parts of speech. As Priscian clarifies, there are only 'partes igitur orationis sunt secundum dialecticos duae, nomen et verbum, quia hae solae etiam per se coniunctae plenam faciunt orationem, alias autem partes "syncategoremata", hoc est consignificantia, appellabant'.[114] As *syncategoremata*, interjections are incapable of fully formed conceptual signification or expression, and instead signify not the abstract concept of an emotion but rather the actual emotion itself: while the noun 'pain' conveys the concept of pain, the interjection 'agh!' conveys the sensation of pain. As a result of this, the interjection is understood to lack deliberation, order and reason. Like a missile, it is 'thrown into' a sentence, and as such is a *vox incondita*. By erupting within a sentence in a manner that is essentially uncontrollable and that compromises linguistic and syntactic order, it indicates both the presence of strong emotion and the absence of rational control. Such aspects are commented upon by Augustine, who uses the interjection as a tool for classifying degrees of sin in outbursts of rage and other forms of immoderate expression.[115] Yet this is far from the only theological engagement with interjections.

Later medieval grammarians and theologians explore its emotional dimension, but draw more upon current understandings of the soul and its powers. Greater attention is paid to the nature of the interjection, its relation to cultural endowment, and its precise connection to the mind.[116] Over the course of the twelfth to fourteenth centuries 'speculative grammar' emerges – an approach to the study of languages influenced by scholasticism and speculative logic. This type of grammatical study posits 'a structural parallel between language, thought, and reality' – in essence that there is a direct relationship between language and ontology.[117] The grammarians who practised this approach became known as the *Modistae*, and they re-categorised the parts of speech under 'modes of signifying'. Interjections signify *per modum affectus* – in the mode of affect rather than concept. In terms of its psycholinguistic structure, the interjection emerges more from the irrational soul and its powers than the rational soul. Roger Bacon (*d.*1294), in his *De signis*, provides a clear analysis of this. He asserts that the interjection is a special type of sign that signifies 'per modum conceptus licet imperfecti, et per modum deliberationis imperfectae' (in the manner of a concept, albeit, an imperfect one, and in the manner of imperfect deliberation).[118] As an imperfect expression, it cannot signify as verbs and nouns do – conceptually – but rather affectively:

Set secundum quod est interjeccio habet (gemitus) vocem absconditam et inperfectam et informem, quia inperfectus est conceptus, et inperfecta deliberacio, et affectus vincit conceptum, *unde dicuntur significare per modum affectus*, hoc est quia homo afficitur dolore, id est, dolet antequam concipiat dolorem, sive antequam moretur circa concepcionem, quia conceptus ejus transit cito in affectum, licet non subito sicut in vocibus que omnino significant naturaliter.[119]

(But inasmuch as it is an interjection it has a vocal sound that is hidden and imperfect and unformed, because the concept is imperfect and the deliberation imperfect and the emotion overcomes the concept. Hence they are said *to signify in the manner of an emotion*, [and] this is because the man is afflicted with pain, i.e., he is in pain before he conceives the pain or before he delays with respect to the conception because its concept quickly transitions into an emotion, granted not suddenly as is the case of vocal sounds that signify completely naturally (emphasis mine).)

The power of grief is such that it overcomes the initial conceptual work of the mind. As a result, the mode of signifying proceeds emotionally, and is dominated by that particular emotion. Language and thought break down to a single cry, and so signification is mediated through affect rather than concept. Any signification *per modum conceptus* is only very limited and incomplete. The commentary on Priscian by the Pseudo-Kilwardby goes into greater detail. He asserts that interjections are uttered when a person is 'seized by the strong motion of something agreeable or adverse, with sense dominating and reason succumbing'. This element of reason, however, is 'almost prostrated or hardly manages to restrain sense and does not control it in its motion, as it is evident in the apprehension of something extremely sad, such as the loss of a father', and as a result 'man breaks into a vocal sound, which truly signifies by institution something which is signified by man almost naturally by means of an interjection, because reason is succumbing and sense dominates'.[120] How passion engages with language, and how it psychologically develops through language, is complex. What this text presents is a model of the way forms of spoken and written language operate on a cognitive level.

Other writers go into more detail, and explore the deeper psychological impact of interjections and how they map onto the powers of the soul itself. In a grammatical treatise, pseudonymously attributed to Robert Grosseteste in Oxford, Bodleian Library, Ms Digby 55, a series of precise connections between the interjection and the powers of the soul are made. As with all other texts, it notes the nature of interjections first, stating that 'Interieccio est pars oracionis indeclinabilis mentis affectum significans voce non disposita. Omnes cetere partes oracionis significant mentis conceptum ('The interjection is the indeclinable part of speech that signifies the affects of the soul with disorganised sound. All the other parts of speech signify mental concepts').[121] From here, the text asserts that specific types of interjections engage with either the concupiscible or irascible powers of the sensory soul, or with the rational soul:

Accidit igitur interieccioni significacio tantum sicut et preposicioni, que dividitur secundum diversitatem affeccionum. Anime vero sensibilis sunt due vires sub vi affectiva, concupiscibilis et irascibilis, conveniencium et non conveniencium racione. Concupiscibilis dividitur in gaudium et cupiditatem. Gaudium quidem est affectus presentis convenientis cupiditas futuri convenientis. Irrascibilis dividitur in dolorem et timorem. Dolor est affectus presentis inconvenientis, timor futuri inconvenientis. Hinc sunt interiecciones euge, hay, atat, heu.[122]

(Therefore, the interjection acquires meaning in the same manner as the preposition, which is distinguished by the difference of the affections. As far as its affective faculty is concerned, there are indeed two faculties of the sensible soul, the concupiscible and irascible faculty, on the basis of convenience and inconvenience. The concupiscible faculty is divided into joy and desire. Joy is the affection for a present convenience, desire for a future convenience. The irascible faculty is divided into pain and fear. Pain is the affection for a present inconvenience, fear for a future one. Hence we have the interjections *euge, hay, atat, heu*.)

The connection between language and emotion runs far deeper here. The four central passions of the soul mentioned in early philosophical and medical texts are combined with the four main interjections from Donatus. The result of this combination is a classificatory schema for the interjections themselves, one that possesses great utility. As Modistic grammar notes, there is a deep connection between language and ontology. This is a key distinction specific to speculative grammar, summed up well in the larger terms *actus exercitus* and *actus significatus*: in other words, certain words only signify while others only express. For instance, a cry of sheer pleasure (*euge*) expresses a mental state that exists at the moment of its articulation, while the proper noun joy only signifies that state and does so without its actual occurrence within the soul. As Knuuttila notes, 'the act expressed as *actus exercitus* by an interjection or by a logical term is an act signified (*actus significatus*) by the corresponding noun'.[123] Thus, the interjections do not simply signify a given emotional state, they also work to evoke it. According to Modistic grammar, the interjections of pain and fear (*hay, atat*) will, when read or spoken, evoke those specific emotions, will engage the irascible power in specific ways. Such ability is of great use in evoking the passions required for sowle-hele: specific forms of language can work to evoke specific emotions within a determined sequence. As this text goes on to note, there are interjections that can engage with the rational soul and others that have a liturgical use: 'Dum tamen pulsus ipse voces non formet ut vocem naturalem gemitus, risus et consimilium, interiecciones erunt ut deo gracias, alleluya, salve et consimilia'.[124]

Bacon clarifies this potential, noting that interjections of prayer can be used to ensure correct intention. As he writes in his *Opus Maius*, the word *Osanna* signifies *per modum affectus*, and so when it is said during mass it works to synchronise emotionally the congregation with the celebrant, ensuring that specific passions are evoked within the persons who speak and hear this word. It is through such words that mankind gains 'et ideo cum verba proferuntur profunda cogitatione et magno desiderio, et recta intentione, et cum forti confidentia' ('profound cognition, great desire, just intent, and the strength of confidence').[125] In this way the interjection is a potent instrument in the evocation of emotion, and so must be used with care. Its utility is also realised in more poetic contexts. According to John of Garland (*c*.1190–1270), 'Interiectiones semper preponuntur, aliquando in oratione inperfecta, aliquando perfecta, et hoc quando exprimitur affectus doloris, uel gaudii, uel metus, uel admirationis' ('Interjections always go first whether in an incomplete sentence or in a complete one. They are used to express a feeling of sorrow or joy or fear or wonder.').[126] Such compositional advice gestures towards the interjection's wider use, and is especially significant for those religious and devotional texts that aim to treat and heal the souls of their readers by evoking powerful emotions. Indeed, the grammatical texts in Digby 55 sit side by side with texts on the soul and two medieval religious lyrics translated into Middle English: 'Candet nudatum pectus' and 'Vox Christi in cruce et Responsus peccatoris'. The theory of language informs the practice of it in poetic contexts.[127]

By using this grammatical and compositional knowledge, it is possible to comment more precisely on when and how a text attempts to manipulate the emotions of the reader, and on what parts of the soul are being engaged. For those texts which are commonly associated with 'affective piety', an appreciation of medieval grammar provides a useful method of seeing into their inner workings with greater precision and detail. Even the *Pore Caitif*, a text which usually relies on arresting imagery to evoke emotions, also deploys the interjection at specific moments to heighten their overall emotive impact. For instance, at the end of an extended section that deals with those who bear false witness, the text moves into a more impassioned register, asserting 'O hou orrible it is a man to forsake his god & bitake him to þe feend in bodi & in soule, and þus doen alle þilke þat witingli & wilfulli beren fals witnesse'.[128] The interjection 'O' is a cry of horror and disgust at those who forsake God which adds great expressive force to the end of this section. In terms of the grammatical theories outlined above, it signifies *per modum affectus*, and as such it evokes a corresponding state of horror and disgust within the irrational soul of the reader. In essence, it works to make them feel a certain way about a certain topic. The pattern is subtle, but deliberate; it also recurs. In a section from a much wider passage on the dangers of the flesh and the sins it commits, language becomes carefully crafted and arranged for maximum impact:

> But þe fleish coueitiþ & shewiþ euere yuel entisyng, þe fleish stiriþ venemous doyng, þe fleish clepiþ wraþ, þe fleish terriþ mansleyng, þe fleish stiriþ spousbreche, þe fleish sittiþ in drunknesse, þe fleish beriþ al courtise of þis world & þe fleish desiriþ al yuels. O, þou wrecchid fleish, not oonli þou sleest þi silf, but also þe soule, þin owne loss sufficiþ not to þi silf but þat also þi soule be drenchid in to helle. Wo to þee soule.[129]

In terms of its composition, this whole passage is a masterful example of rhetorical effects. It is comprised of a structured series of repetitions, and a loose form of parallelism. The constant 'þe fleish' works to generate a form of pathetic fallacy that builds up a gradual emotional charge – an almost breathless presentation of a series of images that implicate 'þe fleish' in all forms and manners of sin. Through repetition, each image merges seamlessly into the next, creating an expansive visual tableaux that covers many of the deadly sins.

From here the imagery moves from the sins of the body to the suffering of the soul – similarly personified, and damned to Hell. The word used to describe this damnation, 'drenchid', is an extraordinarily evocative choice. Its semantic range is wide, meaning 'to be drowned', 'to be sunken', 'to be engulfed', and 'fallen'.[130] Each meaning is at play here, and the result is a violently forceful image of the soul being submerged in or swallowed by Hell. In effect the reader becomes like the soul, swallowed whole by a horrendous procession of images of sin and vice. Yet, before this final image is delayered, the language of the passage changes. After all these images of sin there occurs the interjection 'O' – a cry, *per modum affectus*, designed to evoke and express a specific emotional state. Its use here not only emphasises the point that the flesh is horrible, but also evokes a corresponding emotional state within the reader. There can be no delight in that procession of images, only fear and horror. The force of the interjection is tactically deployed, occurring at the main conceptual shift in the passage from flesh to soul, from sin to consequence. Very carefully, very deliberately, the reader has been manoeuvred into feeling a certain way, has had the horror of the flesh transposed to become the danger and woe of the soul. Such examples are slight, yet they nevertheless illustrate the importance of imagery and language when it comes to understanding the role of emotion within a text. Moreover, they serve

INTRODUCTION 25

as an example for this book's main method of analysis. To understand how texts heal the soul through manipulation of the passions requires a careful analysis of their form and structure, their imagery and language. The texts of sowle-hele are full of powerful poetic images, but also raw cries of emotional force and potency. Understanding the nature and function of these features, these words of 'frute & of fiir', is the key to understanding the therapeutic potential of such texts.[131]

The Ground of Health

> Be contrition we arn made clene, be compassion we arn made redy and be trew longyng to God we arn made worthy. Thes arn iii menys, as I understond, wherby that al soulis come to hevyn ... for be these medycines behovyth that every soule be helyd.[132]

With her customary clarity and force of articulation, Julian of Norwich asserts that the best treatment is a medicine of extremes, not of moderation. Contrition, compassion and longing are some of the most central emotional states of religious life, but they are also some of its most intense. There is no sense of balance to the emotions here, only their increasing potency and force. There is, however, a sense of order. This treatment is inherently a programmatic one, moving from one emotion to another, from one medicine to another. So too will this book. The focus will always be on the texts of the Vernon manuscript, but as this collection of material is too vast to be examined by just one monograph, the book will instead proceed thematically, focusing on a specific medicinal emotion and analysing the texts most associated with it. This principle of selection is hoped to adhere to the manuscript's overall broad function: it offers texts of sowle-hele and, with its extensive index, presents itself as a veritable and searchable pharmacy to the reader.[133] As Gillespie has noted, its focus on sowle-hele 'seems to proceed on three levels' – there is a structure within this manuscript that reveals itself subtly when its function is considered.[134] Julian's course of treatment thus acts as the inspiration for the structure of most of this book. While it is a highly flexible organisational schema, it is not complete. Penance, compassion and longing are medical emotions, but there is one more: fear. All medical treatments have a beginning and an end, and it is fear which operates as the first medicinal emotion of the soul.

This therapeutic movement from *timor* to *amor* requires a caveat – an acknowledgement of the potential dangers of therapeutic reading. To that end there will be a fifth chapter which will survey a process that is itself medically inflected – a process which deals more with the control and moderation of the emotions, with the 'discretion of spirits'. Many of the following chapters share a specific structure that moves from the general to the particular. They will begin by elucidating the medical significance of a given emotion, before exploring precisely how a text within the Vernon manuscript works to evoke it.

Chapter One explores the medicine of fear. It begins by offering an account of fear's medical and theological significance, and explores how medieval religious authors understood this powerful passion as the first step in the soul's programmatic treatment. After this contextual material, the chapter turns to the texts in Vernon which not only show an awareness of this theology of fear, but also strive to evoke it: the *Speculum Vitae* and the *Prick of Conscience* respectively. These pastoral texts are far from simple, and they contain a wealth of vivid imagery designed to make their readers understand the power of fear, and also to dread sin, sickness, and the judgement of God.

Chapter Two explores the medicine of penance. It begins by offering an account of the medical understanding of confession, focusing in particular on how the component emotional states in this practice operate therapeutically. From here, the chapter investigates Richard Maidstone's *Penitential Psalms*, and a selection of thirteenth- and fourteenth-century penitential lyrics, and confessional lyrics from the Vernon manuscript. It explores the importance of the lyrical form as a tool for evoking and sustaining strong passions, and shows how they use structured shifts in imagery and perspective to encourage a penitential complex within the reader.

Chapter Three explores the medicine of compassion. This chapter differs from others as it concerns itself with the complex nature of compassion. It argues that compassion is not, strictly speaking, one emotion of the soul but rather a constellation, a specific configuration of emotions and modes of intersubjective awareness. It begins by noting the medical motifs that underpin compassion in the period, paying particular attention to the Augustinian idea of Christ the Physician, or *Christus Medicus*. It then moves to clarify the essential nature of compassion as one of intense torture for the soul. Finally, it offers an extended analysis of the most evocative and potent Passion meditations in Vernon: the *Prickynge of Love*.

Chapter Four explores the most potent medicine of the soul: longing. This is a chapter of extremes, as this longing is as painful and difficult as it is delectable and desirous. More than an emotion, longing is a complex of contrasting and intensive states all directed towards God. It demands the utmost from the soul, and is the completion of the soul's prior medical treatments: fear, penance, compassion and desire are all mixed and melded together in this state. The chapter begins, therefore, by clarifying what longing essentially is, how it is connected to humility, and the nature of its medical impact upon the soul. It ends with an analysis of the Vernon version of *A Talking of the Love of God*, a text that is lyrical, powerful, visually splendid and utterly compelling – a text that is as extreme as the emotions it seeks to evoke.

Chapter Five pauses from passion, and offers a discussion of a key aspect of any medical treatment: moderation, or the work of discretion. All medicines must be correctly administered, and the virtue of discretion is key to that. It begins by noting how dangerous therapeutic reading can be, and how the emotions it evokes can become pathological. It then moves to consider the precise dangers and difficulties that beset the soul through immoderate reading: madness, a self-destructive sorrow, and the vice of pride. It ends by considering how discretion and a modified penitential subjectivity are the solutions to such dangers. As a result, it moves beyond Vernon and explores the most influential texts of spiritual discernment: the texts of the *Cloud* author, and the *Chastising of God's Children*.

The book ends with a brief Conclusion. It summarises the overall analysis, and makes it clear that one of the crucial aspects of medieval religious texts is the confluence, and contrast, of ideas of health and of harm.

1

Apprehensive Medicine

For Seynt Bernard seyth thus vpon *Cantica Canticorum*: 'I knowe wel that ther may noo man be saued but yf he knowe himself', of the whiche knowynge waxith in a man the moder of his helthe, that is humilite, and also the drede of God, the whiche drede as it is the begynnynge of wisdom so it is the begynnynge of helthe of mannes soule.[1]

Health begins with apprehension, with a composite of knowing and fearing. For this text, a popular fifteenth-century vernacular example of the *ars moriendi* tradition, the health of the soul is intimately connected to the presence of fear, or drede.[2] The imagery used underscores this point, and is at once gentle yet potent. Drede and humility are co-mothers to *salus animae*, able to make it 'waxith' within the soul: images of conception and gestation, of familial connections and relations, all combine here to present both drede and humility as inherently natural. To feel this way is, in essence, the natural state of being for all of humanity. This extends to the medical aspects of the passage, as such an imagistic combination makes the point that treating the soul is a similarly natural process. A sense of progression is also evident here: drede is the 'begynnynge', the very inception of sowle-hele; humility is its 'moder', that which nurtures it. This rich and detailed passage presents the origins and nature of sowle-hele in a manner that is immediately intelligible and which emphasises its natural dimension. It is not, however, the only example. Later in the text it notes the connection between 'loue 7 drede of God and a zele of the hele of mannys soule'.[3] Though it is ultimately a natural state, sowle-hele is nevertheless characterised by a sense of urgency. The text unambiguously states that 'principaly and first of alle other thynges, and withouten eny othir delayes and longe tarienges' one must 'diligently prouyde and ordeyne for the spirituel medicyne 7 remedye of his soule'.[4] The rationale for this is due to the fact that 'as a certeyn decretale saith, bodily syknesse comeþ of syknes of the soule': sin and sickness are connected, as all illnesses suffered by humanity have an ultimately spiritual cause.[5] As a consequence, obtaining sowle-hele is all the more vital a goal – one that can only be achieved through the operation of the first medicine of the soul: drede.

The connection between fear and therapy is, of course, hardly unique to the *Book of the Craft of Dying*, nor fifteenth-century devotional tastes. Drede's therapeutic utility in treating the soul has a long history in medieval theology and a substantial presence in religious texts from the period. One central aspect of that history is the force and power associated with drede. While the passage above presents drede through natural, nurturing and almost gentle imagery, this emotion is anything but tender. As is clear from the very title of the *Book of the Craft of Dying*, such medicinal drede is deeply connected to the reflection on death. Evoking this emotion often requires an intensive, visual, focus on the last agonised gasps of the body, and the first cries of the soul's torment. Suffering and pain are its focus, and yet despite its unremitting intensity, its effects are salutary and begin to provide relief from the soul's sickness – sin. Such complexity is reflected in the word's semantic range, as it can mean 'fear', 'terror', 'anxiety', 'awe/reverence', 'doubt' and 'danger'.[6] Though distinctive, each aspect of drede can be seen as operative in some sense when it comes to treating the soul: to feel drede is not simply to be startled or frightened, but to undergo a complex emotional experience; one that incorporates reverence and awe alongside doubt, danger and a pervasive terror. It is, as an emotion and the first medicine of the soul, potent and powerful. This therapeutic emotion, and the means of evoking it, are the focus of this chapter. It begins with the theology of fear, its complex gradations, and their roles and functions. From here, it considers the medical operation of drede, and how texts from the period understand its medical potential and effects. Finally, the chapter moves to explore the *Speculum Vitae* and the *Prick of Conscience*. Though these texts of pastoral care offer elementary detail and guidance in the faith, they are nevertheless focused on fear, the first medicine in the *cura animarum*.

Feeling Dreadful

Now þou hast seuene manere seknesses, and heore medecynes. After comeþ þe souereyn leche and takeþ his medecynes, þat sauen mon from þe seuene vices and confermen him þe seuene vertues, þorw þe ʒiftes of þe holigost, þat ben þeose: Þe spirit of wit, and of vnderstondynge, Þe spirit of counseil, and of strengþe, Þe spirit of connynge, and of pite, Þe spirit of drede of God.[7]

Drede is a gift as much as it is a medicine. As the text makes clear, virtue and vice exist within a therapeutic schema in which God is the ultimate doctor. His role is to provide all these important medicines for each and every person. In this way drede comes from God but is also ultimately directed towards God: each of these medicines operates to promote the very virtues that lead the soul towards salvation. How each one functions is given interesting and succinct formulation. Drede, despite being the last in this list, operates in the most primary and elementary of ways. As the text notes, 'furst mon moot leue wikkednesse: and þat vs techeþ þe spirit of drede of god'.[8] Drede arrests the progress of sin, while at the same time it spurs the soul on to progress away from sin – it works to halt the illness as well as to hasten the cure. This text, an extremely influential Middle English translation of Edmund of Abingdon's (*d*.1240) *Speculum Ecclesiae*, merges catechetical and contemplative instruction to provide summary engagement with many of the key aspects of religious life and teaching. Its remarks on drede, therefore, draw from both contemporary and much earlier discussions on the theology of fear. All discussions, however, have a shared point of origin: the Bible.

In the Scriptures fear, or *timor*, plays an important role in the soul's relationship with God: only God deserves to be feared, and from that fear comes wisdom, spiritual cleansing, and the perfection of salvation.[9] Patristic theology, building on the disparate mentions of fear in the Bible, subdivides *timor* into two interconnected types: *timor servilis* and *timor filialis*. Each plays a role in a Christian life. The first form is 'servile fear', or the 'fear of a slave'. This is the initial form of fear of God, and is characterised as a fear of God's Law and His terrible punishments for any transgressions. While fear is here directed towards God, the object of focus is nevertheless the self: it is essentially a more spiritual form of self-preservation based upon an aversion to pain and suffering. The second from is 'filial fear', or the 'fear of the son'. It is the more advanced and perfect form of fear, based upon an aversion to sin and a reverence of God, and is characterised as the fear of a son towards his father.[10] The object of focus in this type of fear is God rather than the self. Thus, it is a more inherently selfless form of fear, as it is chiefly concerned with avoiding disappointing God, and with an awareness of the insignificance of the self compared to God's awesome nature.

The specific impacts of these forms of fear are explored by St Basil, Gregory of Nyssa and Gregory of Nazianzus. Collectively, they articulate its utility in perfecting the soul, as the movement from one form to the next works to restore the soul's divine image, to cleanse it from sin, and to alleviate the impacts of *natura lapsa*.[11] *Timor* becomes therapeutic, cleansing the soul and restoring it to a prior and better state. In this way fear is also a process that facilitates better moral behaviour, spiritual cleansing and an increasingly intimate relationship with God. While these are all important developments in the theology of fear, during the Middle Ages *timor* is subject to much more sustained and systematic thought, undergoing further subdivision, classification, and ever more refinement and precision. The most important development is the elaboration of *timor* in the work of Peter Lombard. In his influential *Sentences*, he begins by noting that *timor* is in essence a Gift of the Holy Spirit, and then proceeds to subdivide *timor* into specific variants. The main types are *timor mundanus sive humanus, timor servilis, timor initialis* and *timor castus sive filialis vel amicalis*; and later in the same text he provides yet another division – *timor naturalis*.[12] This becomes a highly influential series of types and they are soon gathered into broad categories that have specific moral valences: morally neutral (*timor naturalis*), morally laudable (*timor initialis timor castus, timor filialis, timor amicalis*) and morally harmful (*timor mundanus sive humanus*) forms of fear.[13]

Morally neutral fear is essentially the inbuilt and reflexive form of fear common to all humanity (and animals) when a real or imagined threat is perceived. From this fear other forms emerge that can lead to moral or immoral ends. For Bonaventure, it is the beginning of all others, and so he terms it *timor-passio* in his commentary on the *Sentences*. Drawing from St John Damascene's *De fide orthodoxa*, he provides a list of individual types: *segnities* (a fear causing laziness or inaction), *erubescentia* (fear of/causing embarrassment), *verecundia* (fear of/causing disgrace), *admiratio* (fear causing awe-filled intellectual immobility), *stupor* (fear causing rational paralysis) and *agonia* (fear causing the complete and agonised breakdown of mental and physical abilities).[14] Each of these has specific causal circumstances and meanings, but they all share a common feature in that the experience of them creates cognitive and physical impairments.[15] To assist in separating the good from the bad, Bonaventure provides a more general classification that deals with the origin of a given type of fear. Fear comes either naturally, from libidinousness, or from grace.[16] With this scheme in mind, the majority of these forms of fear tend to have a negative moral tendency. The reason for this is that they are, in essence, opposed to the more spiritual forms of fear: they are worldly, and focused on the self and its position and status.[17] It is this point that gains considerable currency and is emphasised in other texts. The *Glossa Ordinara*'s commentary on Exodus 15:12–16 is unambiguous:

> Impios etiam hodie terra deuorat, qui semper de terra cogitant, terrena faciunt, de terra loquuntur, litigant, terram desiderant, in ea spem suam ponunt, ad caelum non respiciunt, futura non cogitant, iudicium dei non metuunt, nec promissa eius desiderant.[18]

> (Indeed, the earth today devours those impious people who always think about, make, speak about, argue over and desire earthly things. They place their hope in the earth; they do not look to heaven and they do not think about the future. Neither do they fear the judgement of God nor do they desire his promises.)

Such worldly drede is sinful, as it is utterly self-absorbed and comes from 'libidinousness'. It focuses not on God and eternal things, but on the world and transitory things. However, there are two forms of useful fear: *erubescentia* and *verecundia*. For William Peraldus (*d*.1271), in his vastly influential *Summa on the Virtues and Vices*, *erubescentia* 'is the best passion', while *verecundia* enables all things 'to be upright or honest'.[19] While these forms could easily focus on worldly concerns, they nevertheless force the self into a consideration of its behaviour: they provide not simply a form of self-reflexivity, but of self-scrutiny. As such, they can both shade into morally laudable forms of fear – forms which are inherently 'inspired by a love and respect for God' and which are predicated upon 'the subjugation of physical and temporal anxieties to spiritual and eternal concerns'.[20]

When focused on God and Heaven, fear can be far more useful. For Bonaventure, morally laudable fear was a gift of grace and could spur the soul into reaching higher states of spiritual perfection. Such fear operates differently. In his *Collationes de septem donis Spiritus Sancti*, he notes that such fear arises from a consideration of God's unimaginable power and, by extension, the necessary severity of His punishment.[21] This kind of fear affects the soul in specific ways, causing the person to reflect on the dangers of sin while at the same time appreciating the vast gulf between God and their own being. It fosters not a self-obsession, but a relational self-awareness that generates a salutary humility within the soul.[22] This is one of the key aspects of drede, enabling it to counter pride. The spiritually laudable forms of fear consist of *timor servilis, initialis* and *filialis*.[23] Each is a developmental stage in the perfection of fear, and with each come additional benefits to the soul. The *Glossa Ordinaria* summarises:

> Sciendum etiam praeter naturalem timorem, qui omnibus inest, quatuor esse timores, scilicet mundanus qui maius est, nec a deo. Et seruilis qui bonus est, et a deo, sed non sufficiens. Initialis qui bonus est et sufficiens. Et castus qui bonus est perficiens.[24]

> (Indeed, it must be known that beyond natural fear, which is in everyone, there are four types of dread: *mundanus*, which is evil and does not come from God; *servilis*, which is good and from God, but is not sufficient; *initialis* which is good and sufficient; and *castus* [or *filialis*] which is good and perfecting.)

There is a developmental trajectory within spiritually laudable fear. Each form differs from the last not simply in terms of its relative perfection, but also in terms of what it consists of. *Timor servilis* is still based upon a fear of pain and punishment, still focused on the self, but is directed towards God and heavenly matters. As Bonaventure notes, 'thus servile fear, when someone fears to rush into eternal torments, comes from love of eternal health and blessedness'.[25] The next stage, *timor initialis*, is 'sed tamquam medius'– an intermediary stage characterised by a fear of punishment alongside a greater apprehension of guilt and shame.[26] The focus here is less on suffering and more on offending God.[27] The object of fear is thus more important and more spiritually noble – an 'object of greater principle' is its focus.[28]

The final and most perfect form of fear, *timor filialis*, is characterised not by being frightened by God's wrath over sin, but rather by being struck with reverential awe at His nature: it is deeply connected to *humilitas* or Poverty of Spirit.[29] At this stage it is more akin to a heightened familial love and respect, a sense of wonder that spurs the soul to actively pursue virtue and to flee vice – and its object is exclusively God. Its effects upon the soul, therefore, are extremely potent and extremely salutary, working to cleanse the soul for God. As Bernard of Clairvaux notes, it is 'the fear that purifies, [and] by this purification she [the soul] may be made ready for the vision she longs for. It is a vision reserved for the pure of heart'.[30] The cleansing power of fear, its ability to remove pride and instil humility, is the essence of its therapeutic potential – one fully realised and elaborated in a range of later medieval vernacular texts of spiritual guidance.

In the *Book of Vices and Virtues*, a fourteenth-century translation of the *Somme le Roi*, drede is essential for any progress in the overall improvement of the soul. It is one of the seven gifts of the Holy Spirt, and acts as a targeted treatment for pride:

> Þe ʒifte of drede is þe first of alle þe ʒiftes þat casteþ out al synne of a mannes herte or a wommannes, as we han seid tofore. But propreliche he destroieþ þe rote of pride, and sett in his stede þe vertue of humblenesse.[31]

Drede, an emotion common to all humanity, is the only medicine strong enough to remove the universal sin of pride. It potency is total, and is conveyed here through the combination of powerfully antithetical imagery – it is at once utterly destructive and creative. Drede 'casteþ out' pride, yet it is more than simply purgative as it can 'destroieþ þe rote of pride': it works to obliterate the first sin, not simply counter it. The agricultural imagery is used to convey this potency, as drede works to weed out a stubborn root. Yet the imagery also conveys its creative power – drede removes the root of pride and replaces it with the more desirable and useful 'plant' of humility. Drede thus cultivates virtues within the soul as much as it 'casteþ out' vices. The use of 'propreliche' emphasises this point. This adverb, meaning 'actually, specifically', signals that the passage is using agricultural imagery not as an arch metaphor, but as a functional equivalent for how drede impacts the soul.[32] Word choice and imagery combine to convey the potency of fear and the forceful manner of its operation. Its therapeutic potential is subtly alluded to. The word 'rote' is an obvious reference to plants and planting, and a less obvious reference to medicine: this word can also be a translation of the Latin *radix*, used in medical texts to diagnose the 'root cause' of an illness.[33] This is more explicit elsewhere in the text, when pride is noted to be 'more myschefous þan any oþer siknesse, for certes he is in gret peril þat alle manere of triacles turneþ hym in-to venym'.³⁴ Pride is the ultimate toxin, corrupting everything, turning every medicine – those 'triacles' – into poisons. It can only be purged, therefore, by a treatment that is similarly extreme. Drede is that medicine, and is presented as one of the medicinal gifts of the Holy Spirit:

> But þe Holi Gost is þe goode phisicion þat scheweþ hym his siknesse and meueþ þe humores wiþ-ynne hym & ȝyueþ hym a purgacion so bittre þat he delyuereþ and saueþ hym and makeþ hym hol and turne to þe lif. Riȝt þus turbleþ oure lord þe herte þat he wole hele.³⁵

Like the *Christus medicus*, the Holy Spirit also has a therapeutic role based upon self-knowledge and emotion. Initially, the Holy Spirit provides a form of self-knowledge, highlighting and exposing the illness within the individual soul. After this comes a powerful treatment centred on the emotions. A removal of the illness, a 'purgacion so bittre', is enabled through extreme mental turmoil: the verb 'turbleþ' is rich in meanings, from 'to produce mental/psychological agitation', to 'to torment/afflict'.³⁶ The heart must be tormented through drede before any healing can begin; only this level of emotional intensity is sufficient to remove pride. Such potency is often attributed to drede. For Walter Hilton, drede is a weapon that combats sin: he asserts that one must take that initial desire to sin and 'slee it with the swerd of drede of God, that it schal not dere thee'³⁷. This is but one instance of Hilton's wider – and often more medical than martial – rendering of drede. In a more explicitly medical vein, Hugh of St Victor notes that 'fear cuts out of the soul its attachment to carnal pleasure; and then grace bedews it, purged now and cleansed from its stains, with spiritual joy'.³⁸ Drede works like a surgical instrument, excising sin from the soul with both precision and force. Many texts note this medicinal aspect, but go into greater detail regarding precisely how drede functions:

> Of þe drede of God waxsiþ helful and gret deuocion, and a maner sorew wiþ ful contricion for þy sinnes. Þoru þat deuocion and contricion þou forsakist þi sinne, and perauenture sumwhat of wordeliche goodis. Bi þat forsaking þou lowist þe to God, and comest into mekenes; þoru mekenes þi flescheliche lustis ben distruid. Bi þat destruccion alle vices ben put out and vanschid away; bi putting ouut of vice, vertues biginne to wexe and springe.³⁹

Drede enables a complex psychological response. The experience of this emotion is not simple aversion, but instead the beginning of a layered constellation of additional emotional states and modes of self-reflexive awareness. It both generates and destroys. Initially, drede creates: it 'waxsiþ', a verb with a vast range of meanings, many of which cover ideas of profusion, growth, and intensity.⁴⁰ From this drede of God grows a 'deuocion', a 'sorrow', and a 'contricion' – it is the initial impetus for a wider range of emotional states, all of which are 'helful' or therapeutic. The precise manner of this therapy is then clarified. Drede creates a cascade of different emotional and cognitive responses from within the soul: contrition and sorrow come with greater self-knowledge regarding the presence of sin within the soul. In turn, these additional emotions and modes of self-awareness compel the soul to forsake sin and generate a profound humility, or 'mekenes'. It is this humility that acts as a powerful destructive force. It works to expel, extinguish and obliterate: humility is in essence the 'putting ouut of vice', and brings 'destruccion' to all vices by ensuring that they are 'put out and vanschid away'. Yet, from this complete destruction of sin comes creation and spiritual effusion – 'vertues biginne to wexe and springe' and so generate spiritual health. The passage is, in many ways, a compact summary of the various theological positions on *timor*, as it is only the drede of God that enables such spiritual improvement. At the very start of this section, the text notes the difference between 'drede of þe world', 'drede of seruage' and 'chast drede'.[41] The psychological complexity of drede is presented with clarity, as the passage notes how drede can foster not simply other emotions, but also specific forms of interiority and self-knowledge. Other texts explore these elements of drede's psychological complexity in greater detail. For the *Prickynge*, drede is a key way to remedy pride and is a constant emotional component of all stages of spiritual life:

> We shul hope & triste to be saaf þorou goddis mercy, but we shul ay haue gret drede medlid with-al, & þat is þat we falle not in-to presumpcioun ne in-to fals sikernesse; and we shul commende þe gret pite of oure lord & putte oure triste in his precious blood & in þe prei3eris of his blessid modir & maiden oure ladi seynt marie and so in tristful drede lede oure life.[42]

Fear must persist for more than a mere moment. Its power and medical potential can only be realised through endurance, through its amalgamation with all aspects of emotional and psychological life. Drede must be 'medlid' with the mind. This word has a range of meanings, but they all encompass the idea of complete admixture and combination. Drede must be merged and combined with all aspects of the person. Here it is merged with trust, combined with it to the point that it is indistinguishable. This subtly makes a wider point about the complexity of drede and its layered nature. The drede of God is not simply fear of punishment, but rather an emotional state that includes an inter-subjective aspect: the person fears and trusts God, has a relationship with Him that is based upon an appraisal of what He will and will not do. Through drede one can move closer to God.

Initially, drede works preventatively: it inhibits over-confidence and roots out pride. Later, when it is not only amalgamated with other emotions but also habituated within the soul, it promotes a more expansive awareness of the self and its relationship to God. In this way drede functions as both an emotional constant, and as a catalyst for developing self-awareness. This dual aspect to drede is given sustained attention in texts of contemplative guidance. In *A Tretyse of þe Stodye of Wysdome þat Men Clepen Beniamyn*, an adaptation of Richard of St Victor's *Benjamin Minor*, drede and other emotions are subject to an extensive allegorical treatment. Here, drede is rendered as Ruben, the first child of Leah and Jacob – an infant with particular powers:

> Þis is þe first felt vertewe in a mans affeccioun, wiþoutyn whiche none oþer may be had. And þerfore, whoso desireþ to haue soche a sone, hym behoueþ besily & oft also beholde þe iuels þat he haþ done. He schal on o partye þink þe greetnes of his trespas, and on anoþer partye þe power of þe domesman. Of soche a consideracioun springeþ drede, þat is to sey he, þat Ruben, þat þorow ri3t is clepid þe sone of si3t. For verrely is he blent þat seeþ not þe peynes þat ben to come & dredeþ not to synne. And wele is þis Ruben clepid þe sone of si3t, for whan he was borne his moder cried & seyde: 'God haþ seen my meeknes'. And mans soule in soche a consideracioun of his olde synne & þe power of þe domesman beginniþ þan trewly to se God by feling of drede, and also to be seen of God.[43]

Drede is a 'felt vertewe' – something more than simply an emotional reaction or state. As such, it has a wider impact upon the soul and its powers. Specifically, it generates forms of self-knowledge, and modes of self-reflexive awareness. This is given potent figurative expression through drede's additional appellation: Ruben is drede personified, but he is also called the 'sone of siʒt'. Drede is connected to the power of perception, and functions here as a mode of perception as much as an emotion. Drede of God is truly a form of apprehension – both a knowing and a feeling. Initially, it promotes knowledge of the self before God: it contains an element of penitential awareness, a dawning realisation of the state of the soul and the presence of sin. Yet drede goes further still, and fosters modes of reciprocal perception, creating a relationship between self and God. This is reflected in the figurative family drama of the passage, as Ruben not only sees God, but *is seen by Him*: drede fashions a relationship between God and the soul, as to drede God is ultimately to see, and to be seen by, Him. From this apprehension one more thing is born: meekness. Speaking of the soul, the text notes that 'also by Ruben he is mekyd'.[44] Drede's impact is profound, and works to humble the soul in front of God. Such meekness is an integral part of the therapeutic operation of drede. As Hilton notes in his *Scale of Perfection*,

> [W]hat that thou feelist, seest, or smellest or savours, withouten in thi bodili wittes, or withinne in ymagynynge or feelynge in thi resoun or knowynge: brynge hit al withynne the trowthe and rulis of Hooli Chirche and caste it al in the morter of mekenesse and breke it smal with the pestel of drede of God.[15]

Thought, feeling, sensation and perception are all altered by apprehension. It is this alteration that begins the treatment of the soul. Drede and meekness are connected, presented here as a pair of tools commonly used to prepare medicines. Their interconnection is as integral as their mode of operation: drede and meekness work together to crush and reduce all aspects of the person, while at the same time they combine those reduced aspects with the 'rulis of Hooli Chirche'. Meekness – humility – is a key product of drede, and here the powerful effect it exerts upon the soul is made clear through imagery that alludes to medicine and treatment. As these texts collectively show, drede's therapeutic trajectory begins by removing pride, then bringing the self to an awareness of itself and its sinful nature, before fashioning a more beneficial relationship with God based upon humility. This is a process of many stages, as *timor* does not become *amor* all at once. It begins, as all these texts note, with a servile fear of punishment. To evoke that initial drede requires texts not of contemplative guidance or meditative repose, but of greater visual power and potency, texts which offer lively descriptions of the death and decay of the body, and the torture of the soul. To learn to fear God requires us first to learn of death, and to learn to cower before the consequences of sin: to feel such drede requires texts which begin with our end, which focus on our frailties, and which make us see ourselves in a less than positive light.

Pastoral Passions

>Þe ferthe Werke es of Mercy
>To comfort þam þat er sary,
>Als seke men þat bedde-red lyse
>Or þa þat er in othir anguyse.
>Men suld þam comfort in alle þair bales
>Thurgh gode ensaumples and fayre tales
>To brynge þam out of wrange thoght. (ll. 7687–93)

For the *Speculum Vitae*, a vast pastoral *summae* structured around a line-by-line elaboration of the *Pater Noster*, words can be truly medicinal, can alleviate suffering and compel the mind from 'wrange thoght' to correct thought. This text is a widely disseminated distillation of complex theological concepts in accessible and memorable verse. As its audience is wider than just the clergy, so too is its function more diffuse than simply providing summary information and sacramental guidance. It seeks to treat the soul, to have a medicinal effect, and it outlines the theology of fear and the impacts it can have upon the soul. The very idea of therapy is presented here as the movement of the mind towards the good through the power of words – through 'fayre tales' and 'gode ensaumples'. Such therapeutic texts are not idle and vain romances, but rather treatments that promote correct thought and intention. Subtly, the *SV* is also situating itself amongst the very texts it describes, as it too aims to treat the 'malese of hert' within its readers (l. 7698). Yet it does so through its focus on the 'gode wordes' (l. 7704) of the *Pater Noster*. This prayer is fundamental to the faith and, by extension, the *cura animarum*. Its power lies in its ability to engage the emotions, to make the reader or hearer 'fele' (l. 247) a certain way. As the text notes, the very first word of this prayer – *pater* – 'stirs vs to knawe euen / Thre thynges in Godde, Fader of heuen' (ll. 295–6), and 'askes of vs sex thynges to halde' (l. 370). These six demands cover 'Luf and Drede and Obedience, / Seruyse, Honour, and Reuerence' (ll. 373–4): they encompass emotions and actions, states of being, and modes of subjective and intersubjective awareness. Beyond its meaning of 'fader' the first word of the *Pater Noster* articulates a trajectory from potent emotional states to the performance of morally good actions. It all begins with love and drede:

>Þe first thynge þat Godde askes of vs
>Es Luf, þat we luf hym þus:
>With al our hert in body wroght,
>With al our saul, with al our thoght.
>With al our hert, þat es to say
>Þat we on nathynge, nyght ne day,
>Sette our herte to luf mare
>Þan on Godde. (ll. 375–82)

Body, soul, and thought – luf occupies all aspects of being. It is not a gentle passion here, but an all-consuming engagement of the person in the service of God. The anaphora of 'with al our' stresses the total nature of that love, emphatically connecting heart, soul, and thought together. The result is to generate a sense that luf of God not simply requires such total engagement, but demands it: the stress patterns of the lines and the use of repetition make it impossible to escape the incessant requirement of 'with al'. God can only be approached with such a love. So intense is it that we would 'suld tittar thole, if we war wis, / Our lyues be parted fra our bodys' (ll. 387–8). Death, with all the pain and suffering it inflicts on the body and soul, is preferable to forsaking the luf of God. This luf is a ceaseless form of service, occupying all temporal periods – 'nyght' and 'day'. The references to time paradoxically lend a sense of timelessness, with the endless love of God matched by the endless procession of the hours. Luf here is an active service, not simply an interior state of feeling but a total emotional orientation of the person towards life. This is reflected in the rhyme of 'wroght' and 'thoght': action and emotion are one, the interior disposition a mere beat away from its exterior manifestation; both connected and sustained by luf. Yet, luf is not the only passion mentioned:

> Þe secund thyng es Drede alswa
> To haue in hert, whareso we ga,
> Þat we Godde drede with al our myght
> Thurgh Sones Drede (þan do we right),
> And noght thurgh drede þat men calles
> Carls Drede þat oft falles.
> For carls dredes þair louerdes thurgh awe,
> And noght for luf, als men may knawe. (ll. 399–406)

Drede must be just as present as luf, it too must be a passionate commitment that occupies the heart, body, and soul night and day. Yet, unlike luf, the text goes into more detail regarding the nature of that drede, specifying two forms: 'Sones drede' and 'Carls drede'. The distinction draws from the theology of fear mentioned earlier in this chapter, and the text distills that theology into an easily accessible and intelligible form. The main didactic impulse is not to provide abundant Biblical references for this point or theological authorities; rather, it is to delineate how one should approach God emotionally. Moreover, the text makes it clear that one emotion can be predicated upon another, that to fear as a Son requires the presence of luf. This deepens our understanding of luf: the point made here is not that one emotion counters another, but that one emotion can enrich and augment the other. Luf in this context is a backdrop, an emotion that can at once contain and convey that of drede: *timor* and *amor* are deeply, yet distinctively, intertwined. To love God requires the cultivation of an emotional complex – not just love and then fear, but both together – an emotion set within another that redefines and re-orientates it. The nature of this emotional complex is soon clarified:

> Þe gode sons thurgh luf has drede
> To wreth þair fader in worde or dede;
> Þis may wele be Sones Drede called.
> Swilk Drede in hert suld we halde
> And drede ay mare Goddis greuaunce
> Þan payne of helle or his vengeaunce,
> For drede of payne anely to se
> Es drede withouten charyte. (ll. 407–14)

To explain how one can love through fear, the text employs the familiar domestic context of the relationship between father and son. Immediately recognisable, this relationship allows the various particulars of the idea of *timor filialis* to become clear and intelligible. The ideal manner of approaching God, the emotional complex that it requires, is one intimately familiar to all. The text thereby generates an important relational context integral to its didactic agenda: we are encouraged to relate to God as the very words of the *Pater Noster* suggest – as 'Our Father'. By figuring such a domestic relationship, the text also constructs an important comparative context, in which the fear of pain and punishment are set as nothing compared to the fear of displeasing our Heavenly Father. Word choice supports this, as 'greuaunce' encompasses a range of meanings that include not only offence, annoyance or displeasure, but also injury and sickness. Its use endows the figured domestic relationship with a set of specific dynamics: God is not a remote deity but a parent, someone we can wound, injure and displease by our actions and behaviour, and Whom we are responsible for upsetting. The word implies agency, willed behaviour and considered action – all nuances that place the onus for maintaining this familial relationship with God upon us. In such a setting the concept of sin is likewise reconfigured. It is not an abstract concept, or even a violation of Divine law, but instead an attempt to wound or injure our father – a terrible and unnatural severing of family ties.

Through such careful choice of language specific theological concepts are rendered in more accessible ways, their meanings saturated by emotional tones and hues that lend them both immediacy and expressive force. The use of rhyme is another important poetic device, as 'greuaunce' is rhymed with 'vengeaunce'. Yet here end-rhyme serves not to unite the two forms of drede but rather to emphasise the crucial disparity between them. 'Vengeaunce' conveys the senses of legal, punitive justice and retribution, but also of vindictiveness, fury and power. It figures, therefore, a different set of intersubjective dynamics: God here is not our father but instead a more legalistic, impersonal and remote judge who seeks retribution for crimes against Him. Such a sense of retribution is much less emotionally sophisticated: we are not sons here but law-breakers, not members of a family but fugitives from the terrible force of justice. God is made more abstract here, intelligible and approachable only through the concepts of law and punitive justice. The relational context is less intimate and, as a consequence, less moving. It lacks not simply love, but also that key Christian virtue of charity. While it is not the preferred form of drede it does contain 'litell mede' (l. 415), and so possesses some utility:

> Bot first thurgh ferdnes may Drede bygyn
> Anely for vengeaunce of synne,
> Thurgh whilk men may bygynne do wele
> And afterward a swete luf fele,
> Þat þe Haly Gast with Drede sal knyt
> In þair hertes to stable þair witte.
> Drede mas a man synne forsake
> And Luf mas a man gode vertus take. (ll. 417–24)

Servile fear is a state of 'ferdnes', of pure terror. Yet it nevertheless holds an initiatory or inductive potential, drawing the person into a deeper set of emotional states and cognitive processes. It is the beginning of a higher state, a method to achieve higher virtues and move closer to God in a more familial manner. Though this form of drede begins with 'vengeaunce of synne' it soon turns into 'swete luf'. Emotional states are dynamic and progressive, with the drede of God changing and evolving into ever-increasing degrees of intimacy with God. Through it the Holy Ghost operates upon the soul, healing it: the word 'knyt' meaning both fasten and heal.[46] Drede's therapeutic potential is subtly figured, and exerts a strong force over the soul and its powers. Subsequent lines emphasise this, as drede 'stables' the wit. As a verb this word has a range of meanings beyond simply to pacify or stabilise, and includes the sense of 'to establish', 'to order' or 'to make morally steadfast'.[47] Drede has, therefore, extremely potent psychological and cognitive properties, healing the soul by pacifying and establishing morals within it. The benefits of drede are given succinct and memorable articulation: it causes the person to forsake sin and pursue virtue, with the end rhyme working to convey that sense of the dual properties of Sones drede. Its therapeutic function is elaborated upon later on in the poem, during its exposition of the '*sed libera nos a malo*' line of the *Pater Noster*. Here the text provides further detail regarding what sins drede targets and what virtues it encourages.

> For þe prophete þat Dauid hight
> Says þus in þe Sauter right,
> Þat Drede of Godde in hert to halde
> Es þe bigynnyng of Wisdom called.
> For þe Gift of Drede þat we aske last
> Þe first and þe mast synne may cast
> Out of þe hert þar it es inne;
> Þat es Pryde, rote of al synne. (ll. 3503–10)

In an overt reference to the Biblical authority of the Psalter and King David, the text asserts the connection between drede and wisdom, and specifies how it removes pride from the soul. As one of the Gifts of the Holy spirit, it works to cast out the 'rote' of pride. Drede has, therefore, considerable potency: the use of agricultural terms and images, aside from being a commonplace in the discussion of the seven deadly sins, is an effective poetic choice.[48] The image such a word evokes conveys the power of drede. Uprooting is not gentle or subtle, but violently forceful, ripping out from the heart the embedded sin of pride. The virtues drede establishes are conveyed in much the same way. Such fear 'plantes and settes / Mekenes þat Pryde mast lettes' (ll. 3479–80) in the heart: after the forceful harrowing of the heart, drede gently plants an important virtue. The choice of imagery is instructionally effective, not only being immediately familiar to a medieval audience, but also deftly summarising the main impacts of drede with mnemonic economy and precision. Drede roots out the vice of pride and plants the virtue of mekeness. Much as drede is a dynamic emotional state of love, fear and charity, the virtue of 'meknes' is also processional and programmatic. While a good in and of itself, the nourishment of this planted virtue leads to higher states: through it one may be lead 'Vnto þe parfyte blissedhede / þat es to say of Gastly Pouert' (ll. 3482–3) – to the blessedness of the Beatitudes. Such a point is ultimately derived from the advanced theological treaties on the soul and its powers mentioned in the introduction – that fear, the primary emotion of the irascible might, can lead to Poverty of Spirit. A direct reference to the Beatitude of Matthew 5:3, 'Blessed are the poor in spirit', follows. The connection contextualises and clarifies that enigmatic saying of Jesus, placing it within the more readily understandable and familiar context of the Drede of God. It is a subtle but significant rhetorical move, allowing some of the more abstract sayings of the Bible to be set within a frame that aids and supports their ready explication and application to the life of faith. Yet all this is begun through the words of the prayer and the proper filial disposition they evoke:

> Yhete þis worde, when we it rede,
> 'Qui-es', stirs vs to haue Drede.
> For al-if we Godde our Fader halde
> And we be here his childer called,
> He es rightwys and sothfast
> And wil yhelde vs at þe last
> Aftir our dedes (and þat es skille)
> Be þai gode or be þai ille. (ll. 1453–60)

The prayer is a dynamic force, stirring those who hear or read it to feel a specific way. In this sense it operates just as rhetoric and poetic were understood to do, dispelling apathy and moving its audience towards a specific state of emotional engagement. In this instance the words are held not only to evoke fear, but also to construct a specific relational context regarding God – they encourage us to see him as our father. Within a single couplet the text emphasises this point, explicitly delineating the specifics of that filial relationship: 'Our Fader halde' and 'His childer called' are held together rhythmically – the key Christian relationship rendered here as a poetic as well as divine unity. Yet the idea of being stirred by words is not confined to the emotional; actions are also mentioned. The text itself is quick to move from the state of drede to the performance of morally good actions. Good deeds are never far away, and the *Pater Noster* is presented as the vehicle by which these states are enabled – providing, of course, that it is correctly understood and explained. This is achieved not through dry exposition, but vast poetic expansion and extension of the prayer's meaning and referential content. All this is designed to address that central problem referred to at the beginning of the text (ll. 140–50): that many know the words of the *Pater Noster* but few feel the proper savour and sweetness of them. The text's careful poetic presentation of the prayer works to defamiliarise and revivify it. Drede is given extensive treatment, and is seen as a key emotional state to be evoked in the person via the proper understanding of the prayer. The *SV* is clearly concerned with the power of drede and, over its course, outlines the importance of drede in the life of faith and in the treatment of the soul through words. Yet, it is not the only text in the Vernon manuscript to show a preoccupation with the power of apprehension.

The *Prick of Conscience* is another text of pastoral instruction that has similar interests to the *SV*, but takes them to new levels of emotional intensity. Unlike the *SV*, the pastoral nature of this text is not so concerned with the various sacramental and catechetical issues of Lateran IV. Its focus is more practically orientated, concerned less with 'instructional programmes' and more with evoking in its audience a 'visceral' horror and fear.[49] It is the earlier of the two texts, and the *SV* draws from it in places. Yet the positioning of the *PoC* is after the *SV* in the manuscript. This could be significant: the *SV* provides summary instruction that outlines the power of fear, while the *PoC* acts as a spur to evoke it. Throughout this text, vast amounts of vivid and detailed images are layered to bring the reader into the very drede the *SV* describes. The *PoC* is altogether much darker in tone and more forceful in nature; the images it deploys are a source of immediate, emotional potency. From the outset it notes the crucial importance of 'þe way of mekenes principaly / And of drede and luf of God almyghty' (ll. 141–2). Over its course the text attempts to evoke and sustain this crucial emotional state through abundant imagery. Its goal is to teach, but this consists not simply of the provision of information; feeling and fact must come together:

> For an unkunnand man thurgh leryng
> May be broght til undirstandyng
> Of many thynges, to knaw and se
> Þat has bene and es and yhit sal be,
> Þat til mekenes myght stir his wille
> And til lufe and drede and to fle alle ille. (ll. 177–82)

Pastoral instruction must be more than the sum of its epistemic parts. Information must lead somewhere (ll. 229–30): it must 'stir' the person, move them to a greater engagement with the key issues of the faith and to that salutary complex of luf, drede and meekness. The knowledge imparted and the feelings evoked are practically orientated, are meant to work in unison to guide the person in behaviour and outlook. To that end the text shows an acute awareness of the variegated nature of audience psychology. Initially, it makes the broad classification of all persons into two classes: one 'þat can noght suld haf wille / To lere to knaw bathe gude and ille', and another who 'þat can oght suld lere mare / To knaw alle þat hym nedeful ware' (ll. 174–6). Not everyone possesses the same level of knowledge, willpower or even disposition. As such there exists a potentially problematic issue of variation. The audience is not intellectually nor emotionally homogeneous, and so the act of teaching must be able to overcome that barrier. The form that teaching takes is therefore paramount. Instruction must cut across differences in ability, intellect, and even psychology to further one goal:

> Bot som men has wytte to understand,
> And yhit þai er ful unkunand
> And of som thyng has na knawyng
> Þat myght styrre þam to gude lyfyng.
> Swylk men had nede to lere ilk day
> Of other men, þat can mare þan þay,
> To knaw þat myght þam stir and lede
> Til mekenes and til lufe and drede. (ll. 151–8)

Irrespective of whether those addressed have sufficient 'wytte', all teaching must achieve one aim. It must provide knowledge that can 'styrre' the person towards that emotional complex of meekness, luf and drede. The souls of all persons must be moved, universally, in specific and directed ways. Knowledge has, therefore, an important emotional function, it must lead 'wythalle til mekenes and drede' (l. 230). In the context of pastoral care, 'defaut of knawyng' (l. 279) is as much an emotional problem as it is one of inadequate instruction. On this the text is emphatic, asking the rhetorical question 'What wonder es yf þai haf na drede? / For what þai suld drede, þai knaw noght' (ll. 276–7). Beyond this division of intelligence and ability, however, the text makes three finer gradations regarding the psychological nature of its audience. Each constitutes an exemplary type that, in sum, are the central problems faced by all pastoral teaching. The text is quick to use the authority of Scripture in its taxonomical endeavours, with each type of person connected to a Biblical quotation. The first type in many ways poses the most difficult pastoral problem:

> Yhit som men wille noght understande
> Þat þat mught mak þam dredande,
> For þai wald noght here bot þat þam pays
> Þarfor þe prophet in þe Psauter says
> *Noluit intelligere*
> *Ut bene ageret.* (ll. 281–6)

Those who are in this group are characterised by a stubborn refusal to believe despite instruction. They actively refuse to listen to teaching, and are wilfully disobedient and unreceptive: they 'wil noght undirstand ne lere / To drede God and to do his wille' (ll. 290–1). Such wilful ignorance consists not simply of an aversion to teaching but also of a relentless self-involved focus on their own pleasure. It is their guiding principle and the entirety of their moral compass (l. 292). The pastoral care for this type is difficult as they refuse to engage with instruction in any sense – there is neither knowledge nor the desire to know. The second classification is more complex:

> Som understandes als þai here telle,
> Bot na drede in þair hertes may dwelle,
> And thurgh defaut of trouthe þat may be;
> For þai trow nathyng bot þat þa se,
> But groches when þai dredful thyng here.
> Þarfore þe prophet says on þis manere:
> *Non crediderunt*
> *Et murmuraverunt.* (ll. 293–300)

An emotional malaise, not a default of knowing, is the central problem here. Persons in this grouping know and understand what they are being told, but they have no belief due to their lack of drede. In terms of pastoral care, they are receptive to teaching in that they are capable of understanding what they hear, yet they do not believe in it. The reason for this is twofold. On the one hand they are incapable of believing in anything that is not immediately present to them. Things they cannot see are, for them, impossible to believe in. There is a problem of sense knowledge, as they require not logical proof but sensory stimuli: for them to believe in something requires it to be put before their eyes. The second reason is that whatever teaching they receive generates an incorrect emotional response. Instead of pastoral instruction causing a salutary drede, unresponsive anger is generated – they 'groches gretly and waxes fraward' (l. 305) when they hear things they dislike. There is no savour in their instruction, only active contempt. Teaching this type is difficult, as the initial receptivity is soon contorted and twisted into something spiritually useless.

In the third classification there is yet a further understanding of the intricacies of human psychology in the practice of pastoral care:

> Som can se in buk swilk thyng and rede,
> Bot lightnes of hert reves þam drede,
> Swa þat it may noght with þam dwelle,
> And þarfor says God þus in þe gospelle:
> *Quia ad tempus credunt, et in tempore*
> *Temptacionis recedunt.* (ll. 307–12)

Instruction and learning are not issues for this group, as they are keen to know as much as possible, and may in fact be able to read pertinent material themselves. What they read or hear also provokes the correct emotional reaction of drede. Initial receptivity soon changes though. The drede that is evoked only lasts a short time, and soon fades. As a result they are in spiritual danger, believing themselves to be advancing in virtue when in fact it is the reverse. The text provides a precise psychological reason for this. They have a problematic disposition – 'lightnes of hert': they are frivolous or fickle in their affections, easily changeable from one state to another. After deploying another scriptural quotation to support this diagnosis, the text asserts that 'swilk men er ay swa unstedfast' (l. 324). This word means not simply infirm of purpose or belief, but also unstable.[50] There is, therefore, an instability about these people that makes all teaching useless. Memory is singled out as a contributing factor. Initially they believe and feel, 'but tyte þai had don, and forgat / His werkes and thogt na mar of þat' (ll. 322–3). This is a significant detail that has broad implications: to forget pastoral instruction is a fault of both the audience and of the nature and form of their instruction. With great subtlety, the text is figuring here the importance of poetic persuasion in pastoral care, as only this can address all three of these problematic issues.

Regarding the first, a good poetic argument is forceful, containing arresting images and rhetorical figures that command the attention of those who do not wish to listen or know. In terms of the second, it can also present vivid and sensorially rich depictions that can make present before the eyes of the mind that which is described. Poetic arguments can mimic sense data, simulating reality for those who refuse to believe what they cannot sense, and delimiting the range of emotional responses to them. Finally, good poetic arguments are memorable ones, and can impress themselves upon the hearts and minds of their hearers due to their poetic nature. It is no coincidence that the text presents itself as the means of addressing these problems immediately after highlighting them:

> Bot whaswa can noght drede may lere,
> Þat þis tretice wil rede or here;
> Yf þai rede or here til þe hende
> Þe maters þat er þarin contende,
> And undirstand þam al and trow,
> Parchaunce þair hertes þan sal bow,
> Thurgh drede þat þai sal consayve þarby,
> To wirk gude werkes and fle foli. (ll. 328–35)

Whether read or heard, the contents of the text are arranged so that a specific emotional response is achieved. Through the text's metre and tones a salutary drede can be evoked and sustained in the audience that can compel them to pursue virtue and flee vice. This pastoral agenda is directly connected to and achieved by both the form and content of the text. It is designed for 'laude men þat er unkunnand' (l. 338), and can be either read or recited. Its effects on any who engage with it will be potent:

> To mak þam þamself first to knaw
> And fra syn and vanytese þam draw,
> And for to stir þam til right drede,
> When þai þis tretisce here or rede.
> Þat sal prikke þair conscience withyn,
> And of þat drede may a lofe bygyn. (ll. 340–5)

The text is designed to stir and move, to bring about that emotional complex of 'lofe' and 'drede'. It will not be subtle in this endeavour, and will use some degree of force. As the text asserts it will 'prikke' the reader – a word which possesses a range of interconnected meanings. On one level it means 'to pierce or penetrate', and on another 'to disturb', 'to unsettle', 'to inscribe' and 'to incite or urge'.[51] The text, therefore, will make an almost surgical incision on the reader, cutting into 'þair conscience withyn' to evoke those passions of fear and love. This process is not going to be gentle but rather disturbing and unsettling. The use of 'prikke' gestures towards the tone and tenor of the anticipated reading process. With great economy, the text sets up expectations of intensity and potency within the audience. The secondary meaning of prikke – to incite or urge – is integral here, as the text will deploy a vast range of poetic images to compel the reader into specific emotional states. It will do this via highly vivid descriptions, offering the reader a sensory overload of details and textures that make present before the eyes of the mind the things, states and penalties described. The imaginative syllogism, discussed in the introduction, is on full display throughout this text, with the reader being placed into an increasingly rich sensory world that aids in evoking and maintaining specific emotional responses. For instance, the description of conception and birth:

> Þar duelled man in a myrk dungeon
> And + a foul sted of corrupcion,
> Whar he had na other fode
> Bot waltsom glet and loper[d] blode
> And stynk and filthe, als I sayde ar;
> With ther he was first norisshed þar. (ll. 456–60)

This is simply horrific. One of the most familiar and familial aspects of life becomes reconfigured as something horrendously strange and vile. Conception and childbirth, while not unsafe activities during the Middle Ages, are nevertheless stripped of any normative emotional tenderness. The images here are at once shocking and forceful, compelling the reader to feel a certain way. The womb is no longer the site of generation but rather incarceration – the child a prisoner within a ghastly flesh jail. It is a place of almost punitive torture, relentlessly assaulting all the senses. For the reader, sight, smell, touch and even taste are all evoked in this description. Not only is the womb a dark and sinister dungeon, but it is also a filthy pit full of noxious odours and slimely substances. Corrupt matter – coagulated blood and oozing slime – encircle the infant in a torrent of filth and vileness. Yet the text does not stop here. Lest any should be inured to this poetic rendering, its potency goes one sense further. The infant is force-fed this waste matter as its first and only sustenance. Our first food was not mother's milk but her own filth and corruption: we are not simply put in a prison, but put in one that we are forced to consume. This is a nightmarish, but effective and memorable, image. The emotive potential here is quite obvious, each imagistic impression carrying with it a fragmentary feeling, working cumulatively to build up a thick picture of both sense and horror. The use of hypotactic constructions makes it difficult to rush through this description; it forces us to hold images and the sense impressions they evoke in the mind. Through its syntactic structure, this poetic moment becomes attenuated and extended into an immersive space of image, sense and sound. The evocation of drede is therefore not far behind.

Imagery is not used simplistically in this text. Throughout, there is a subtle poetic sophistication and comprehensive understanding of the effects on the mind of images and the sounds of words. Contrast and counterpoint are deployed to make their effect all the more potent:

> Herbes forth bringes floures and sede,
> And tres fair fruyt and braunches to sprede,
> And þou forth bringes of þiself here
> Nites, lyse, and other vermyn sere.
> Of herbes and tres springes baum ful gude
> And oyle and wyne for mans fude;
> And of þe comes mykel foul thyng,
> Als fen and uryn and spyttyng.
> Of herbes and tres comes swete savour,
> And of þe comes wlatsom stynk and sour. (ll. 648–57)

This description, much like the prior passage, is drawn from Innocent III's *De Miseria Condicionis Humane* (Books 1.3–1.7), and is underpinned here by strong and evocative contrasts.[52] From plants and herbs come all good things, useful and beneficial; from man comes all filth, vile crawling creatures, vermin and corrupt emissions. The fruits of each are juxtaposed, but they share a common sensory register. The trees and things of nature generate not simply visually beautiful flowers, but also medicinal and nourishing food and sweet odours – they please sight, taste and smell. In contrast man is an affront to all these senses, emitting disgusting substances and creatures. The layering of these strong contrasts is both striking and engaging. Instead of placing an extended description of each in opposition, the text interweaves them together, constantly contrasting one image directly with another. The rapid oscillation between contraries generates a jarring and dizzying effect, as the reader's focus shifts from one to the other in a process of ideational augmentation. Point and counterpoint ricochet off each other in specific ways, making the images and sense impressions fall into sharper focus and relief. The reader is held within these rapid oscillations, immersed within the verse and what it describes. Constant shifting of images, and of the senses, substances and creatures they portray gives this passage an intense and restless energy.

In terms of psychological impact this is a very effective choice, as it prevents the images from becoming stale or dull. Such variety is itself a principle of medieval aesthetics, the idea that strong contrasts and antitheses are the hallmarks of good artistic craft.[53] Sharp contrasts maintain the emotional potency of the images, making the reader see them afresh each time. In each contrast the reader is permitted a moment of brief relief from the horrors of the human body and its rancid emissions, but this moment serves only to add yet more emphasis to the next series of horrors. Psychologically, the mind's eye cannot rest on an image long enough for it to become commonplace or for it to lose its initial cognitive and sensory impact. Such rapid variety and contrast are, however, not the only weapons in the text's poetic arsenal. It also makes use of what could be considered the artistic opposite: the gradual and careful extension of imagistic intensity and detail. This is yet another way in which the text seeks to compel the reader.

In less than one hundred lines after the above passage, the text moves into an account of the decay and ageing of the human body (ll. 761–805). It operates in a very different manner, using different techniques to convey its emotive images:

> His mynde es short when he oght thynkes,
> His nese ofte droppes, his hand stynkes,
> His sight wax[es] dym þat he has,
> His bak waxes croked; stoupand he gas.
> Fyngers and taes, fote and hande,
> And alle his touches er tremblande.
> His werkes forworthes þat he bygynnes,
> His hare moutes, his eghen rynnes,
> His eres waxes deef and hard to here,
> His tung fayles, his speche es noght clere.
> His mouthe slavers, his tethe rotes,
> His wyttes fayles, and he ofte dotes. (ll. 774–85)

Instead of variety and oscillation there is intensity and focus – an unrelenting attention to the details of decay. The central image is the rotting of man, but the whole image is unfolded gradually and with potent precision. Over the course of these lines the man described slowly crumbles, each line a successive though subordinate imagistic flash that further augments that central image of decay. New details and new textures come to the fore for a brief moment, before being succeeded by yet another stage in man's inexorable decomposition. Yet, while there is no rapid fire of contrasting images, the passage is not static or slow. The paratactic profusion of detail is relentless and generates a sense of fluidity, of coursing or streaming decay. Man diminishes and disintegrates before our very eyes. Much like the arming scene of Gawain, or the initial presentation of the Green Knight in *Sir Gawain and the Green Knight*, the precise but modulated use of detail causes the passage to deepen, to gain an intensity through the gradual release of the various subordinated images of decay. It is supported by the use of anaphora throughout most of the passage, which not only binds the images together, but also makes each resonate with the others. Each repetition of 'his' strikes the ear in a way both familiar and distinct, adding new tones to the decomposition of man. The whole passage itself mirrors this on a structural level. It moves from external sense impressions – the general stench of man – to increasingly specific and interior observations. It numbers the body's extremities before moving to the interior: we hear first of the trembling hands and feet, before viewing the running eyes, nose, rotten teeth and the failing tongue. Eventually, the poem moves into describing the now faulty emotional responses, cognition and judgement of this man – his inability to think clearly and without prejudice (ll. 795–800). The overall effect is again one of an inescapable immersion in decay.

Image and its articulation are key to this text, and to the ways in which they evoke and sustain the emotions of the reader. All of its images are potent. In one translation of St Bernard, the text notes that the human corpse soon rots into ever greater foulness: a dead body goes from corpse to 'vermyn . . . and aftir vermyn stynkand uglynes' (ll. 916–7). As medieval psychology maintains, each image evokes a specific emotional response or tone; this one is no exception. However, the broader linguistic presentation of the images in the text must also be considered. The poetic arrangement of the text's striking images allows greater possibilities for evoking and sustaining specific emotional states, as language can magnify and extend the images in effective ways.

When the text moves to a more general section on *contemptus mundi*, its use of images is significant. It compares the world to four different things: the sea, a wilderness, a forest and a battle (ll. 1214–47). Each different metaphorical comparison evokes new imagistic registers, each of them sinister and frightening, that cause the reader to view the world in new ways. Within each comparison, however, a further set of images is delayered. We hear of the ebb and flow of 'tydes' (l. 1215), of 'stormes þat blawes'; of a wilderness populated 'ful of wild bestes' (l. 1227); of a forest 'ful of thefs and outlawes' (l. 1237); and of a 'feld ful of batailles' (l. 1247) that consists purely 'of enemys þat ilk day men assayles' (l. 1248). A chain of images is created here, each one with its own emotive potential and range. As such they are all harmoniously linked together as sub-sets of the overarching metaphorical context, and constitute a polyphony of emotive response. There is, therefore, a layering not simply of the images but also of their specific cognitive effects. This is a consistent example of the rhetorical device of *amplificatio*. Yet the text goes beyond this as the layering of images is both mediated and played with via language. Images are not simply presented, but presented in specific ways. In a section that deals with the vagaries of fortune, the text notes that rapid changes are the everyday occurrence of the natural world: 'Now es day, now es nyght; / Now es myrk, now es light' (ll. 1434–5). Such change is a token of all aspects of life in the world:

> For now es mirthe, now es murnyng;
> Now es laghter and now es gretyng;
> Now er men wele, now er men wa;
> Now es a man frende, now es he faa;
> Now es a man light, now es [he] hevy;
> Now es he blithe, now es he drery;
> Now haf we ioy, now haf we pyn;
> Now we wyn and now we tyn;

> Now er we ryche, now er we pur;
> Now haf we or-litel, now pas we mesur;
> Now er we bigg, now er we bare;
> Now er we hale, now seke and sare. (ll. 1450–61)

This successive list of contraries and contrasts is relentless, and is a key moment in the *contemptus mundi* theme of the text. It is comprised of small imagistic flashes that work cumulatively to enact what they describe. Yet, they do this only due to their poetic arrangement. The technique and method of narration here is crucial to this, as it offers rapid comparison between diametric opposites. The effect is subtle at first but quickly picks up force, as the reader begins to lurch from one extreme to the next, shunted from one thing to another again and again. In many ways this enacts the earlier metaphorical presentation of the world as a sea of troubles, as the reader now follows the ebbs and flows of the narrative tide. The metre is key to this effect, maintaining a constant beat that at once controls the passage of time and provides an aural contrast to the constant shifts and variabilities it describes. The consistent and the contrasting are brought into play both metrically and visually. The move from 'wele' to 'wa' is, while varied, essentially consistent – a constant variability in fortune and circumstance embodied by the verse itself. There is the use of *amplificatio* here, but it is of a different order, providing not diversity and abundance but rather depth. The constant reiteration of changes in fortune is a method of deepening the emotional potential of the images described: the reader is immersed in a succession of imagistic and aural impacts that extend the force of the verse into new depths of emotive intensity. All these images have a similar emotive potential, but they are all held together in such a way that maximises that potential and builds it up into a constant process of emotive evocation. The poetic arrangement of the passage sustains and maintains all emotive sense impressions, enriching and deepening them as much as possible. Such effects are at work throughout the whole text, often in more extended form than here.

In the account of the pains of purgatory, nearly 400 lines (ll. 2900–3280), the narrative becomes deliberately slow. The various details of torment are set out in a manner that is neither swift nor brisk, but gradual and recursive: these lines are effectively slight variations on a theme, the reader bombarded with the same basic fact in different but modulated ways. In the passages dealing with the judgement of the soul after death by fifteen accusers (ll. 5420–640), the narrative is potent and visually excessive, and is made to race ahead via the constant use of the conjunction 'alswa' for each of the soul's accusers. This has the effect not only of quickening the narrative, shaping it into a tumultuous chorus of accusation, but also to bind the various units of the passage together into one larger emotional chain of signification. In all cases the effect upon the reader is designed to be inescapable: drede is meant to be evoked. Towards the end of the text this goal is made all the more explicit. The text asserts that 'whaswa of þis wil take hede / May be stird til luf and drede' (ll. 9482–3):

> For if a man it rede and understandes wele
> And þe materes þarin til hert wil take,
> It may his conscience tendre make
> And til right way of rewel bryng it bilyfe,
> And his hert til drede and mekenes dryfe
> And til luf and yhernyng of heven-blis,
> And to amende alle þat he has done mys. (ll. 9549–55)

Engagement with this text – either reading or hearing it – will have profound psychological and behavioural effects upon the person: this text seeks to make those who encounter it flee the bad and pursue the good. The word 'dryfe' is a key signal. It means 'to chase', 'to purse', 'to compel', 'to push'.[54] The reader, therefore, is to be compelled and forcefully moved by the text's poetic arguments and images, made to feel drede at the sinful origins of mankind and at the punishments that await in Hell and Purgatory. Powerful persuasion is key to this. The text will 'stirre lewed men til mekenes / And to make þam luf God and drede' (ll. 9595–6), evoking specific emotional states. In turn, these states encourage morally good action: through the text the reader wil 'be stird þarby til ryghtwyse way, / þat es, til the end of gude lyfyng' (ll. 9607–8). That word 'stirre' has a similar set of meanings as 'dryfe', but includes the more medical sense of enliven and invigorate.[55] Overall, this brings about that crucial apprehension – a state of both knowledge and affection that is given articulation in moral action. The most repeated word here, 'stirre', signals the principal effect of the text. It is not something passive but rather intensely active, urging the reader into feeling and being a certain way.

The use of anaphora in the above passage adds emphasis to this: each 'and' a successive addition to the range of effects the text exerts upon its readers, and each a recapitulation and reformulation of the various effects of the poetic images it presents. Such is the potency of the poetic argument that the text is sceptical about those who are not moved by its persuasive power. While it does acknowledge that some will 'noght þarby stirred be' (l. 9601), it makes it clear that such persons must therefore suffer from a cognitive deficiency: they are 'wittles' (l. 9603) and so psychologically incapable of being moved by poetically arranged images. Those who are unmoved and yet not mentally incapacitated must be the hopelessly reprobate – 'over-mykel hardend in wikkednes' (l. 9603): the text, with all its incisive power, cannot 'prike' them. These persons are the outliers, those who exist at the extremes and fall outside normal categories of human response and psychology. For everyone else, with their variegated but normative mental states, the text will operate in similar ways, stirring the conscience, evoking emotion, and compelling action or 'ryght way of lyfe' (l. 9571). However, this is not all the text does; there is an additional cognitive state it enables. Drede of God's judgement and punishment begets other states:

> May make a man knawe and hald in mynde
> What he es here of his awen kynde
> And what he sal be, if he avyse hym wele,
> And whar he es for to knaw and fele.
> Yhit may he se, when he it redes,
> What he es worthy for his dedes;
> Whether he es worthy ioy or payne,
> Þis tretice may make hym be certayne. (ll. 9558–65)

Drede is dynamic, and causes not simply the removal of pride but also a profound sense of introspection. Through the text's numerous poetic images, the reader is encouraged not simply to feel a certain way, but also to reflect upon those emotional states in a guided manner. The form of introspection here is almost confessional in its range, its modes of assessment, its quantifications and comparisons. The conscience, newly pricked by the text, is now enabled to gaze upon and into itself in a manner that is essentially confessional. Drede begets an introspection predicated upon assiduous self-scrutiny into deeds, motives and their ultimate consequences. Self-scrutiny gives way to a sense of self-diagnosis: an assiduous attention to the conscience, to its careful modulation and the emotional registers it evokes, sustains and is predicated upon. This attention to the diagnostic will become ever stronger in medieval religious culture, and as others have shown, it is a distinctive feature of lay spirituality after the 1380s.[56] It begins, though, with the stirring of the emotions, with that initial pricking of conscience. From this inceptive phlebotomy all else develops – it is the first cut in the surgery of the soul. Of course, this incision is certainly not the deepest: other texts are required to continue, augment and intensify the treatment of the soul. The next chapter will look at perhaps the most potent form of versified writing that can generate specific emotional and penitential states: the medieval moral and penitential lyric.

2

Lyrical Treatment

> Or hastow som remors of conscience,
> And art now falle in some devocioun,
> And wailest for thi synne and thin offence,
> And has for ferde caught attricioun?
> (*Troilus and Criseyde*, Bk. 1, ll. 554–7)[1]

While Chaucer sets the words of Pandarus to Troilus within the courtly context of love-sickness, these words nevertheless offer an important insight into medieval understandings of emotional response and psychology.[2] Emotions are never static, but instead move and progress into deeper and/or different states. Fear is an important emotion for 'sowle-hele', but is not the only one. The force of fear ultimately moves in different directions, into different and layered emotional states. Here it leads to an almost confessional self-awareness, dynamically changing into an emergent state of attrition. The whole scene dramatises confessional introspection, not only in the respective physical postures of Troilus and Pandarus, but also in the states of emotional response it is predicated upon. Fear does not stand alone, but is connected to remorse of conscience, devotion, attrition and the presence of sin. Emotion stirs and shifts in a dramatic cascade or progression, changing and layering into deeper states of penitential awareness. It is this emotional progression that is the essence of sowle-hele, moving from a salutary drede to a more purgative penance.

The pastoral materials mentioned in the prior chapter are ways of enabling the 'ground of hele', but the fear and drede they create cannot be static or remain at the level of servile fear of punishment. They must move into penance, through the fear of attrition and into the sorrow of contrition. The penitential lyric is one means of enabling such a therapeutic movement. The lyric form itself operates as an 'affective catalyst' that can be used to evoke more potent and directed emotional states.[3] While the pastoral materials discussed in the prior chapter make sustained and extensive use of mnemonic verse, the lyric is distinctive for its ability to generate both intensity and engagement. Verse can aid the memory to be sure, but the use of exegematic narrative, anaphora, complex rhythm and rhyme, the rhetorical potency of stanzaic arrangement, and alliteration and metre, all have physiological and so psychological impacts. The lyric will, through reciting it, control both thought and breath, allowing emotion and its articulation to coalesce into specific temporal moments arranged and circumscribed in a lattice-like structure, one designed to amplify the emotions its performance is predicated upon. This chapter explores that genre of writing. It begins by looking at the highly medical understanding of confession and contrition during the Middle Ages, before exploring how Richard Maidstone's *Penitential Psalms* works to evoke and sustain sorrow for sin. The chapter closes with an analysis of a range of medieval penitential lyrics from Vernon, assessing how they function to evoke sorrow for sin and encourage their readers to perform a simulated confession.

Confession as Medicine

In the *Twelve Profits of Tribulation*, a popular fifteenth-century Middle English translation of the *Tractatus de tribulacione*, the sacrament of confession is given a highly medical rendering:

> For as the body is purged by medicinalle drinkis of euell humoris, ryght so is the soule made clene by tribulacions sent from the souereyne leche oure lord god of veyne affeccions and euell maners . . . the secund purgacion of mannys body for euel humoris is by crafty blood-lettynge, and that is of two manners, as by openynge of þe veyne, or els by boxynge or ventusynge. Openynge of the veyne is properyd to confession, and boxynge or ventusyng, to tribulacion.[4]

Penitential work is like a form of medical procedure – phlebotomy via needle. As the practice of venesection requires some skill, this metaphor endows penance, and by extension the priest who carries it out, with a specialised role and agency. It is a targeted treatment for sin, a 'crafty blood-lettynge', that is itself much subtler than the medicinal drink of tribulation, or the procedure of 'boxynge or ventusyng'. Such an understanding of penance is dominated by ideas of penetration and precision. Through penance the soul is in effect punctured and drained of sin – 'the veyne be the which blood or syne ys voided oute, is the mouth . . . þat is to sey, be confession'.[5] Auricular confession is less an act of self-disclosure than it is a medical act of incision and excavation. Its precision is emphasised through this medical metaphor. Just as one should 'voyde oute wicked blood for the purgynge of his body, and kepe his good bloode for his norrisshynge', the act of confession should 'shew all his synnes, and with-hold and kepe preue all his good dedis'.[6] Confession is not a general cleansing effected by a similarly general discursive act, but instead a specialised procedure that purges only sin from the soul; one predicated upon specific linguistic acts and their attendant emotional states. Such a medical understanding of penance is, however, far from novel. While the Fourth Lateran Council of 1215 presents the priest in 'the manner of a skilful physician' and as 'the physician of souls', the medical rendering of confession pre-dates this by some time.[7] The concept of the *medicus animarum* dates back to the Cappadocian Fathers of the early church and the idea of the *Christus medicus*, and appears in early medieval penitentials.[8] The idea of the medicine of the soul is so frequently employed in religious contexts throughout the period as to be something of a hackneyed commonplace.[9] It is from this broader metaphorical context that confession comes to be seen specifically as a medical procedure, as the purgative removal of sin.

For Hugo of Fouilloy (*c*.1096–*c*.1172), writing in the early twelfth century, purgation is the dominant conceptual paradigm: 'Sicut enim in quolibet infirmo aperiuntur carnis pori, ut per sudorem fiat purgatio morbi, sic per confessionem peccati fit laudabilis purgatio animi' (Indeed as in every sick person the pores of the flesh open so that by means of sweating a purging of the disease shall be made, thus by means of confession of sins commendable purging of the soul should be made).[10] Sweating, according to medieval medicine, is a form of natural and involuntary purgation that occurs to combat disease.[11] It is employed here as a conceptual analogy for how the work of penance ought to be understood. The sacrament is rendered as an inherently natural and defensive process directed towards the ultimate health of the soul. It is a treatment that is conceived of in terms of removal and extraction only. The disease of sin cannot be managed, only removed – literally sweated out. Sin here is highly physical, possessing a fluid quality as something internally present within the body yet ultimately inimical to it – much like a disease or poison. Its treatment, therefore, operates within exactly the same therapeutic parameters. William De Montibus (*c*.1140–1215), in one of the most influential pastoral texts from the period – the *Peniteas Cito* – has this to say about treating the soul:

> The Spiritual Antidote
> As doctors cure the body with various medicines
> (He does not heal a fever as a wound or tumour),
> So sickly souls demand various treatments.
> You should impose the contraries of the soul's diseases:
>
> The avaricious man should give away his possessions;
> The lustful man should castrate himself.
> Envious man, put aside jealousy; proud man, put aside your puffing up.
> Sobriety restrains gluttony; patience, anger.
> Self-criticism removes resentment; sadness, sloth.[12]

Allopathic treatment, or the medicine of the contraries, is one of the foundational principles of all medieval medicine. It is used here in a highly literal sense to explain the treatment of the soul: the venomous affections of sin are cast out through their opposites. Such treatment is highly specialised, and there is here a sense of the adaptability of the treatment to the particular illness. The careful differentiation between fever, wound and tumour conveys the idea of confession as a personalised form of treatment and care. By extension, the act of enjoining a penance participates within that framework – it is the result of considered medical skill. The medical metaphor allows this degree of complexity, and is not merely being used for rhetorical flair; there is the sense here that the separation between the metaphorical and the literal is far from absolute. William of Auvergne's (*c*.1180–1249) understanding of confession comes to similarly somatic conclusions:

> Quoniam ergo vomitus est juxta literam evacuatio ventris corporalis, aut in parte, aut in toto per os, sive ministerio oris; evacuatio inquam ventris corporalis in parte, vel in toto, quam inducere solet, vel indignatio stomachi vel ventris, vel abominabilitas alicujus, quod in ventre est: sic per os, sive ministerio oris evacuatur, sive exoneratur venter cordis, sive conscientia a vitiis; et peccatis, ea scilicet dicendo, ac manifestando sacerdoti.[13]

(Vomit, literally speaking, is the emptying of the belly, either partly or fully, via the mouth or by the agency of the mouth; I repeat, the emptying of the belly partly or wholly, which an upset stomach or belly or something inimical to them inside the belly usually induces. In the same way, the belly of the heart, or conscience, is emptied or relieved from vices or sins, by the agency of the mouth, by speaking or revealing these things to a priest.)

This more vivid image of purgation conveys the mechanics and intended outcomes of penance. It is presented as a medical procedure, to be induced and monitored by the priest. The metaphor is quite detailed and maps bodily organs and interior states onto each other. Such use of metaphor is significant, and works not as a form of rhetorical persuasion but as a careful articulation of the functional dynamics of confession. Through this choice of language confession becomes an act of some intensity, requiring the specialist administration of a priest-physician. Metaphor works not just to connect medicine and confession, but also to clarify how penance functions. In much the same way, Robert Grosseteste, the influential thirteenth-century bishop of Lincoln (*c*.1175–1253), connects spiritual and physical illnesses:

Curabit namque ut medicus, immo super quam medicus, lepram heretice pravitatis, ydropisi cupiditatis, ciragram tenacitatis, podagram pigricie, et superacutas febres luxurie, et ut ad unum dicam, omnem morbum spiritualiter curabit, et curatos in sanitate conservabit.

(For he will cure as a physician, nay, somewhat above a physician, the leprosy of heretical deformity, the dropsy of greed, the hand-gout of niggardliness, the foot-gout of sloth, and the highly scorching fevers of luxurious living; in a nutshell, he will cure all spiritual ills, and preserve his cured patients in good health.)[14]

Sin and sickness operate in much the same way, and share more than a surface similarity. They are equally debilitating and dangerous. By combining the two, Grosseteste also combines the method of their treatment. His pastoral handbook, the *Templum Dei*, makes this clear, stipulating that priests ought to consider the complexion of each penitent.[15] In this way the priest really needs to be a skilful physician and effectively use the knowledge of physiognomy to aid in the overall pastoral treatment of those under his care.[16] Yet, while the assessment of complexion is important, it is made only to further the efficacy of the penitential treatment. In this Grosseteste is unambiguous. To return to a quotation referenced earlier in this book, he makes it clear that penance, the ultimate treatment of the soul, operates as a purgative:

In hac tabula est tota cura officii pastoralis, ut obstetricante manu per vinum et oleum contra vulnera et infirmitates educatur coluber tortuosus, et preambulis preparationibus detur medicina purgativa inducens sanitatem, et inductam conservet quousque pro infirmitatibus dotes et pro vulneribus beatitudines inducantur

(In this table there is all the duty of the pastoral office, that the twisting snake is to be taken out by the hand of the obstetrician with wine and oil against wounds and illnesses, and a purgative medicine is to be given during the preliminary preparations, a medicine which induces health, and once induced it conserves it until gifts and blessings are brought about instead of illnesses and wounds.)[17]

Grosseteste conveys the centrality of purgation by a complex and unexpected analogy, comparing the healing work of the pastoral office to the work of the obstetrician. However, he then reconfigures the central function of obstetrics from parturition to purgation, making it refer not to the delivery of a child but to the removal of a toxic presence. The goal of the priest-physician is to apply the required purgative medicine which removes the venomous worm or snake from the soul; only then can virtues be established and, eventually, the blessedness of the Beatitudes be attained. This purgative medicine must counter and remove the venom of sin through penitential states. As such the operation of the medicine is purgative, but its essential nature is wholly affective. As the *Peniteas Cito* made clear, the procedures for removing sin from the soul operate in accordance with the medicine of the contraries. As sin is the inevitable and aggregate product of disordered emotional states and responses, the judicious evocation of contrary emotional states will provide a means of combating and expelling those sins from the soul.[18] One of the early writers on confession, Alanus de Insulis (*d*.1202), offered the first definition of the difference between two types of penitential sorrow – attrition and contrition:

> Similiter malum, quod est in homine, ut fornicatio, vel aliud criminale peccatum, aut continuatione augetur, si homo perseveret actualiter in peccato; aut attritione remittitur, ut quando aliquis dolet se hoc commisisse, cessans ab opere, quamvis non poeniteat perfecte; aut contritione dimittitur, quando plenarie de peccato convertitur. Sunt enim multi, qui dolent se peccasse, et corde atteruntur, non tamen plene conteruntur, nec firmum habent propositum non relabendi, nec ore confitentur. Isti minus mali fiunt, sed desinunt non esse mali, nisi perfecte conteruntur.[19]

> (Similarly, an evil that is in a man, such as fornication or another criminal (deadly) sin, either is continually increased if the man perseveres actively in the sin; or is diminished by attrition, as when someone sorrows that he has committed it, ceasing from the deed, although he is not perfectly penitent; or else it (the sin) has been struck down by contrition, when he is completely turned away from sin. Indeed, there are many who sorrow that they have sinned, and who are worn down in their hearts, yet still are not completely ground down (i.e. contrite), nor do they have a firm resolve not to relapse, nor have they confessed aloud. These persons become less evil, but they do not cease to be evil unless they are completely contrite.)

These two emotional states constitute the essential work of confession, and are in effect the only ways of purging sin from the soul. The difference between them lies in intensity. Attrition, from *attritio* – to rub away, is a general sorrow for sins committed and an indistinct sense of not wanting to repeat them. This stage is in many regards connected to the servile fear of God, of punishment for sins committed. While salutary, the sorrow arising from this is nevertheless limited in its therapeutic efficacy. Sin has been diminished, not destroyed. Therein lies the problem: the emotional medicine is not sufficiently strong enough to effect lasting change. Only the next stage, contrition, can do that. This stage, from the word *contritio* – to grind down, is vastly more potent. It is still a sorrow for sin, but is far greater in intensity. The choice of word itself reflects this distinction: attrition merely wears away; contrition reduces to dust. William de Auvergne offers a more arresting image of the differences between the two: 'I say therefore that attrition is thus to contrition as a nonlethal wound is to killing'.[20] This image brings their relationship into a stark contrast: attrition is a mere prick of the flesh, contrition a fatal laceration that immediately kills. The emotional states, while related, differ sharply in terms of their intensity. Nevertheless, to ensure that the next stage in the treatment of the soul is carried out, the penitent must move from the fear of God and fear of punishment, to a deep sense of sorrow that crushes sin out of the soul.[21]

Such understandings of sin, and of the emotional processes by which to get rid of it, are deeply embedded within a wide range of Middle English religious texts. For Richard Rolle, sin is likened to a toxic fluid that must be purged before any attempt to move closer to God. It is, in the *Ego Dormio*, 'venemus synne' that is 'bitterer þan þe gall, sowrar þan þe atter'.[22] The *Oelum Effusum* also renders it as a toxin. Referring specifically to the healing power of the name of Jesus, Rolle asserts that

> Sothely nathynge slokynns sa fell flawmes, dystroyes ill thoghtes, puttes owte venemous affeccyons, does awaye coryous and vayne ocupacyons fra vs. This name Ihesu lelely haldyn in mynde drawes by þe rote vyces, settys vertus, insawes charytee, inȝettis sauoire of heuenly thynges.[23]

Such language recalls the theological understanding of sin and its extraction mentioned above. Here, the soul is poisoned by the venom of sin, a state that must be remedied to avoid spiritual and moral death. The treatment consists of immediate extraction: sin must be put 'owte' of the soul, drawn out 'by þe rote'. Ideas of extraction and removal, of purgation, govern Rolle's understanding of sin. In his *Incendium Amoris*, quoted here from Richard Misyn's (*d.*1462) Middle English translation, he asserts how vital it is that 'syn is pourgyd', and warns of the spiritual dangers if 'couetyes, þe rote of synnes, is noȝt drawne owte'.[24] At its core, sin is an emotional disorder that begets 'coryous and vayne ocupacyons'. By asserting that the emotions are venomous, Rolle connects sin to the emotional capacities of the person. As a result, he conveys both sin's universality to mankind, and the difficulty of its removal. Any extraction of these 'venemous affeccyons' must, therefore, be a forceful process that is emotionally mediated: as he notes in his *Form of Living*, what 'clenseth vs of þat filthede . . . is sorowe of hert ayeyns þe synnes of thoght'.[25] Intensity is key:

> Puchase the þe wel of gretynge, and sese nat til þou haue hym, for in þe hert where terys spryngeth, þer wil þe fyre of þe Holy Gost be kyndled, and seþen þe fyre of loue þat shal bren in þi hert will bren to noght al þe roust of syn, and purge þi soule of al filth, as clene as þe gold þat is proued in þe fourneys.[26]

This is writing of emotional extremes, as Rolle deploys an arresting set of images to articulate the force required to purge the soul. Sorrow and love are presented as elemental opposites – a perpetual spring and an all-consuming fire. Both of them operate upon the soul in an intense manner. Images of metallurgy are then introduced as functional parallels for the cleansing work of these emotions: they act as a furnace upon the soul, blasting the rust of sin away and purifying the soul into a precious metal. The point made here, with Rolle's signature poetic skill, is that only emotional intensity will suffice: only sorrow to the point of tears and a love that burns can purge the soul of its venomous sins. Such statements refashion elements of books 22 and 23 of Gregory the Great's *Moralia in Job*, and Anselm of Bec's idea of compunction: that complex blending of love and fear that leads to a deep sorrow for sin and a profound love of God.[27] Such passions are important tools in the treatment of the soul, an idea that is also evident in more widely disseminated texts.

In the second book of the *Scale of Perfection*, Hilton makes the therapeutic importance of intense emotion very clear. The soul can only be 'heeled of goostli sikeness' when all those 'bittir passions and fleschli lustis and othere oodle feelynges aren brente oute of the herte with fier of desire, and newe gracious feelynges aren brought in with brennynge love'.[28] The subtle use of prose rhythm makes the importance of affective strength all the more compelling. The couplets 'brente/herte' and 'fier/desire' not only endow the emotional states with an elemental potency, but also reinforce their conceptual connection: the heart's 'bittir passions' must be scorched away by an all-consuming fire of emotion. These comments regarding treatment are set within the more general discussions of sin and its nature in Book One. Here, Hilton asserts that 'unclene affeccions . . . owthere bynemen the liyf of the soule bi deedli synne, or ellis thei feble the soule and maketh it seek, yef thei ben venial'.[29] Sin is a toxic presence constituted by a corrupt emotional nature: in essence sin is 'a fals mysruled love unto thisilf. Oute of this love cometh al maner of synnes bi sevene ryveres, the whiche aren thise: pride, envie, ire, accedie, coveitise, glotony, and leccherie'.[30] Emotion is the main constitutive element in all the deadly sins. Moreover, they are the product of a common emotion, a shared self-love that has festered and polluted the soul. This shared nature is the key to their treatment. Penitential states, that sense of sorrow and shame for the self and its actions, are the natural medicine for the poison of self-love. Attrition, and more specifically contrition, will both work as effective medicines for sin. This is not a gentle process, however. As Julian asserts in her *Revelation of Divine Love*, God's desire to treat and heal the soul is a process of some force:

> I shall al tobreke you for your veyn affections and your vicious pryde; and after that I shal togeder gader you and make you mylde and meke, clene and holy, by onyng to me.[31]

The potency of this treatment is intense. It consists not of gentle and tender forgiveness, but rather of grinding down the essence of sin – those poisoned emotions. It is, in effect, the primary operation of the medicine of penance, specifically contrition. It will not simply remove sin, but also promote that key virtue of meekness. As she notes towards the end of the text, 'we shall be made ashamd of ourselfe and broken downe as anempts our pride and presumtion . . . throw contrition and grace we shall be broken fro all things that is not our lord'.[32] Beyond the drede of God lies the crushing sorrow for sin evoked by true contrition. It is this complex and layered emotional state that constitutes the next stage in the treatment of the soul; exemplified and evoked by a particular form of writing: the penitential lyric. These lyrics are key in evoking and sustaining the crucial forms of sorrow that sowle-hele requires; a feature they owe to their poetic forbears: the penitential Psalms – texts which not only offer medieval writers a vivid psychodrama of penitential self-awareness, but also formulas for evoking it.

Vessels of Affect

The Book of Psalms occupies a dominant position within medieval religious life and thought, used not simply as a tool of the liturgy but also as a rich creative and personal resource. For Richard Rolle, they are multipurpose and multimodal, able to evoke contrasting and intense affective states as and when required. When commending the benefits of his own translation of the Psalms to the nun Margaret Kirkeby, he states with his signature audacity and confidence that

> In þaime is so mekeil fairehede of vnderstandynge and medicyne of words þat þis boke es called garth enclosed, wele enseled, paradys fulle of appelles. Nowe, with halsom lare, druvyd and stormy saules it bringes in tille the clere and peesfulle lyf, now amonestand to forthink synne with teres, now hyghtand ioy.[33]

First and foremost, the Psalms are the implements of passion. Not only do they record the 'vivid psychodrama of David's relationship with God' – his yearning for forgiveness and joy in the Divine – but they also model that emotional trajectory.[34] They function as the poetic apparatus or mechanism by which both penitential sorrow and jubilant joy can be evoked. Their rendering here as a 'medicyne of words' is a succinct articulation of their instrumentality, of their status as tools of feeling rather than expositions of knowledge. In this sense Rolle is drawing from a long tradition on the effects of reading the Psalter; his main sources being Cassiodorus and, to a lesser extent, Peter Lombard.[35] Rolle's prologue is, in many respects, a composite paraphrase from these two sources. Yet, while Cassiodorus notes the healing power of the Psalms, he also provides some other comments on their nature.[36]

> Quorum virtutes ut breviter divinus sermo concluderet, in septuagesimo psalmo dicturus est: Ego autem confitebor tibi vasis psalmorum veritatem tuam. Revera vasa veritatis, quæ tot virtutes caplunt ... hydriæ quæ vinum coeleste recipientes, puritatem ejus in novitate semper custodiunt ... Apotheca valde copiosa, de qua cum bibant tam magni terrarum populi, ubertas ejus nescit expendi. Quam mirabilis autem ex ipsis profluit suavitas ad canendum.[37]

> (To put the seal briefly on the virtues of the psalms, God's word is to say in Psalm 70: 'But I will confess to thee thy truth in the vessels of the psalms.' Truly they are vessels of truth, for they contain so many virtues ... They are the water-jugs containing the heavenly wine and keeping it ever fresh and undiluted ... They are a most abundant store, the fecundity of which cannot be exhausted, although so many peoples of the earth drink of it. What a wondrous sweetness flows from them when sung!)

The Psalms' primary function is articulated in the broadest instrumental terms. They are vessels of emotion, operating as the poetic receptacles which contain and convey the passionate freight and potency of David's relationship with God. Their presentation as water jugs adds to this: they contain something vital and, by extension, they can pour these contents out. They hold those emotional states 'ever fresh and undiluted' – at once useful and to some degree forceful, as they contain something potent. As an inexhaustible store, they have a sense of quantity and depth. There is something limitless or unbound about them; the emotional states they contain at once immeasurable and infinitely useful. The mere recitation of them is enough to access this potency – in essence this is their primary function: 'Melos siquidem blandum animos oblectat, sed non compellit ad lacrymas fructuosas; permulcet aures, sed non ad superna erigit audientes. Corde autem compungimur, si quod ore dicimus' (True a charming song delights our minds, but it does not impel to fruitful tears; it soothes the ears but it does not direct its hearers to heavenly things. But we are pricked at heart if we can heed what our lips say).[38]

The emotional reach of the Psalms is simply greater than anything ordinary music can evoke. While normal music can soothe, the Psalms can pierce and provoke. They possess here a forceful, somatic dimension, impacting upon the body's most vital organ and centre. What they evoke is far from gentle. Only emotional states of the greatest intensity – penitential sorrow or jubilant joy – come from them.[39] In this way they function to both contain and convey: the reader can both draw from these vessels and be carried by them. Such an impact upon the person is parsed medically in both Cassiodorus and Rolle. The phrase 'medicyne of words' is, for Rolle, far from a rhetorical ornament: the Psalms are actually therapeutic and can in fact operate as a method of treating the soul. In his commentary of Psalm 37:5 he clarifies the nature of their therapeutic importance:

> Thai rotid and thai ere brokyn, myn erres, fra the face of myn vnwit. Myn erres, that is the wondis of my synnes, hale thurgh penaunce, rotid whils I eft assentid til syn. And thai ere brokyn when I synned eft in dede; and all this is fra the face of myn vnwit.[40]

Sin for Rolle is a rotting of the soul, something that breaks and corrupts it. The remedy is to be found in penance, as only penance can work effectively to destroy the rot of sin. Such penitential medicine is deeply connected to the work of the Psalms. As Rolle asserts in his Psalter prologue, these vessels of emotional force can be used to make the reader 'forthink synne with teres'. Within them lies the ability to enable the key therapeutic emotion within the penitential process: contrition. Their function, therefore, is to evoke, intensify and perfect specifically modulated emotional states; a goal most vividly realised in later medieval verse translations of the Penitential Psalms (and penitential lyrics). One widely circulated example is the version by the Carmelite Richard Maidstone.[41] The translation of *Psalm L* is found in the Vernon manuscript, and so was understood to have a role to play in the overall provision of sowle-hele. The reason for this is due to the text's emotive power. In its complete form, this text is written in the eight-line ballade stanza form, and mixes loose glossing with more extensive devotional elaborations. As such, it loses none of the original force of the Penitential Psalms, and realises and accentuates specific emotional modulations throughout.

From its opening poem, the text notes that its entire purpose is 'for synne in man to be fordon'.[42] Yet, this is a purpose that is often articulated in medical terms.

> Mercy, lord, for I am seke;
> Hele me, forbrused beþ alle my bones,
> My flesshe is freel, my soule haþ eke
> Ful greet matere of mournynge mones. (ll. 17–20)

Sin is intensely physical – it subsists in the flesh and the bones as much as it does in the soul. This is a subtle but important move. The initial acknowledgement of sin in the proem has now shifted into a specific register that presents sin as an illness. Sin, both in terms of its nature and impacts upon the person, has been carefully re-narrated in a medical way. This has the initial effect of lending urgency and import to the whole purpose of the text, and allows the reader to conceptually apprehend the function of the Psalms in a specific way. Christ becomes at once the Divine Judge and the doctor of souls – the 'lowely leche' (l. 131) – or *Christus medicus*. Yet the text goes much further than simply referencing Christ as a doctor and sin as an illness. The medical register is used as part of an overarching structural presentation of penance. Throughout, there is the constant and deliberate attempt by the text to engage the reader in specific ways and to facilitate the emergence of specific emotional states, and specific postures of self-analysis:

> Hem nedeþ not, þat bene in wele,
> Þe water þat vs wassheþ here;
> But we fro him al day stele
> And greuen God þat haþ no pere;
> We mow not fro harme vs hele,
> But if we wepe in water clere. (ll. 147–52)

Integral to the presentation of sin as a pathological state is the idea of its remedy – the medicine that will cure the illness of sin. Time and again the text interconnects both concepts. Penance is here a therapeutic bath, a treatment designed to wash away filth. Such a rendering of penance's function infuses the sacrament with a range of additional meanings and senses. It is seen here less as a form of quasi-legalistic examination and punishment, and more as an hygienic and to some degree gentle activity designed to be beneficial. Ideas of ritual cleansing and medical treatment come to the fore here, but only for a moment. The lyric soon shifts, with penance becoming all the more abstract and distinctive – the cleansing bath is made of tears, its water the result of considerable sorrow. That initial, and essentially gentle, image of the bath now becomes vividly strange and surreal: the reader must wash themselves in their own tears, in the product of their own pain and sorrow. The emotional force of penance is made most explicit here, and is keyed into its therapeutic efficacy – only by washing oneself in one's own tears will one's sick soul be healed. The idea of medicine, and by extension its broader connotations of health and harm, of life and death, are being used by the lyric to simultaneously articulate the importance of penance and the manner of its operation. The reader is left to hold a crucial point in mind: that without pain and sorrow to the point of tears, there can be no healing of the soul. Yet all is not focused on the emotional here. These tears, shed in sufficient quantities to saturate the soul, are also the product of self-accusation and self-scrutiny. The lyric is careful to assert the importance of specific modes of self-knowledge.

The passage opens with a comparative judgement: the reader is presented not with their own diseased interior, but instead with the knowledge that there are some who do not need the healing work of the *Christus Medicus*. It is an inherently intersubjective move, an acknowledgement that not all suffer the same condition. This socially directed form of comparative analysis is augmented by the verse into a form of self-analysis that shades into self-accusation. The lines 'But we fro him al day stele / And greuen God þat haþ no pere' delineate both the specific sin of theft, and its consequence of hurting God: the narrative voice moves from an understanding of others, to an understanding of its own condition due to its own actions. The mention of healing in the following line connects such self-analysis into the overall treatment of the soul and the work of penance. Specific states of emotion and self-knowledge are connected together through a medical motif into the sacrament of penance. The lyrical form aids in the transferral of such states, allowing the reader to literally rehearse them through the act of reading. In this way the text bears witness to the sickness of sin, and at the same time offers the means of treatment: the soul's anguished cry to God. Over its course, emotional states are given considerable imaginative attention, and the text evokes those same states in its readers, enabling the precise treatment of the soul. This is one of the key abilities of the lyrical form – emotional focusing – and it is evident throughout the text. However, it begins with the careful use of the narrative voice. After opening with that anguished cry to the *Christus Medicus* for aid, the text moves deeper into the interior state of the narrator figure:

> And my soule is destourbled sore,
> But, lorde, how longe shal hit be so?
> For if I synne more and more
> Þenne mot I suffere pynes mo.
> I lede a lyf aȝeynes þi lore,
> So wrecched, þat me is woo,
> But þi mercy may me restore;
> Þer is no helpe whenne þat I go. (ll. 25–32)

The use of exegematic narration – or 'I-voice' narration – generates a sense of introspection and interior reflection. Through it, the text establishes a psychological interior as a landscape for the reader to co-inhabit. For what follows this is a vital move, as it simulates one of the key aspects of penance: it enables the reader to enter into a specific mental state, to situate his- or herself in a particular position. This structural device is used to enhance the emotive potential of the passage. It begins with a sense of fraught angst, of restless searching. The opening line comprises both an astute self-analysis of state of the soul, and a direct question to God. A dramatic energy is constructed here, as introspection turns to prayer, and through the careful use of narrative voice the reader is incorporated into the emotional ambit of this pattern of analysis and questioning. The careful use of alliteration and end rhyme – 'soule/sore, synne/suffere; sore/more, and mo/woo' – establishes a series of powerful interconnections here, linking pain and suffering into the lyrical presentation of the soul. Assonance between 'woo/mo/so' and 'sore/more', creates a particular sonic impression of impassioned wailing and lament. The opening turmoil and trouble attributed to the soul becomes part of the verse form, its affective state carried and conveyed via structural form and the use of repetition and rhyme, into the interior of the reader. In the same way the treatment of the soul is also subtly figured: the connection between 'lore' and 'restore' works to present God's law not as a static absolute, but as the only remedy for the soul's inner turmoil. The direct address to God, itself a subtle imitation of prayer, is made much more explicit in the next passage:

> Turne þe, lord, my soule outwynne,
> Make me saf for þi mercy;
> For foule wiþ feþer ny fische wiþ fynne
> Is noon vnstidfaste but I.
> Whenne I þenke what is me wiþinne,
> My conscience makeþ a careful cry;
> Þerefore þi pite, lord, vnpynne,
> Þat I may mende me þerby. (ll. 33–40)

The verse carefully constructs a moment of self-reflection, focusing and exploring the inner state of the narrator's soul. Self-analysis becomes self-accusation: of all creation, here birds and fish, the narrator alone occupies the exclusive category of 'vnstidfaste'. Perspective shifts and twists in upon itself, as the line 'Whenne I þenke what is me wiþinne' dissolves the relations between subject and object, compelling the reader to try out a complex form of self-reflexivity. Crucially, nothing specific is mentioned by the verse. The much-maligned inner state is essentially devoid of concrete description. Through the careful use of silence, the text generates a hollow space that works to augment the effect of the verse. All that exists in this passage is a vague but nevertheless atmospheric sense of the horror of conscience. It is left to the reader to imagine what exactly would cause one's own conscience to 'makeþ a careful cry' to God. The reader is being very skilfully manipulated here in terms of perspective, yet is given great imaginative freedom in terms of detail. Within the verse there is a sense of tight control, the careful movement from one state to another. Through rhyme a series of opposites are held in suspension: 'outwynne/wiþinne/vnpynne' occur at key points in the verse, and work not simply to structure its rhythm, but also the rhythm of the concepts it deals with – it moves, deliberately, outward then inward, then outward again. Ideas of interiority become augmented and enhanced with additional ideas of containment and release. The reader's perspective is confined to their interior – the verse ensures that the reader cannot look away from the inner state of the soul. Yet, there is no precise delineation of that inner state, it is a blank canvas for the reader to project their own inner state onto. The verse has very carefully positioned the reader into a specific mental posture, one predicated upon a groundswell of emotional energy that will lead into prayer.

From this intense focus on the inner state of the soul, and the indistinct sense of horror that it generates, the verse then moves into an anguished 'careful cry' to God. The shock of self-knowledge compels the soul to speak to God, and to ask only for pity – 'Þerefore þi pite, lord, vnpynne / Þat I may mende me þerby': emotion begets emotion, anguish working to unlock God's pity. Yet this pity has a medical and restorative power to it, as it works to 'mende' the horrendous inner state of the soul. It is a deliberate strategy aimed at manipulating the reader's psychology. Though subtle here, the importance of emotion is a theme returned to time and again in this text. It seeks to evoke contrition, to reduce sin to dust with the weight of intense feeling. Over its course it deploys a range of techniques to further that process. One of the most frequent is the constant connection it makes between mercy and intense sorrow. As soon as the narrator asks God to be allowed to 'wasshen in mercy welle', the reader is confronted with a scene of great internal turmoil:

> I have trauailed in my waylynge,
> My bed shal I wasshe euery ny3t,
> And wiþ þe teres of my wepynge
> My bedstre watter, as hit is ri3t.
> Synne is cause of my mournynge,
> I fele me feynt in gostly fi3t;
> Þerfore I wepe & water out wrynge,
> As I wel au3te and euery wi3te. (ll. 49–56)

The image of the bed so saturated with tears that it is washed by them, is both abstract and evocative. It has a certain charge that endows penance with real potency. This charge comes from the strong contrasts that constitute the image. The nocturnal moment of rest, the still silence of the night, is essentially rent asunder by both the narrator's wailing cries and the flood of his emotions. Such contrasts convey a deep sense of inner anguish, presenting a total absence of rest and quiet in the location within which they are most closely associated. The image also has repetition built into it: as the text asserts, this scene plays out 'euery ny3t' – the inner bedchamber becomes the locus of a very interior and recursive torment.

The narrator soon specifies the cause of such suffering – sin. Yet instead of moving into an analysis of a specific sin or set of sins, the narrator only goes further into the nature of his emotional anguish. His lament that 'Synne is cause of my mournynge, / I fele me feynt in gostly fi3t' provides no supplementary detail on this sin, but only emphasises his condition. The reader learns that the sin, whatever it is, causes an emotional crisis so strong that he faints and swoons in his soul. The detail the verse gives is sparse, but it is nevertheless potent: there is a rawness to the stanza, a sense of an inescapable sorrow that is accentuated by a relentless focus on the emotional and psychological consequences of sin in the abstract. It causes nothing but pain and spiritual death. The verse form furthers this sense of menace and restless confinement. End rhyme connects 'waylynge/wepynge/mournynge/wrynge' over the course of the stanza, making connections and associations of mourning and sorrow that magnify the narrator's anguish; the last 'wrynge', syllabically shorter than the words it rhymes with, works to punctuate the verse faster than expected, layering a suddenly breathless quality to the pain and suffering the word naturally evokes. While the rhyme scheme is relatively simple, it is quite flexible, allowing the central image of the soaked bed of tears to be unpacked and extended over the whole stanza. The initial mention of the image is superseded by the narrator's swooning, but through the line 'Þerfore I wepe & water out wrynge', it recurs again, though now with added import. The reader's exposure to it is refreshed, as the central perspective is maintained for as long as possible. This is the contrition mentioned earlier, the deep sorrow for the presence of sin. But the text goes further. The next stanza builds on the emotional force created here, and moves into a prayer to God for mercy (ll. 62–4). The movement from anguish and self-knowledge to heartfelt prayers for mercy is repeated over the course of the text in various different forms. The next two stanzas also comprise prayers for mercy, yet the evocation of emotional states is still paramount.

> Oure lord haþ herkened my prayere
> And receyued myn orisoun,
> For alle þe bedes þat we sayen here
> To him þei beþ ful swete soun;
> Now lorde þat bou3test man so dere,
> Wiþ blody bak & body broun,
> Þou vouchesaf so vs to here,
> Þat neuer synne vs drawe adoun. (ll. 73–80)

The use of imagery in this stanza is tactical in its subtlety. While prior stanzas focus on a central image and then work to extend and magnify it, this stanza begins with only the most general statement that prayer is delightful to God. Yet after the mention of the 'swete soun' of prayer, things begin to change rapidly. The stanza shifts from a focus on sound to a focus on sight, as the visual details of the Passion are mentioned with increasing frequency. These details are confined to strange levels of perspective, and details of colour. The lines 'Now lorde þat bou3test man so dere / Wiþ blody bak & body broun' introduce the redemptive work of the Passion, and then focus only on specific imagistic aspects of it. The reader does not see Christ torn and in agony completely or all at once; instead, the bloody back is the first thing mentioned. Narrative perspective alights only on one detail initially. The focus on such a visual detail is jarring, creating the impression of seeing Christ from an unusual angle: the reader is behind Christ yet close to Him, seeing only His bloody back and not His face or front. Yet, within the next beat of the line, the perspective has shifted again and moved out in the distance to view Christ's whole body. The shift is discordant, as is the specific detail of the body being brown: the reader is confronted with imagery that is at once specific in detail yet indistinct in the aggregate. The two mentions of Christ's suffering offer little more than two sense impressions, yet they both paint the narrator's prayer for mercy in the textures and colours of the Passion. Their function is to insert the emotive force of the Passion into the prayer for mercy.

The verse form supports this, as the use of alliteration and end rhyme draws connections between the prayer and the Passion that are potent and inescapable. The 'bedes' of prayer are connected to the other plosives in the passages – 'beþ/bou3test/blody bak/body broun' – as alliteration works here to forge links between sound and sense that interpose the notes of the Passion into the prayer of the narrator. In much the same way the end rhymes of 'orisoun/soun/broun' also work to reinforce this connection. The result is a very carefully constructed, albeit subtle, emphasis on the Passion that makes the prayer for mercy all the more arresting. This is done to further the emotional goals of the text. The mention of the Passion is tactical, occurring at a narrative moment when the emotional intensity generated by penitential self-scrutiny may normally begin to dissipate. In effect the prayer for mercy cannot be made without the consequences of sin being subtly re-inscribed through the mention of Passion imagery: penitential feelings are not allowed to ebb, but are instead buttressed and enhanced to a new level of lyrical intensity. Emotional states become layered, interconnected and complex – a technique that is used frequently over the course of the text:

> My gilt to þe I haue made knowen,
> I haue not hid fro þe my wrong;
> Þrourȝe shrifte wol I fro me þrowen
> Al my mysdede & mourne among;
> For certis, lorde, we truste & trowen
> Þe welle of grace wiþ stremes strong
> Out of þi faire flesshe gan flowen,
> Whenne blood out of þi herte sprong. (ll. 121–8)

The stanza is essentially a confessional formula designed to locate sin within the narrative I-voice, and thus to be rehearsed by the reader. Penance is the focus here, presented in a manner designed to increase its emotive potency. It is rendered as a throwing away of sin, and as an engagement with the 'welle of grace'. Both are images that are easily understood. Yet, therein lies the danger: the metaphorical rendering of penance here is inimical to mood, as these images are not themselves predicated upon or even evoke intense sorrow. To ensure that the reader is not inured to or loses that key sense of sorrow, the stanza quickly establishes a connection between penance and the Passion. The image of the well of grace with its 'stremes strong' is soon twisted into something much more forceful. It becomes indistinguishable from the blood emerging from Christ's heart. The Passion, with all its emotive force, is carefully layered over the verse here. The alliteration of 'stremes strong' and 'faire flesshe/flowen' with the sibilance and consonance they create, simultaneously slow the pace of the verse while fusing the two central images together: water becomes flesh, flesh that flows with the heart's blood. This connection between prayer and Passion accentuates the emotional impact of the text. Sin and the consequences for Christ are forever held in suspension.

As both Passion and penance fuse, so too do mercy and grace become inseparable from the torrents of Christ's blood – from the physical consequences of sin. By mentioning Christ in this way, we move from the penitential state of fear of punishment and the desire for mercy, to a sense of pity and an implicit sense that sin's consequences are not simply self-focused. Again there is a shift in perspective: the stanza offers an interior moment of self-scrutiny that quickly turns into a consideration of the wider consequences of sin. In this way the pity for Christ is used to guard against self-pity, and to deepen the sense of shame and horror. By layering emotional states through the use of interconnected key images, the stanza catalyses in its own form and content a subtle movement towards a deeper sense of contrition. This is seen most clearly in stanzas that are also found in Vernon:

> More-ouere þou wasche me fro my synne,
> And fro my filiþis clense þou me;
> Enserche my soule wiþoute & ynne,
> That I no more defoulid be;
> And as þin herte cleef atwynne
> Wiþ deolful deeþ on rode-tre
> So let me neuere werk bi-ginne,
> Lord, but ȝif hit like þe![43] (ll. 17–24)

Jesus' cleansing of the soul, itself a gentle image, is used to figure the work of confession. The words of the narrator have a confessional quality to them, a sense of introspection coupled with a desire for forgiveness and regeneration. Yet, this image, and the mood it generates, soon gives way to a more aggressive visual landscape. The Passion, with all the violence it entails, erupts into the verse in two interconnected images. The first is the split heart, rent asunder by sin; the second, the Cross. While there is little vivid detail here, the aggregated image of a split heart on a Cross is nevertheless powerful. The level of detail is descriptive enough, and strange enough, to fix the reader's attention – we move from Christ bathing the soul to the stark form of a Cross with a split heart on it. The overall image is at once physical and emotive, conveying not simply the actual heart but also the pain of sorrow and heartache. Its use here thus merges the emotive force of the Passion with the desire to confess, as the cleansing of the soul and the Passion of Christ blur into one. The initial cry for mercy becomes one of anguish at the result of sin: the end rhyme of 'synne/atwynne' fosters a sense of interrelatedness between sin and its consequences. There is here a layering of image and its emotive impact. Both have independent potencies, but those forces are weaved together in a specific manner: the cleansing of sin is imbued with gravity; the Passion with a sense of personal immediacy. The overall emotional charge of the verse becomes augmented and deepened, as the reader is forced to make specific ideational associations that add intensity to that initial prayer for mercy. Such a technique is not confined to the Passion however:

> Bi-hold hou in sunne I was conceyued
> Of my Modur, as Men beon alle,
> And of my ffadur nouȝt receyued
> Bote flesch ful ffrele and fayn to falle.
> Bote seþþhe þi flesch, lord, was parceyued
> And for vr sake strauht on stalle,
> Was neuer sinful mon deceyued,
> Þat wolde to þi merci calle. (ll. 41–8)

A burst of self-accusation, of lament for the filth of the world and of conception, is immediately followed by the mention of Christ's nativity. The arrangement is jarring and unexpected, causing shifts in the reader's engagement with the verse. Until this point narrative focus has rested on the idea of the horrors of sin – its presence the source of all sickness and weakness. The heavy use of alliteration in 'ffadur /fleshe/ful/ffrele/fayn/ falle' makes uncomfortable associations between family and corruption: the sudden string of those alliterative units reconfigures the idea of family as the locus of filth and weakness. This highly critical mention of father and mother is thrown into sharp relief by the sudden mention of Christ as an infant. At this point the verse slows down, rapid hyper-alliteration giving way to a more deliberate and measured focus on the nativity of Christ.

The juxtaposition of a harsh image with a tender one does more than simply garner attention. Its function is to deepen in the reader the sense of shame and guilt articulated by the initial stanza line, as the sense of self-accusation and lament is overlaid by the tender image of Christ. Such an overlay operates by strong contrast not antithesis. Sin's ubiquitous presence and its fundamental connection to the family is meant to evoke a certain sense of lament that is indirectly magnified by mention of Christ's nativity. The line 'for vr sake strauht on stalle' makes a direct connection between Christ and mankind, forcing the reader to think not only of the corrupting presence of sin but also of the unconditional love for that gentle child. The narrator laments not just sorrow for sin and the pain of his own inner state, but also for the loss of innocence – the figure of suffering changes from the narrator to the innocent and silent child. With this change comes a range of newly heightened emotional states. Sorrow, pity, self-accusation, and the foreknowledge of the Passion become interconnected and layered, imbued with a compelling new depth and potency due to their complex interconnection. Through the layering of emotional states, the stanza moves gradually into generating a sense of contrition – each line offering an increase in the emotional weight and gravity of the situation described, and linking it back to the reader. Other sections of the text do this with greater speed and intensity:

> Make in me, god, myn herte clene,
> Þat rihtful gost in me þou rewe.
> Ffrom seuen sunnes þou make hit schene,
> Wher so þou go I may þe suwe.
> Allas þi tormentes for tene,
> Þi bodi blak, þi bones bluwe!
> Mekeful lord, þou make hit sene
> Wiþ-Inne myn herte, þat hidous hewe. (ll. 81–8)

At its emotive peak, this passage combines confessional self-awareness and a cry for mercy, with a tactical reminder of the potency of the Passion. The narrator's desire for spiritual cleansing and renewal makes reference to the damaging effects of the seven deadly sins. From the stanza's outset there is a carefully modulated confessional aspect that is broad and encompassing in its generality, but which is also quickly overlaid by the images and impressions of the Passion. The interjectional cry of 'Allas' marks a rapid shift in tone and imagery. The verse moves from the seven deadly sins and the narrator's pursuit of Christ to the vivid sense impressions made by the crucifixion and the desire to have them imprinted upon the heart. Metrically it signals an abrupt move to a more compact and rapid form, with alliteration becoming tighter and more concentrated. The sudden 'tormentes/tene', 'bodi/blak/bones/bluwe', and 'herte/hidous/hewe' all structure the passage of narrative time much more than in the prior lines. The verse becomes faster but also concentrates upon the Passion with great intent. The interjection thus inserts a sense of shock and horror/sorrow into the verse, which is extended throughout the remaining lines by the use of alliteration. The layering of emotional states here is complex, as the stanza allows multiple senses of pity, regret and sorrow for sin to be configured and reconfigured in patterns that evoke and sustain the contrition of sin. The narrator moves from sorrow at the lamentable state of his inner being to sorrow for the crucified Christ, from a form of self-pity to a pity for Christ and profound desire to have the image of His Passion imprinted upon the heart. Self-knowledge furthers a self-less concern for Christ: through careful shifts in narrative perceptive, the reader is brought into and out of specific delineated moments of self-reflection, self-accusation and concern for others. Considerable emotional energy is built up and sustained here through oscillations in narrative perspective, allowing the emotional impacts of each to overlap and develop. The result is a potent backdrop for the reader to imaginatively inhabit:

> Weore sacrifice to þi likyng,
> I hedde hit ȝiue wiþ herte fre;
> But, certeynly, no such þing
> As in him-self plesaunt may be.
> Þi-self were offred, a child ful ȝing,
> And afturward on Rode-tre,
> Whon of þin herte þe blod con spring:
> Þerfore myn herte I offre ro þe. (ll. 129–36)

Images of Christ's Nativity and Passion are interwoven here to add further emotional weight to the stanza. The initial narrative perspective – the narrator's own desire to make an offering to Christ – shifts to that of a 'child ful ȝing', before moving by the end of the next line to the 'Rode tre'. Such rapid oscillations between key moments in the life of Christ provoke pity and sorrow, merging Christ born with Christ crucified: within the space of one full line, the reader must hold the image of that 'child ful ȝing' with that of 'blod con spring'. It is a technique of augmentation that operates by layering contrasting images over each other. Rapid oscillation makes the emotional impact of the nativity blur into and thus accentuate the emotive potency of the Passion: through rhyme the reader must now see the Passion as the crucifixion of a young child, must associate the Nativity with streams of blood. The stanza thus layers emotional states in ways that move the reader to sorrow and contrition: the result of sin is essentially a form of infanticide.

Each of these aspects of Christ's life add depth and gravity to that opening desire to make an offering to Christ, as they form an emotional backdrop that makes the final line of the stanza all the more potent. After the appearance of each of these images the narrative perspective shifts back to the opening, as the narrator offers his own heart to Christ. Such a sudden shift moves the emotional force generated by those images onto this final act of self-giving: it draws from prior lines to accentuate its own image of pity and compassion, and draws the reader into that particular posture. These shifts and the emotional layering they produce allow the text to evoke new depths of feeling. Contrition is the goal of these penitential Psalms – not a gentle sorrow for sin, but rather one that is crushing in its potency. The recourse here to a range of images designed to reflect and magnify emotional states is proof that the text is concerned with evoking more than a basic regret for sin. The text uses the lyrical form to more precisely modulate and maintain the emotional impact that each image offers. As a result, the reader is brought into ever increasing degrees of layered emotional response. With the rhythm of the verse these layered states stagger the movement from a servile fear of God and punishment (attrition), to a more complex and contrite sense of sorrow for sins (contrition). These verse Psalms are vessels of emotion, able to contain and convey intensive emotional states to the reader in specific ways and with specific purposes. To aid in crushing sin out of the soul, these Psalms use the power of images and verse form to catalyse the reader's emotional response to new levels of intensity. However, their emotional nature is not left unmanaged: this text does not simply evoke a set of feelings, but instead a confessional self-awareness. Time and again the verse places the reader into a confessional posture, into increasing moments of self-analysis and accusation:

LYRICAL TREATMENT 69

> For I was stille, þerefore my boones,
> Eldede whil I shulde crye alday;
> I cryed & ȝitt mut more þan ones,
> To gete foryeuenesse if I may.
> I haue matere of greuouse grones,
> Þat haue made many a wylde outray;
> I crye þe mercy, kynge of trones,
> I haue trespassed, I say not nay.[44] (ll. 105–12)

Interposed between stanzas of great emotive potency are ones that offer a moment of self-reflection. The narrative I voice is here utterly focused on itself and its inner state. Sentiments expressed in an earlier stanza 'Hele me, forbrused beþ alle my bones / My flesshe is freel, my soule haþ eke' (ll. 18–20), are now revisited with an intensity and clarity of exposition. Again the narrative goes ever inward, focusing on the urgent need for mercy. End rhyme makes a direct connection between those diseased 'boones' and those 'greuouse grones' and 'wylde outray'. The entire stanza is set within a narrative context of gaining mercy from God. The only treatment for the sickness of sin is a prayerful cry to God: a confessional posture that the text will accentuate and revisit time and again. Mercy is what is needed, and the narrative I voice ensures that the reader is also bound up in that careful movement inwards, simulating those very cries of prayer. Elsewhere the narrative focuses intently on that inner state, and the damaging nature of sin on the soul:

> For in my flesshe is þere no hele
> In prescene of þi worþi face,
> My bones wanten pees & wele
> For synnes þat me þus deface.
> My wilde wille, my wittes frele
> Encombre me whenne I trespace;
> Þerfore whenne deeþ shal wiþ me dele
> I see no helpe but only grace (ll. 217–24)

The verse moves beyond introspection and into self-diagnosis. The narrator does not simply lament his condition, but provides an analysis of its principal cause: within flesh and bone lies the ever-constant, and ever-damaging, presence of sin. It is presented here not in the pastoral taxonomies and categories of self-analysis, but only in terms of its primary function: it works to 'deface' – to disfigure and deform. Such a rendering shifts narrative perspective into a more carefully delineated interior landscape. The narrator presents not simply the existence of sin but also its work within the soul. This figure at once objectifies, localises and personalises the impacts of sin; and by extension it allows the reader to occupy a similar posture of self-diagnosis. Yet, the stanza does not stop here but proceeds further inwards.

The damaging impacts of sin are not confined to the body, but reach into the soul as well. The line 'My wilde wille, my wittes frele' moves into the deformed psychology of the narrator, and presents a soul as corrupted as the body it inhabits. Imagery here is striking: the will is out of control, yet the wits are frail and feeble; both are trapped – 'Encombre' – due to sin. The simultaneity of these images offers a glimpse into the complexity of sin – it is something that deforms in the most striking, and to some extent paradoxical, of ways. Alliteration is used here to convey that sense of complexity and strangeness: 'wilde/wille/wittes' sets up a pattern of expectation that is denied by the use of 'frele'. This small stylistic choice generates an oddly haunting quality, enabling the verse to perform in itself the same inner discord it describes. Through the narrative voice, the reader is brought into this carefully created interior, forced to rehearse the same scene of critical and diagnostic introspection.

> My woundes beþ alle roten & ranke
> Tofore þe face of my folye,
> For, siþen I firste in synne sanke,
> To late I gan for mercy crye.
> But Crist þat quykedest him þat stanke,
> Þe broþer of Martha & of Marye,
> So brynge me fro þis breery banke
> To bene in blis aboue þe skye (ll. 234–8)

Through the voice of the narrator, the reader is once again placed into a posture of confessional introspection and diagnosis. The wounds of sin are compared to the stench of the dead, specifically Lazarus, and can be healed only through the intervention of Christ. Over the course of the stanza, the reader is brought not only to the acknowledgement of sin's damaging effects within the body, but also to the fact that only Christ can help. Self-diagnosis shades into prayer, as the final lines 'So brynge me fro þis breery banke / To bene in blis aboue þe skye' move the reader into begging Christ for mercy. The alliteration here of a string of plosives creates a gentle slowness in the verse, evoking the sense of a prayerful state. The confessional overtones of this, though subtle, are nevertheless potent. From beginning to end, the reader moves carefully into a position of penance and prayer. Such techniques are inseparable from the text's ability to evoke and sustain strong penitential feelings. These versified Psalms layer the emotional states required for contrition, and compel the reader into confessional self-examination and prayer. They are vessels of emotional force and potency, allowing the reader to be moved in specific ways and into specific states. Yet, the Psalms are not alone in this function. Many medieval penitential lyrics also enable similar forms of emotional manipulation.

These texts differ from the Psalms in a key way – length. Maidstone's verse translation of the penitential Psalms is quite long; in comparison, medieval penitential lyrics are not. Their comparative length allows for greater narrative focus and intensity on specific topics and situations, offering tightly controlled and localised instantiations of the emotive power of verse. Glosses and translations of the Psalms can prove very useful in training a reader in the methods of the *lectio divina* – in forging a complex web of associations and links between other Biblical texts.[45] Penitential lyrics do not have this specific didactic agenda, and so they possess none of those constraints and can freely move into areas and scenarios that are not covered in the Biblical texts. While the Psalms are confined to the specifics and particulars of David's relationship with God, the lyrics are free to dramatise other relationships and scenarios that may speak much more directly to the imaginations and psychologies of their readers. Though they may use the techniques and formulas of emotional manipulation found in the Psalms, they push that unique ability of verse to new levels of complexity.

Tools of Treatment

> Gods servants, holy church, shal be shakyn in sorows and anguis . . . for he seith: 'I shall al tobreke you for you veyn affections and your vicious pryde; and after that I shal togeder gader you and make you mylde and meke, clene and holy, by onyng to me'.[46]

For Julian, sorrow and anguish are not purposeless or useless, but are medicines of the soul that have a direct function in its eventual restoration. Her remarks here are set within the broader context of a vision God grants her, which reveals the purpose of suffering and tribulation. While she does not directly refer to penance, nor to contrition, she does highlight the central function of intense sorrow – to crush the vain affections from the soul. As her remarks show both the importance and purpose of intense emotional states in the reformation of the soul, they thus clarify how the penitential process operates. In much the same way, the penitential lyrics seek to aid in crushing sin and humbling the prideful will by augmenting the emotional responses of their readers. As mentioned earlier, they are 'affective catalysts' and 'proforma prayers' that have a deep connection to the penitential Psalms, but which nevertheless operate differently.[47] Freed of the narrative limits of David's relationship with God, the lyrics can establish broader and more engaging moods by dealing with aspects of human psychology and life not covered in the Biblical text. A sense of regret, itself central to the penitential process, can be powerfully evoked in just a few short lines. This is evident in the signal stanza lyric 'Miri it is while sumer I-last'[48]

> Miri it is while sumer I-last
> With foules song;
> Oc now negheth windes blast
> And weder strong.
> Ei, ei, what this night is long,
> And Ich with wel michel wrong
> Sorwe and murne and fast.[49] (ll. 1–7)

Without mention of confession, mercy from God, or even explicit reference to sin, this one-stanza lyric can still generate penitential feelings through its focus on retrospection. It carefully manipulates the passage of time, and the reader's perception of that temporal passage. The lyric moves from the distant and merry summer to the long and cold night, before finally resting on a reflection of the course of a whole sinful life: rapid oscillation between temporal expansion and contraction is played with here in the course of this single stanza. The movement is both highly structured and discordant. The distant past moves seamlessly into a present tense reflection on the nature of misspent life, and a sense of regret thus bleeds through into the current narrative moment. The opening word 'Miri' is soon echoed hauntingly in the opening of the second sentence with its interjectional cry of 'Ei, ei'. Such a mood is established without direct reference to anything in particular, and the lyric is almost empty of any concrete things. There is mention of 'sumer' and 'foules song', but these references are forcefully contrasted with 'windes blast', 'weder strong', and 'michel wrong'. In comparison to the versified penitential psalms, and their vivid psychodrama between David and God, this lyric is essentially empty. There is no personal relationship presented by the verse, no interpersonal dynamic with God. All that is present is a consciousness reflecting upon the passage of time and upon itself in a manner that is part lament and part introspection. It does not approach the levels of self-diagnosis and moral castigation of some of the Psalms, but it does nonetheless generate a penitential mood. The last lines, 'And Ich with wel michel wrong / Sorwe and murne and fast' constitute both the introduction and exit of the narrative voice, and the only mention of affective states.

While short, these lines do express a regret so general as to be poignant: they create a narrative space so open that anyone can enter into it. In this way the lyric works by its lack of imaginative bounds. The verse scenario is one without any real limitation, one any reader can readily inhabit. The 'Sorwe and murne and fast' is a part of this general sense of regret, and while it is connected directly to the 'michel wrong' carried out by the narrator, the verse makes no mention of specific sins. All that is left is a universal regret at a universal state of being. The brevity of the lyric is part of its potency, as its shortness endows it, and the regret it speaks of, with a haunting quality. Its comparative shortness enables it to be both memorable and potent. It can be repeated easily, yet by virtue of that shortness it never loses its tight focus on a specific topic and the emotional states it evokes. Though brief, it establishes a general mood of regret, one that can feed a penitential self-consciousness.

Other lyrics work to similar ends but emphasise the penitential aspects of the verse, shading into a prayer-like form. In 'An Orison of Penitence to Our Lady', the boundaries between prayer and lyric are almost indistinct.[50]

> Hayl mari!
> Hic am sori,
> Haf pite of me and merci,
> Mi leuedi,
> To þe I cri.
> For mi sinnis dred ham hi
> Wen hi þenke þat hi sal bi
> Þat hi had mis hi-don
> In worde, in worke, in þoith foli.
> Leuedi, her mi bon! (ll. 1–10)[51]

The whole stanza is in effect a petition to the Virgin for mercy and grace. By opening with a formal address to Mary, the whole tone of the lyric is more closely patterned upon a prayer. This is reflected in the rhyme scheme which, as Furnivall and Brown note, is strange and most likely derived from an as-yet unidentified Latin hymn.[52] The lyric develops from strongly liturgical sources, and its content is unambiguously penitential. The first six lines are repetitions of the same basic cry for mercy and forgiveness. The alliteration between the first three clauses not only connects the address to Mary, the acknowledgement of guilt, and the desire for mercy together, but also extends that opening cry for as long as possible. The reader is held by the verse in a penitential position that is immediately reinforced by the following two lines. The rhyme scheme here is hypnotic and recursive, circling around that central cry for mercy. The next full sentence of the lyric focuses on sin, and is keyed into the speech, deeds and thoughts of the narrative I voice. However, no particular sin is specified, allowing the reader that crucial narrative space to embody the prayer by inserting their own individual sins. This section has a complex mono-rhyme, with 'mis hi-don' connecting with 'her mi bon': such echoes forge theological links between sin itself and the work of Mary as intercessory with God. The last line, another cry to the Virgin, is reiterated with slight variation by the first line of the next stanza: the 'Mi bon þu her' echoes the prior stanza, and serves to fuse the two together. This feature is repeated for each successive stanza and generates a complex form of ideational and emotional concatenation: each stanza is a link in a penitential chain, and each link feeds back into the opening emotive tone of the lyric. The effect is powerful, as the reader is brought constantly back to that opening cry for mercy and the sense of sorrow and regret it evokes.

Subsequent stanzas focus on different subjects for emotional import, such as protection from demonic agents, and the sacrifice of Christ:

> Þi face to se,
> Þu grant hit me,
> Lefdi ful-fillid of pite;
> Þat hi may be
> In Ioy wit þe
> To se þi sone in trinite,
> Þat sufferid pine and ded for me
> And for al man-kyn.
> His flesse was sprade on rode-tre
> To leys us al of sine. (ll. 31–40)

There is an increasingly emotional tone to the lyric, drawing in the Passion. The whole stanza is predicated upon the strong contrasts of heavenly joy and earthly suffering. The 'sone in trinite' is the first mention of Christ the reader is exposed to, and it serves to magnify his pain when the verse presents his Passion. This aspect of Christ's life is given an arresting visual treatment – his flesh spread out – but it is an image that is not elaborated. Instead it is mentioned by the verse only to augment penitential feelings. The mono-rhyme of 'man-kyn/sine' stresses the connection between humanity and the presence of sin, while encapsulating the Passion. This makes a subtle theological point – that only the Passion can come between humanity and sin, and that it is the result of sin. It is the final mention of sin that dominates rather than the Passion: the central feature here is the focus on penance, as the line 'To leys us al of sine' emphasises the primary function of the Passion. Throughout the lyric the importance of penance is never diminished. Given its prayer-like form it could easily be memorised and used before undertaking the sacrament. Its function is thus to augment penitential states into new and more vividly realised emotions – to intensify the reader's sorrow for sin to the point of contrition.

Some of the lyrics appended to the Vernon manuscript are an excellent example of this. As has been noted, these lyrics encapsulate the core themes of the various texts of the manuscript – catechetical, pastoral and devotional.[53] They work not simply to summarise, but to concentrate and catalyse the core essence of the texts of sowle-hele in the rest of the manuscript, and consist of a wide array of thirteenth- and fourteenth-century materials. A number of them are penitential lyrics and, like others in that genre, they seek to intensify feelings of contrition through verse scenarios that encourage feelings of regret or act as prayerful cries for mercy. In accordance with this focus on 'sowle-hele', there are specific lyrics in the manuscript that move from dread of punishment for sins, to penance and contrition. The common 'Ubi sunt' lyric 'Where ben they beforen us weren', has a number of manuscript witnesses; Vernon is one of them.[54] This version, though, is part of the longer text 'Sayings of Saint Bernard: Man's Three Foes'.[55] It begins with our end, with the assertion that 'mon is worm & wormes Cok' and moves to consider the decay of the body (ll. 7–12), and the difficult relationship it has with the soul (ll. 13–48). The damnation of both is given sustained attention (ll. 79–150), and provokes a certain degree of dread and fear of punishment. However, the text soon moves into a more penitential section, one full of regret at the passage of time in a misspent life.

At this stage, the text evokes a rich and varied landscape. Highly specific and sumptuous detail is carefully deployed to generate a striking and glamorous scenario: the reader hears of 'houndes' and 'haukes', of 'riche ladies in heore bour' resplendent in 'gold in heore tressour', all bearing attractive countenances (ll. 181–6). Such detail is immediately more accessible than the remote past of King David seen in the Psalms, and permits greater levels of engagement and identification. Narrative focus rests on specific objects and people but only fleetingly. As in the prior lyric, the passage of time is carefully controlled here. The opening line with its 'Where ben heo þat bi-foren vs weren' evokes a distant past that is made vividly present through the rich imagery. The next stanza soon generates an abrupt temporal shift. With the lines 'Ac in a twynklyng of an eiȝe / Heore soules weren for-loren' (ll. 191–2), narrative perspective lurches into a present moment. Narrative time oscillates rapidly between two temporal periods over the course of the next two stanzas: the reader hears of 'þat gomen and þat song' (l. 193) before being confronted with 'Heore weole is comen to weilawei' (l. 197). Such a contrast between past luxury and present suffering does more than simply illustrate a moral point; it also generates a level of regret and menace. Time moves quickly, and with it comes disastrous consequences:

> Heore paradys þei hidden hyr,
> And now þei liggen in helle-fyr
> Þer pit and peyne is euere;
> Strong is þere in peyne and wo,
> Ac hopen þar hem neuer-mo,
> ffor out ne comen þei neuere. (ll. 199–204)

Mention of 'paradys', of 'helle-fyr', establishes a more overtly religious context for the narrative. Once again, narrative time moves from the distant past to the immediate present, and vividly realises the relationship between cause and effect. Regret thus becomes a dominant present condition: the hellish sufferings of the characters stand in stark contrast to their decadent prior lives, and add greater emphasis to the consequences of sin. In contrast to the earlier stanzas, present sufferings are given more focus here. The opening mention of paradise is brief, while the torments of hell are given more attention. The use of end rhyme in 'wo' and 'mo' serves to extend the narrative focus on suffering: the reader cannot pass over the pains of Hell quickly, but must linger in their sonic extension. There is little concrete detail, or enumeration of the torments of Hell. All that is present is a cry of anguish reiterated and mirrored through two lines of the stanza. Suffering is focused on here in a manner that evokes a sense of depth, but leaves much of the ideational work to the reader's imagination. Functionally it is contrasted with the earlier mention of Christ and the sorrow for His suffering, as regret has in effect two temporal periods:

> Þou take þe crois to þi staf
> And þenk on him þat þeron ȝaf
> His lyf þar was so lef;
> Wite wel þi fot wiþ staues ord
> And mak þe traytur speke þe word
> And wrek þe on þat þef. (ll. 163–8)

The use of passion imagery is understated and subtle, confined to 'þe crois' and Christ's own act of self-sacrifice. The theological import of this is passed over in favour of a more direct and compelling focus on the need for revenge for this unlawful killing. The notion of spiritual combat is rendered as an actual combat against the 'traytur' of the Devil. The use of images in the verse are much more accessible and relatable, as they reference human relationships, feelings and proclivities rather than theological abstractions. Until this point, the verse has been concerned with presenting the inevitable punishment for decadence; now it moves to the regret for the death of an innocent. This adds depth and urgency to the emotional reach of the text: it situates the consequences of sin in a broader social context that shows its terrible impacts upon others. The use of the present tense verb 'wrek' signals a move to the immediate present, as the verse moves forward with a new resolve and a sense of exhortation. Yet, from here, the verse moves back into the past – this time of the narrative voice. Exhortation shades into the introspection and regret of the following stanzas. Despite all this, there is still no direct mention of sin itself. This begins to change in the final two stanzas.

> Allas, þat þei euere were boren or bred,
> Þat heer on eorþe such lyf han led
> And deserued such meedes,
> To brennen in þe fuir of helle,
> Euer-more þer-Inne to dwelle
> And glowen in þo gledes! (ll. 205–10)

Regret becomes all the more immersive here, all the more suffocating. The opening cry of 'allas', a tactical use of the interjection, is an expression of emotional force that moves the reader toward powerful sorrow. The entire stanza is a single sentence, a breathless enumeration of the consequences of a misspent life. This sense of sorrow is made manifest through the careful manipulation of narrative time: the whole stanza contrasts origin with final damnation, images of being 'boren or bred' with those of living forever 'in þe fuir of helle'. This is accentuated through the rhyme of 'meedes/gledes' and 'helle/dwelle', as each pair manipulates narrative time. The rewards or 'meedes' of such a 'lyf' are the burning hot coals of Hell – those fiery 'gledes'. A misspent past turns into an endlessly painful future, just as the horrors of 'helle' now become a perpetual dwelling. Domesticity becomes damnation, and so the whole stanza also evokes a liminal dread, a fear of pain and punishment that is subordinated to the overall concern with regret and sorrow. The potent emotional energy of that opening cry is augmented and channelled by the imagery and language of the stanza, moving from dread into sorrow, and from here into a prayer for mercy:

> Ac Moder & Mayden, heuene-Qween,
> As we hopen þat þou wol ben
> Vr warant from þe fende:
> Þou help vs dedly synne to fleen,
> And þat we mote þi sone seen
> World wiþ-outen ende. Amen. (ll. 211–16)

Sin enters into the verse in a manner that is extremely general and open, but far from fleeting: it is mentioned here in a climactic way, the first and only direct request made of the Virgin by the narrator. Though no specific sin is mentioned, therein lies its evocative power: it refers here to any and all sin. This allows the verse to have the widest impact upon the reader. Sin is here an empty space within which the reader can place the recollection of their particular sins. The request for defence and protection – Mary is the 'warant' or 'defender' – is the key feature of this stanza.[56] In this way it operates much like a prayer: the reader beseeches Mary for guidance and support in fleeing his or her 'sinne'. The images of decadent living in the prior stanzas are sharply contrasted here with the image of Mary as Queen of Heaven. Subtly, a penitential movement is crafted here that exerts a considerable mental pull. The emotional energies of the prior stanza are carefully manipulated here into a prayer-like state for heavenly assistance: the verse moves the reader into a penitential context predicated upon regret and sorrow. Over the course of these stanzas regret becomes more complex and layered. It begins with regret over misspent youth and self-indulgence, before gradually shading into the regret for the consequences of sin on others and on one's self. The last line loosely translates the doxology of the *Gloria Patri*, and culminates in a direct prayer which ends with Amen. It thus posits an eternal temporal period that contrasts with the mention of Hell in the prior stanza. The reader is swept along by this current, directed into a specific frame of mind: to cry, eternally, for mercy in prayer. While the move to prayer occurs only in this last stanza, other lyrics give more attention to it.

The Vernon lyric 'Merci God and Graunt Merci' is one such example – a later lyric that also offers a vivid imaginary scenario for the reader to occupy.[57]

> As I wandrede her bi weste
> ffaste vnder a Forest syde,
> I seiȝ a wiht went him to reste,
> Vnder a bouȝh he gon a-byde;

> þus to crist ful ȝeorne he criȝede.
> And boþe his hondes he held on heiȝ:
> 'Of pouert, plesaunce & eke of pruide,
> Ay Merci, God, And graunt-Merci!'. (ll. 1–8)

The lyric opens in the exotic and evocative spaces familiar to romances and the *chanson d'aventure* genres.[58] Through the narrative I voice, the reader is immediately drawn into a vividly realised landscape and into a specific posture. Images do not linger here, but are fired off in rapid succession. Each line has a dominant imagistic object that is immediately replaced by the next line – the opening 'weste' is followed by the 'Forest', a 'wiht' and a 'bouȝh'. Narrative focus is shifting, moving from one object to another, delaying any imagistic intensity and building up a sense of narrative urgency. Through this technique the reader is led, step by step but with increasing force, towards a penitential display. While the initial setting of a leafy forest is as far removed from the sacrament of confession as can be, penance soon erupts into the verse. Before the end of the stanza's first sentence, there is mention of Christ and the cry of supplication to Him by a lonely figure. It is this cry – a penitential cry – that constitutes the relentless focus of the narrative. Each stanza ends with it, or a variant of it, and four stanzas begin with a near repetition of the line: the cry of Mercy constitutes both the focus and form of the narrative. Moreover, through the method of narration, this reported speech is performed by the reader. The verse presents a model penitential display that the reader inhabits in carefully delineated sequences of confessional self-knowledge and self-accusation: 'God, þat I haue I-greuet þe' (l. 9) and 'I am vnkynde, and þat I knowe' (l. 25) are lines that construct a deep sense of inner self-awareness. The initial setting of a forest is now completely replaced with a series of stanzaic prayers, each one dealing with a different confessed sin or circumstance of sinning, but never losing that focus on mercy:

> Merci þat I haue mis-spent
> Mu wittes fyue! Þerfore I wepe.
> To dedly synnes ofte haue I asent,
> Þi Comaundemens couþe I neuer kepe;
> To sle my soule In sunne I slepe,
> And lede my lyf in Lecheri;
> ffrom Couetyse couþe I neuere crepe;
> Ay Merci, God, And Graunt Merci. (ll. 41–8)

This is a model confession, and covers the broadest and most common infractions in the most general terms. While specific sins are mentioned, there is a tantalising openness in the 'mis-spent' of the first line and the 'dedly synnes' of the third. The stanza, though particular in its purpose in crying for mercy, is nevertheless extremely generic and formulaic: any and all misuse of the senses, or any of the deadly sins, could be inserted here. The same openness is applicable to the mention of the Commandments. Yet, the verse form changes subtly here, as alliteration becomes tighter, and interacts with end rhyme to slow the pace of the narrative. The reader cannot rush into and out of the confessional formula, but must slowly work through the subtle menace of the sibilance in 'To sle my soule In sunne I slepe', and the sharp, percussive self-accusation in 'From Couetyse couþe

I neuere crepe'. Forced to linger in a penitential frame of mind, the reader is presented with comparisons and contrasts through the use of end rhyme: 'mis-spent/a-sent' connects volition with sin, while the 'Lecheri/Merci' pairing works to oppose sin with mercy. Mention of the Passion, of the emotive touchstones of Christ's life, receive little attention beyond 'þat for my sunnes þi blod gon schede!' (l. 12): this ends a sentence and sense unit, as the verse immediately moves onto other topics. The Passion enters for only the briefest of moments, its emotive potency carefully controlled and moderated by the verse form. The main focus is not Christ but rather the penitential awakening of the narrator and by extension the reader. Over its course, the lyric becomes an extended and concatenated prayer. More self-accusation follows, more self-diagnosis:

> Of oþes grete and Gloteny,
> Of wanhope and of wikked wille:
> Bacbyte my neiʒhebors for enuy,
> And for his good I wolde him culle,
> Trewe men to Robbe and spille,
> Of Symony and with surquidri;
> Of al þat euere I haue don ille
> Ay Merci, God, And graunt Merci! (ll. 49–56)

This stanza is a near repetition of the prior one, and as such it operates as a means of extending and deepening confessional self-awareness. It articulates a specific form of self-analysis that keeps the reader locked into a comprehensive confessional posture. The whole stanza is one complete sentence, and offers an unbroken focus on a moment of confessional discourse that deepens the intensity of the reader's understanding of its procedural operation. All emotive force and potency are directed towards that cry for mercy. There is no focus on an image that induces sorrow, but instead on a procession of various instances of sin. This parade of sins is carried out over the emotional backdrop created by the constant refrain of 'merci' in each of the stanzas. The reader is meant to follow the pattern: cries for mercy spill out into yet more self-accusation, which in turn fuel further cries for mercy. This reaches a climax in a later stanza:

> Soþast god, what schal say I say?
> How schulde I amendes make,
> Þat plesed þe neuere in-to þis day,
> Ne schop me nouʒt mi sunnes forsake?
> But schrift of mouþe mi sunnus schal slake,
> And I schal sece and beo sori;
> And to þi Merci I me take –
> Nou Merci, God, And Graunt Merci! (ll. 73–80)

Penance is the ultimate and only solution to the effects and presence of sin discussed over the course of the prior stanzas. With stunning brevity, the stanza now articulates the potent efficacy of confession in a mere two lines. After nine stanzas that explore the nature and presence of sin, the verse now asserts that all manner and extent of wrong-doing is cured with a single act. The play here between the multiplicity of sin and the singularity of confession is striking, and underscores the importance of the sacrament and its principal components: auricular confession and sorrow of heart. Confession is presented here as the sole answer to the two direct questions posed to God – a rhetorical presentation which moves the reader into accepting the inevitability and exclusivity of penance as the cure for sin. The last lines assume a more prayer-like form, a pattern enhanced in the next two stanzas and their address to 'ffader & sone and holigost' (l. 81), and 'Only God in Trinite' (l. 92). The result is subtle but powerful, as the reader gradually assumes a penitential posture before actually performing a penitential act – an articulation before God of the presence of sin and the need for mercy.

The lyric has fulfilled its function, and aided the reader in evoking and sustaining those core aspects of the sacrament – sorrow and speech. Yet, while the whole text is moving, it lacks the relentless focus and emotional range of the earlier examples mentioned above. On the whole it is much more restrained and restraining, as the lyric evokes specific emotional states and immediately channels them into acts of prayer. It catalyses emotional states, but it does so in a more measured way, allowing the reader to focus more on themselves and their own relationship with sin than on the horrendous physical consequences of sin for Christ and for others. Sorrow is in a sense less intersubjective, and more directly concerned with interiority and self-diagnosis. Emotion does not run rampant, but is more tied to the emergence of a specific form of self-awareness that these lyrics establish. They are vessels of emotion that aid in the treatment of the soul. Through the sorrow they evoke, the soul is purged and its poison removed. The phlebotomy and purgation of sin from the soul mentioned earlier is not simply a rhetorical extravagance. Rather, it speaks to what is actually happening in the reading and recitation of these texts: they literally draw sin out of the soul, by forcing their readers to perform a simulated confession based upon a constructed groundswell of sorrow. However, this is not the end of the soul's emotional treatment. After purgation there is yet another medicine: compassion – the presentation of, and co-participation in, the emotional agony of Christ's suffering. The next chapter explores such texts: the Middle English accounts and elaborations of Christ's life, suffering and death.

3

Compassionate Healing

> Loke man to Iesu crist
> hi-neiled an þo rode,
> and hi-pitz his naked bodi
> red hi-maked mid blode,
> his reg mid scurge i-suunge
> his heued þornes prikede,
> þo nailes in him stikede
> þuend and trend þi lords bodi
> þurch wam þu art i-boruhe
> þer þu mit hi-uinde blode and sorwe (ll. 1–10)[1]

Though only a single stanza long, this early fourteenth-century lyric *Respice in Faciem Christi* offers a relentless engagement with Christ in His agonies. This is achieved through extraordinary control of the narrative gaze – a series of highly focused images and details that increase in force and potency. In the first line the reader glimpses Christ with no other adornment, before being presented with Him nailed to the Cross. From here there are careful and structured movements in image and detail: a naked body, red blood, scourged flesh, thorns, and then nails again. The whole stanza is dominated by two main movements. Initially, the image of Christ on the Cross is presented as a whole before being pulled apart into its constituent sections. The reader must move through these specific cross-sections of the image, with new details emerging each time. Christ, whole in the first two lines, is split into a series of segments. The technique makes the horrors of the Passion fresh and arresting: the entire scene cannot be compassed in one movement, but instead must be slowly and carefully moved through. The emotive impact of the image of the crucifixion is strung out, extended and elongated in a manner that forces the reader to see it afresh line by line.

The second movement of the stanza is one of dizzying compression. Once we return to 'þo nailes' in Christ, the sectional images all merge together again into one aggregate whole, and the reader is instructed to 'puend and trend þi lords bodi'. Christ is no longer a procession of tortured parts but instead a fully realised three-dimensional body, one that the reader must hold and turn about in the mind. It is a technique of meditative focusing, of training the mind to consider one central thing through its constituent parts. It is also, however, a technique of emotional focusing. Through this procession of tortures, the reader is immersed in the image as each line builds up emotive force and potency. The overall scene the lyric depicts evokes a complex range of emotional states. While the images in each line, though horrific in their local and specific detail, can generate fear, there is also a penitential aspect to the stanza. The last two lines – 'þurch wam þu art i-boruhe/ þer þu mit hi-uinde blode and sorwe' – offer a simulated moment of self-awareness, a forced realisation that the whole scene is effectively our doing. Yet the focus of the whole verse is not the self, either in its penitential agonies or fear of hellish pains to come, but rather on the sufferings of another: Christ. It is compassion that the lyric seeks to evoke and sustain, something beyond fear and penance yet nevertheless incorporating them. Such compassionate engagement with Christ is the next stage in the soul's treatment. As Julian of Norwich notes, compassion not only makes the soul 'redy' but is one of it 'medycines'.[2] Through compassion the soul undergoes a healing process, administered and performed by Christ Himself:

> Here to acordyng spekeþ Seynt Austyn þus, Goddes son toke man & in hym he soffred that longeþ to man & was made medicyne of man. & this medicyne is so mykell þat it may nouȝt be þouȝt. For þer is no pryde bot þat it may be heled þruȝe þe mekenes of goddis sone. Þer is no Couetyse bot þat it maye be heled thorgh is pouerte. No Wrath bot þat it may be heled throw his pacience. No Malice bot þat it may be heled þrowȝe his charite.[3]

The mystery of the incarnation is, at its core, a pharmaceutical process. God becomes not just flesh and blood, but medicinal flesh and blood. For this text, a classic of Middle English devotional prose, Christ is the source of a medicine so powerful and so plentiful that it defies categorisation and analysis. He heals all things, specifically the Seven Deadly Sins ('Malice' being another name for avarice during the period). In this way He functions like those earlier medicines of fear and penance, though here He treats multiple spiritual illnesses. His healing work is understood in terms of the medicine of the contraries, yet He goes beyond this to counteract many states at once. He is the ultimate medical compound, able to confer a range of benefits through one medicine: Himself. It is a presentation of Christ that, as Love notes, can be traced back to Augustine; specifically his elaboration of the trope of 'Christ the Physician' or *Christus Medicus*. Yet, what is most significant here is the connection between that medicine and suffering: Christ 'soffred that longeþ to man & was made medicyne of man'. It is His pain that brings our relief and cure. Engagement with the 'medicyne of man' is thus in effect and in essence engagement with the suffering of Christ – with the compassionate response to His pain, torture and death. Through compassion, the medicines generated by Christ's sufferings can be accessed; through compassion, the goal of sowle-hele comes ever closer. This chapter focuses on compassion as the next medicine of the soul, and explores how compassion was understood to operate medically with reference to Christ's therapeutic role. It pays particular attention to the most extensive meditation on Christ's suffering in the Vernon manuscript – *The Prickynge of Love* (hereafter *Prickynge*).

Compounded Passions

> Lo þe spiceris shoppe is openyd to þe, ful of al swete spiceri & ful of medicinable oynementis Gracia dei. And saue is þere inouȝe. Go in-to hit & gete þe medicine for to hele the and restore þe, & kepe þe in holynesse. Wat spiceri þat þe liketh & wat letuarie þat þou coueytist þere take hit. Mekenesse & myldenesse, prescience & soburnesse, chastite & clennesse, charite & softenesse, & seuche oþere delicate confecciouns. Ȝif þow loue hem þere mai þou haue hem. Al suche swetnesse is plentiuously hid in ihesu.[4]

The compassionate engagement with Christ provides a specific course of treatment: a series of 'delicate confecciouns'. This term has a precise meaning in medieval medicine, referring to medical compounds. During this period, medical drugs fall into one of two categories: simples or compounds. A simple medicine is a drug made from one ingredient only; all therapeutic effects are contained and conveyed within that one ingredient. A compound medicine, however, combines several ingredients specifically selected to interact together to offer greater therapeutic effects.[5] The medicinal effect of the compound is many times greater than the sum of its parts, as it can deal with multiple aspects of the disordered body. Compassion for Christ, the emotional result of engagement with the 'blod of his herte' (l. 18), is best understood as a compound medicine for the soul. It is not a single emotional state, but rather a complex blend of fear, penance, pity and sorrow alongside a precise configuration of intersubjective awareness. Christ's Passion, in both its general and specific details, can evoke fear as well as penance, can make one recoil in horror at the same time as eliciting penitential feelings of culpability for the torture and execution of another. As Christ's sufferings were manifold, so too is the compassion for them. Such complexity is reflected in its definition, which conveys this dual sense of emotion and intersubjectivity. The word itself in Middle English – *compassioun* – means 'the sharing of sufferings with another; commiseration'; its etymology also conveys this sense, coming from the Latin 'com-patior', meaning to suffer with.[6] Yet the word both in Latin and Middle English is also used in medical contexts to understand the interconnection between the various parts of the body:

> Þe membres beþ so isette togedres þat, for þe byndinge and knettinge togedres, eueryche haþ compaciens of oþir. Þerfore þe membre lesse igreued haþ compaciens of þe membre þat is more igreued. And þerfore if on membre is ihurt, þe humours of þe oþir membres renneþ and comeþ to þe sore place.[7]

Compassion is a relationship as much as it is a series of emotional states. In this sense compassion figures models of physical incorporation: to be compassionate towards Christ means to be, in a sense, inside His body, to suffer with-in Him. An intense intersubjectivity is thus at the very core of compassionate response – an intimacy predicated upon pain and penance, upon an awareness of one's self and another, upon an enhanced penitential subjectivity. To share in the sufferings of Christ is not to have a vague sense of sorrow for Him, but rather to cultivate an empathic capacity that is layered, complex and intense. These aspects of compassion are integral to its therapeutic role, and are ultimately derived from the concept of the *Christus Medicus*. It is through compassion for Christ in His agony that we become his patients – itself a word derived from the Latin *pati* (to suffer)

– those who must suffer with Him. While this idea of Christ's medical role occurs in the Bible and in the writings of the early Church, it is Augustine who develops the most influential elaboration of this concept that figures both the ideal doctor and ideal patient.[8] Over the course of his writings he presents Christ as the ultimate physician, who cures through the use of pain. There is nothing gentle or easy about the care of Christ the Physician:[9]

> Timor Dei sic vulnerat, quomodo medici ferramentum; putredinem tolliet, et quasi videtur vulnus augre. Ecce putredo quando erat in corpore, minus erat vulnus, sed periculosum: accedit ferramentum medici; minus dolebat illud vulnus, quam dolet modo cum secatur. Plus dolet cum curatur, quam si non curaretur; sed ideo plus dolet accedente medicina, ut nunquam doleat succedente salute.[10]

> (The fear of God wounds like the knife of the physician: it takes away the festering, and seems to enlarge, as it were, the wound. Behold, when the purulent matter was in the body, the wound was smaller, but dangerous. Then comes the knife of the physician: that wound hurts less than it hurts now when it is cut; it hurts more when it is treated than it would, if it were not operated upon; it hurts more under the healing operation, but only that it may never hurt again after the healing is effected.)

His is a treatment of extremes, worse than the pain of the sickness itself. The whole passage is dominated by paradox, comparisons and quantifications. Christ cures suffering through even greater suffering, removes the wound by making it much larger; in effect He heals by harming. Here the image of the Lamb of God becomes conflated with that of the surgeon and his knife, and has a shocking, visceral power. Given the pre-anaesthetic nature of Classical and Medieval medicine, there is a deliberate potency to Augustine's choice of simile. The treatment of Christ the Physician is meant to do more than make the reader wince. Fear and pain come together here in a manner designed to elucidate the intensity of the cure: to heal you, Christ will cut you open. This medical role is wholly predicated upon His Passion – the best and bitterest medicine: 'the cup of the passion is bitter, but it cures thoroughly all diseases. The cup of the passion is bitter but the Physician drank of it lest the patient hesitate to drink of it.'[11] The therapy Christ offers is, for Augustine, understood within a shifting nexus of the most severe medical procedures and terminology – surgery, cautery, purgation, and even violent death.[12]

The influence this forceful and visceral conceptualisation exerts throughout the Middle Ages is considerable. For Gregory the Great, to follow Christ was to undertake an important life-long journey that could transform the individual's soul. It was, however, far from gentle. Following Christ meant taking up his Cross, engaging with His Passion in the experience of compassion. It is a process he presents in striking terms. Following the Latin etymology for the word cross (*crux*), Gregory notes that it comes from *cruciare* – to torture: compassion for Christ is, at its very core, the torture of the soul through emotional extremes.[13] Writing much later in the period, Bernard of Clairvaux states that those persons in the second and third degree of spiritual ascent – the animal and spiritual persons – torture their souls with the fear and love generated by meditation on Christ's Passion.[14] In a more explicit vein, William of St Thierry asserts that the fear generated by meditating upon Christ's Passion pierced his soul.[15] Compassion, like surgery, cuts.

Such understandings of compassion's potent and difficult nature underpin Middle English textual engagements with this emotional complex. When Richard Rolle writes that Jesus' name not only means health, but that He provides a 'sorrowyng medicyne', it is this idea of pain and intensity that he is expressing.[16] For Christ to heal him, he must suffer, he must be emotionally tortured. His *Meditation on the Passion A* aims to do that by focusing not just on Christ but also His Mother – a technique of 'wexenge manyfold, with hepynge sorewys'.[17] So too when Julian, during her sickness, asks for the 'wound of kinde compassion', what she requests is not something simple and gentle but instead expressly difficult and painful.[18] Her entire text shows how the compassion she initially asks for thickens and deepens into a much richer and complex self-knowledge, that eventually reveals Christ's compassion for her and all creation.[19] For both, the compassionate engagement with the *Christus Medicus* is a severe encounter that goes beyond a general sorrow for Christ's agonies to embrace fear at their horrific brutality, and a heightened penitential self-awareness of the role of sin in creating them.

In submitting to the intensive care of the *Christus Medicus*, in experiencing the torture of compassion at its utmost, both are following the example of His most famous patient: Paul. As Augustine notes, Paul is the greatest proof of the power of the *Christus Medicus*:

> Si Paulus sanatus est, ego quare despero? Si a tanto medico tam desperatus aeger sanatus est, ego cur vulneribus meis illas manus non aptabo? Ad illas manus non festinabo? Ut hoc dicerent homines, ideo Saulus factus est ex persecutore apostolus. Quia quo venit medicus, quaerit aliquem ibi desperatum, et ipsum sanat: et si pauperrimum inveniat, tamen desperatum inveniat; non ibi quaerit mercedem, sed commendat artem.[20]

> (If Paul was cured, why do I despair? If so desperately ill a patient was made whole by such a great Physician, why do I not put those healing hands on my wounds? So that people would say this, Paul was made an apostle out of a persecutor. Is it not the case that when a doctor comes to town, he looks for a desperate case to cure: and if the patient is penniless is not the despair even greater? He's not looking for money, but how to commend his skill.)

The conversion of Saul to Paul is, at its core, a rhetorical act: a demonstration of skill designed to persuade and convince. Saul, the worst sinner and most zealous persecutor of the church, is seen here as the most debilitated patient. His conversion becomes a miraculous cure that shows the power of the *Christus Medicus*. Underpinning this narrative arc from woe to well is the dynamic between madness and self-knowledge, humility and pride. As Augustine notes elsewhere, Saul is essentially mad – ignorant of his own self: 'Having lost his mind and being desperately ill, [Saul] persecuted [the Church] fiercely in his madness.'[21] Yet, when he receives the care of the *Christus Medicus*, all this changes: Christ 'struck him down, a raging man, and raised him up whole'. Sanity and knowledge of his true self come to Saul through Christ's medical intervention. Being healed by Christ promotes a deep and abiding humility, a health of the soul that must be preserved from boasting and self-aggrandisement. This specific mention of pride is far from unique in Augustine's writings, and is especially evident in his further engagement with the medical treatment of Paul. While Saul's conversion cures him, he still receives constant treatment from Christ as Paul; specifically for the 'tumour of pride':

> Illud est vitium capitale, quod cum quisque bene profecerit, superbia tentatur, ut perdat totum quod profecit. Denique omnia vitia in malefactis timenda sunt; superbia in benefactis plus metuenda est. Non itaque mirum quia sic est humilis Apostolus, ut dicat: 'Quando infirmor, tunc fortis sum'. Nam hoc vitio ne ipse tentaretur, quale sibi medicamentum dicit appositum contra tumorem, a medico qui sciret quid curaret? 'Ne magnitudine', inquit, 'revelationum extollar, datus est mihi stimulus carnis meæ, angelus satanæ, qui me colaphizet. Propter quod ter Dominum rogavi, ut discederet a me; et dixit mihi: Sufficit tibi gratia mea; nam virtus in infirmitate perficitur.'[22]

> (It is a capital vice since pride tempts anyone making progress so that all progress is lost. In short, all vices are to be feared in doing evil, pride is more to be feared in doing good. It is no wonder that a humble Apostle would say: 'When I am weak, then I am strong'. For lest he himself be tempted by this vice, look what sort of medication he said was placed against the tumor by the doctor who knows what cures? 'And lest the greatness of the revelations should exalt me, there was given me a sting of my flesh'.)

Beyond conversion lies compassion: continued progress in the Christian life requires continued pain. For Paul, despite being an Apostle, there is the constant danger of succumbing to pride, of falling into a sickness of the soul again. To remedy this, he is given the *stimulus carnis* – the sting or prick of the flesh – designed to quell any and all prideful urges. It treats Paul's emotions through the pain it causes, eliminating pride and promoting humility: as Augustine asserts 'Behold how merciful God was, conquering all [Paul's] affections'.[23] This understanding of Paul as the model patient, treated through pain, becomes foundational for subsequent medieval engagements with the workings of compassion. As Peter Damian, Odilo of Cluny and Bruno of Segni all note, Paul is the exemplum of someone who 'followed the Cross' – whose soul was tortured by compassion.[24] The *stimulus carnis* thus allows Paul to experience compassion for Christ without the need for physical crucifixion: his soul can be tortured in a way that permits him to follow Christ's Cross to the utmost. His pain becomes paradigmatic, not only for the ascetical and disciplinary practices of monasticism, but also for the process of Passion meditation. True compassion for Christ will, therefore, exert a remedial force upon the soul and its emotions in a manner similar to the operation of the *stimulus carnis* upon Paul. The sting of compassion – the essence of the work of the *Christus Medicus* – will treat the emotions, will promote the health of the soul through inflicting pain on the soul. It is a dynamic given potent articulation in a range of Middle English religious texts. For instance, Julian's own vision of Christ's gruesome and bloody head leads to a profound inner self-awareness, and a sense of the importance of pain in life:

> And this vision was a lernyng to myn vnderstondyng that the continual sekyng of the soule plesith God ful mekyl; for it may do no more than sekyn, suffrin and trosten ... And thus was I lernyd to myn vnderstondyng that sekyng is as good as beholdyng for the tyme that he will suffer the soule to be in travel.[25]

Pain begets perception. As Gillespie notes, this is yet another example of Julian's ability to ventriloquise a range of Middle English spiritual writings; here the genre of tribulation literature.[26] Ever allusive, Julian plays with the semantic range of words through puns and homophones in ways that merit meditation, and enable her text to continually refresh itself. Pain is at the centre here. The importance of 'suffrin' and 'travel' is evidenced not simply by repetition, but also the vivid descriptions of Christ's agony. Yet each word contains other meanings: 'suffrin' (to wait/to suffer), 'travel' (to journey/to endure; and also to endure labour pains/to suffer).[27] Such layers of meaning contribute to the intensity of her prose, and connect her with the torture of compassion. The word she chooses, 'travel', has an etymology in the Latin *trepalium*: a three-pronged implement of torture. She too, like Paul, is subject to the treatment of the *Christus Medicus*, who suffers her soul to endure the torture of compassion.

Her words reflect upon the importance of endurance, of patience in pain, and are integral to her wider understanding of the medical impact of compassion. Her use of the registers and terms of tribulation literature here and over the course of her text is by no means accidental. For her, the medicinal power of compassion lies in what it does to the soul. As she makes clear, 'be compassion we arn made redy': it orders the soul, prepares it for higher levels of spiritual growth, and to receive God.[28] Yet it does so in a highly specific way. When truly felt, compassion will make the soul ready by promoting specific emotions and modes of self-awareness within it. Much like Paul's *stimulus carnis* and even tribulation itself, compassion's intensity and potency are merely the means; the therapeutic ends are different. Being tortured with Christ in Passion meditation will, therefore, treat the passions of the soul, promoting not simply pity but also forms of cognition and relational subjectivity. Christ's meek suffering on the Cross becomes a paradigm to share in, and doing so becomes a therapeutic moment. Of course, in this regard Julian is hardly unique. Many texts from the period assert the medicinal importance of patience, pity and humility to the soul, and of Christ's healing pain in compassion. The influential *Twelve Profits of Tribulation*, makes this clear:

> So Crist, þat in holy chirch is clepid oure moder for þe gretnesse of hys tendyr love þat he hath to vs, he chewed for vs bitter paynes, hard wordis, repreves & sclaundrys, with bitternesse of his passione þat he suffered for us, to noryssh vs & strengh us gostly by ensample of hyme to suffer tribulacions & aduersitees of þis world. As wyne þat is clensed þorrow a bage-ful of spicis, chaungith his owen sauoure, drawynge to hym the sauour of þe spicis, so a man suffrynge tribulacion oweth to clense hyme by the blessed body of oure lord Ihesu, considerynge þe passyon þat he suffred for hym; & so schul it be swete & tollerable, þat to-fore semed full bitter & vntollerable.[29]

Christ feeds His pain to all mankind in a striking moment of maternal nourishment and consumption. The tender bond between mother and child is now endowed with potent and unpleasant connotations, and it is used here to illustrate proximity and equivalency. The metaphor conveys a sense of connectedness, of a reciprocity that is as natural as it is uncomfortable: the sufferings of one become those of another, just as milk passes from mother to child. As the *Prickynge* notes in a more direct way, tribulation and compassion are indistinguishable: by suffering tribulations 'myldely softly & gladly with-owten grucchynge, pleynynge, or misseyinge ... þenne art þow crucified wiþ crist'.[30] Compassion to the point of co-experience is only possible by suffering tribulation in the manner of Christ.

The next metaphor in the passage, the cleansing of wine through a bag of spices, extends this sense of connection. It is an image of fusion: the wine is changed by the 'spicis', merging with them and taking on their distinctive 'sauour'. This use of flavour and taste to describe shared pain is a subtle but clever move. Metaphysical aspects of sensation are used to articulate the nature of compassion and its relation to the self – it is something integral to the self, as flavour is to wine. The overarching point is that Christ's sufferings become indistinguishable from our own through the process of Passion meditation. Yet the process is, at its core, a therapeutic one. The mention here of wine and 'spicis' also overlaps with a medical register. During the period, both wine and spices are seen as integral parts in medical preparations and treatments. The key word here is 'clense': the fusion of wine and spice, of pain and selfhood, is a process of cleansing, of purification. Its ability to treat the soul is made clear at the end of the preceding chapter. Citing the book of Job, the text asserts that 'tribulacion sauith the soule, as Iob saith: *Ipse vulnerat & medicinat*, he wondyth & he helyth; for he woundeth the body, & helyth the soule'.[31] This is the treatment of the *Christus Medicus*. As Christ was tortured, so too is the person who meditates upon his passion: the pain and tribulation born in compassion torture the soul, and in so doing purify it. The profits of tribulation are therefore akin to compassion's medicinal effects, working to foster specific emotions, forms of cognition, and relational subjectivity. To 'suffre paciently aduersitees & tribulacions, & in þi suffring þinke mekely in god' is key to 'þin helth & þi saluacion'.[32]

Patience in suffering is often understood in a medical way. As the *Pore Caitif* notes in a whole section dedicated to the virtue, 'þoruʒ veri pacience eþir meke suffring ... synnes ben purgid'.[33] Patience acts as a purgative, purifying the soul by removing sins – or 'þe filþe of þis world'.[34] In the *Chastising of God's Children* its therapeutic range is extended: 'in al tribulacions and temptacions it is nedeful to be pacient as for a principal remedie aʒens al diseasis, bodili and gostl'.[35] Patience in suffering is something more diffusely therapeutic than a purgative or cleansing agent. Its ability to counter all possible 'diseasis' asserts a far greater medical potential. Yet this potential consists not simply of endurance; patience, as a medical force, encompasses much more. Its therapeutic operation is deeply connected to penance and penitential modes of self-awareness. The key line, 'Eche man, if he serche wele his defautes', asserts that a heightened introspection is an integral part of this process.[36] Through it, 'al diseasis, bodili and gostli' become easier to bear. The word 'serche' can also mean the examination of a patient or of wound with a surgical probe.[37] The virtue is, therefore, more medically and psychologically complex. It is beyond a mere state of practised insensitivity – the text makes it clear here that such 'diseasis' are keenly felt. Patience is a virtue that, as part of its remedial effect, requires a deep self-awareness to be operative. As one of the paradigmatic examples of patience throughout the period is Christ crucified, proximity to Him through Passion meditation thus connects patience and its medicinal effects to compassion. Patience in suffering is, ultimately, born out of compassion, and engenders modes of cognition as much as modes of feeling. Such medicalised presentations of patience are mostly summary, and do not go into great detail or elaboration. Nevertheless, they make the point that the virtue of patience is understood within a medical frame, deeply tied to the medical work of compassion.

Other states that are central to compassion are understood in similar ways, and exert similar effects upon the soul. Pity, in many ways the key constituent emotion within compassion, is given a medical rendering. In the fourteenth-century *Book of Vices and Virtues*, pity is understood as one of the gifts of the Holy Spirit, a gift with medical properties:

þe second [gift] makeþ þe herte swete and debonere & pitous, and þerfore it is cleped þe ȝifte of pite, þat is propreliche a dewe and a triacle aȝens al vilenyes, and nameliche aȝens synne of enuye.[38]

As a medicine, pity possesses considerable potency. The comparison made by the text connects it to one of the most famous medieval medicines – the 'triacle' or *theriac*. This elaborate medical compound was held to be a universal antidote to poison, and was made from the flesh of snakes. It often occurs in reference to Christ and His Blood or Passion.[39] The key word here is 'propreliche', an adverb that makes it clear that the text is not being metaphorical but rather literal: pity operates exactly like a medicine, within the same therapeutic parameters.[40] The connection to Christ is also important, as it underscores the therapeutic work of His Passion. Pity is often seen as vital for an authentic compassionate response to Passion meditation. It is an integral part of compassion as it is itself an emotional state. In medieval psychology, pity is understood as a passion of the soul that is open to rational persuasion.[41] It can be evoked and sustained by argument and, while it originates in the irrational part of the soul, it is not shut off from the rational soul. Pity as an emotion, therefore, contains a deliberative and cognitive component that serves in Passion meditation as the psychological basis for establishing a form of intersubjectivity. It enables an awareness of others and their emotional pain, especially as it relates to the self.

In the *Prickynge*, such pity has formidable effects: 'Þourȝe þis ȝifte of pite a man is made like to criste crucified. For-wy al þe chesoun of his death was for worship of his fader, and for hele of mennys sowlis'.[42] The simile used in this context affords more than simple comparison: through pity we share in His agony, we truly suffer with Him. It is in this shared torment that the gulf between God and mankind diminishes. The passion of pity is so powerful that the boundaries between self and God begin to blur. In that moment the therapeutic parameters of pity, and by extension compassion, open up: as we become like Christ we share His desire to heal mankind. Selfhood becomes expanded and interconnected, aware not simply of itself but of others: through pity 'þenne is his herte stired & opened to alle his euen-cristen and filled so ful of reuthe & of pite þat he þynketh, ȝif nede were, hym-self redi for to suffre and die for hem as crist died for vs.[43] Pity's emergence within the soul is deeply connected to the Passion, and to compassionate response. Once again it enables the self to take the place of Christ, to seek the same horrendous death in a moment in which the distinctions between God and mankind become less absolute. It is an intersubjective moment, as the self relates to God in a direct manner.

In many ways this is a standard expression of the idea of *dilatio cordis* – the heart expanding due to profound meditation on Christ's Passion. However, more precisely, pity enables a radical expansion of the self and its horizons: as the text asserts, pity makes the self 'opend to alle'. Through it, boundaries between self and God, and self and others, recede. Pity is here so profound that it encourages the person to want to die for everyone in the same way Christ did: the emotional ambit of the self expands and extends, encompassing others. It is an intersubjective moment that begets an even greater intersubjectivity, as the self considers itself, then God, then creation. Such an expansion of subjectivity is borne 'wenne aman thenkith inwardli' – a form of introspection developed and practised in penitential contexts, and the essence of the prior emotional medicine of the soul.[44] The subjectivity this fosters is ultimately confessional, but through the operation of pity it moves into a more relational mode: thoughts begin 'inwardli' but end by moving outwards to consider mankind. Cognition is central here. It is not just passions that are mentioned, but also forms of thought: the text is clear that this process occurs when one 'thenkith' on Christ. Pity, as an emotion amiable to rational persuasion, can engage both the irrational and rational soul, offering moments of thought and feeling. Such a process is intensive, as 'pite wondirli fryȝeth a mannys herte and tendrith hit al-so'.[45] This is evident not simply in the imagery used here, but also in the choice of words. The adverb 'wondirli' has a wide semantic range, and can mean miraculous.[46] Yet, in addition to these meanings, the word can also mean 'dreadfully' and 'awesome': there is an element of fear, of intensity, of something related to pain alongside that sense of reverential drede, or awe, at God deigning to die. Pity is a gift so strong and forceful that it torments the heart.

Given the context of Passion meditation, there are unmistakable resonances here of the healing work of the *Christus Medicus*: compassion for Christ begets pity for all that is pure torture, a torture which treats the soul. This pity, however, moves outwards and begets 'a brennande þirst to hele of odir mennys soules as crist hadde'.[47] Once again the boundaries between self and God blur, as the person assumes the therapeutic intentions of the *Christus Medicus*. This complex web of associations between pity, compassion and relational subjectivity are given succinct articulation in the *Speculum Vitae*. Focusing on the virtue of pity it notes:

> It mas a man to sighe sare
> For othir mens here illefare,
> And to haue ioye and solace
> Of othir mens happe and grace.
> Als ilk lym feles what othir aylles,
> When oght it greues or auaylles,
> And ilk lym til hymseluen taas
> Bathe gode and ille þat othir hase.
> For if men smyte outhir fote or the,
> Þe mouthe says 'þou hurtes me'.
> By þe lymes of þe body
> We may knawe Pyte verrayly. (ll. 4543–54)

Beyond emotional correspondence there lies interconnection and incorporation. Pity enables us to understand each other in the most profound and intimate of ways, facilitating the emergence of a relational subjectivity. Yet, the intersubjectivity it fosters becomes something more intensive – a deep and abiding interconnection. Much like the medical understanding of compassion mentioned earlier, pity figures models of physical incorporation: it is akin to the interconnected nature of the body, with each limb sharing to some extent the pain of another. Through pity there is a reciprocal sensation between disparate parts of a larger interconnected system. Pity tortures, but in so doing dissolves differences, making all common in universal pain. This is the wider impact of compassion. It is, at its core, the basis of interconnection between all the various parts of the corporate body of the Church: pity is key to the *Catholic* Church, as it allows the pain of Christ and the pain of others to be universally shared. However, this is not the final aspect to compassion's medical potential. Patience, pity and the prior emotional medicines of the soul all constellate together in compassion to create its final medical effect: humility.

As was evident in the treatment of Paul through the *stimulus carnis*, humility is one of the key medicinal effects of compassion. This appears in Augustine's writings as the 'cup of humility', a parallel to the bitter cup of the Passion that Christ had to drink. Such an idea persists into the Middle Ages. For Rolle in his Psalter commentary, the 'chalice of hele' is in fact 'pyne and passion that is kalde chalice, for it is a plesand drynke to halymen of hele'. Through compassion, an act that allows us to 'folous his passion', this medicine of humility will be unlocked.[48]

Later medieval texts take up similar themes, stressing the connection between thinking on the Passion and humility. As the *Prickynge* notes, 'bi-holde ay his mekenesse & þat shal nedely breke doun þi pride & make þe sum-wat meke.[49] In his *Scale of Perfection*, Hilton provides some clarification. Meekness is one of his abiding concerns, and he divides it into two levels. The first meekness is that 'whiche a soule feelith in sight of his owen synne or frieltees or wrecchidnesse of this liyf, or of the worthinesse of his evene Cristene'; it is understood as 'soothfast and medicynable' but nevertheless 'boistous and fleschli'.[50] The central feature of this meekness is that it consists of a relational mode of self-awareness: the self perceives its defaults and weaknesses in relation to Christ's pain and those of mankind, and that knowledge forms the basis for a radical reassessment of the nature of the self. The second stage is 'loveli mekenesse' or perfect meekness: it is the complete and utter emptying of the self, a kenotic outpouring of love and humility that makes the soul worthy of God.[51] It is the meekness of 'longynge' – the final medicine of the soul, that is explored in the next chapter of this book. The meekness of compassion differs:

> And so bi grace of Jhesu Crist thorugh devoute biholdynge on His manhede and His mekenesse schalt thu mykil abate the stirynge of pride, and the vertu of mekenesse that was first in the nakid wille schal be turnyd into feelynge of affeccion.[52]

Virtue must be cultivated; it does not spring out of the soul suddenly. By considering Christ's torture and death, compassion will be evoked, torturing the soul with the consequences of sin. Such compassion creates an initial meekness that exits within the will rather than the affection. It is a form of self-knowledge – a penitential awareness taken to a new level and situated within a new context. This is the essence of meekness and comes from the tribulation of compassion. As the *Twelve Profits of Tribulation* asserts, 'the fyfte profet of tribulacion is þat it reuokith or bringeth þe to þe knowynge of þi-selfe', and it is this tribulation, this torture of the soul, that 'meketh þe hert & makith hym to be-hold his freelte & to know God'.[53] It is this meekness which will treat the soul in the most intense of ways. Just as the *stimulus carnis* tortured St Paul, and through that pain treated his 'tumor of pride' with a medicinal cup of meekness, so too will the compassionate response to Christ's torture treat the soul. It operates, therefore, like a compound medicine: compassion goes beyond simple fear or penance, combining and exceeding their therapeutic reach to torture the soul with tribulation, evoking a relational subjectivity and a medicinal patience, pity and meekness to push the soul further towards the goal of sowle-hele. Accounts of the Passion, those vivid and arresting engagements with Christ's pain, offer exactly this course of treatment. As Augustine notes in his *Enarratio in Psalmos*, the

Christus Medicus can treat the soul through the *verbi medicina*, or medicine of the word (Ps 93:7); a textual medicine he refers to as the *fomenta verborum*, or poultice of words:

> Conscientia tua saniem collegerat, apostema tumuerat, cruciabat te, requiescere non sinebat: adhibet medicus fomenta verborum, et aliquando secat; adhibet medicinale ferrum in correptione tribulationis: tu agnosce medici manum; confitere, exeat in confessione et defluat omnis sanies.[54]

> (Your conscience had gathered up evil humours, with boils it had swollen, it was torturing you, it suffered you not to rest: the Physician applies the fomentations of words, and sometimes He lances it, He applies the surgeon's knife by the chastisement of tribulation: do thou acknowledge the Physician's hand, confess thou, let every evil humour go forth and flow away in confession.)

The first course of treatment offered here is explicitly textual. Words, arranged and combined like medicines, treat the soul in the most direct and shocking of ways. They work as a poultice, but are also connected with the surgical treatment of the soul, with the torture of tribulation. Christ, who is Himself the Divine Word, is thus a medicine too and operates within similar therapeutic parameters. As the short *Tretise of Ghostly Battle* notes, 'for as the swerde peryssheth, kutteth and maketh separacion, so goddys worde be prechyng, redyng or heryng cutteth and maketh separacion be-twene the soule and synne'.[55] Texts of the Passion, those accounts of Christ's violent death and suffering, partake of this medical power. Such texts seek to torture the soul, to use vivid and arresting images of death and agony to evoke compassionate states of disturbing intensity.

Compassionate Intensity

The *Prickynge*, a popular fourteenth-century prose Passion meditation – most likely translated by Walter Hilton from the widely influential *Stimulus Amoris* of James of Milan – aims to evoke a powerful compassion within the soul. It is a text not of compression but expansion, taking the historical moment of the Passion and transforming it into an immersive, complex and intense narrative sequence. It differs from the *Stimulus Amoris*, offering the Middle English audience a leaner and more compact text.[56] As Jennifer Bryan notes, the translator is 'direct, concrete, sensible, and moderate' in that 'he carefully shapes, prunes, and reorients his material'. Christ is rendered less as the provider of Divine punishment and more as the 'good shepherd, and kind healer'.[57] It is also a text of sowle-hele, and is the Vernon manuscript's longest and most emotionally intense Passion meditation. What it lacks in subtlety it makes up for in detail and force. It is a text deeply concerned with evoking an emotional response, and sustaining it over its course. It seeks to treat the soul and its affections not gently, but with all the brutal force of the *Christus Medicus*. The emotions are one of its key preoccupations, specifically as they relate to the complexity of compassionate response:

> If þou wolt haue compassioun of crist crucified, first shape þe ȝif þou may to be onyd to hym þorouȝ feruent disire, for-whi þe more feruently þat þou louest hym, þe more pite þou shalt haue on his passioun. And þe more compassioun þat þow felest þe more shal þi loue be, for loue & compassioun shullen so wexen ti-gidere in thi thouȝt þat þou shalt come to the tastynge of þis. (p. 14, ll. 5–11)

There is more to compassion than simple sorrow for another. It is, instead, the aggregate of a range of constituent emotions that all exist coterminously. Desire, pity and love are all confected within compassion, and are integral to its proper emergence within the soul. In this way, compassion is not pure but rather a complex blend of other emotions. It is a precise mixture, and as such is much like a compound medicine. Compassion's existence within the soul is given a dynamic and organic quality: as the text asserts, 'loue & compassioun shullen so wexen ti-gidere in thi thouȝt'. The emotional states within compassion emerge and grow together, augmenting and reinforcing each other through their sophisticated interrelationship. Emotional reciprocity and magnification are key to its emergence. This relationship is specifically delineated, the 'more feruently þat þou louest hym, þe more pite þou shalt haue', and the 'þe more compassioun þat þow felest, þe more shal þi loue be': each emotion engages with and stimulates another, which in turn magnifies the overall compassionate response. Emotions become layered, held within a specific configuration that permits compassion to flourish. This extends to the prior medicines of the soul. Vital to the full emergence of compassion is 'clennesse of conscience', which requires that 'man thenke hym-self wicked and vnclene & vnworthi to þis werk' (p. 14, ll. 16–18). Contrition and penitential self-awareness must be a part of compassion. When considering the pain endured by Christ, readers should be 'ferde for to lifte vp oure yȝen to hym-ward & smyte we on oure brestes & sey with þe pubplican, Lord god haue reuthe on me synner' (p. 53, ll. 20–3).

An integral part of the proper psychological response to Christ's Passion is sorrow for individual sin, as well as sorrow for His agony. So too the medicine of dread:

> Ouermore þow mai fille þyn affeccioun of drede with mynde of his passioun. Sith hit is so þat crist god & man, in whom myȝt no synne be, was so peyned for oure trespaces, how moche more we shul drede to by punysshed for oure synnes þat mown no lyue with-outen synnes. For ȝif þe grene tree were so brent & baken vp-on þe harde crosse wat shal þenne worthe of vs dryȝe stockys, þis drede is god, so þat hit be medelid with hope, þat hit kest vs not in despeir. (p. 37, ll. 4–13

Compassion for Christ generates as much fear as it does sorrow. His agonies and suffering constitute the basis for a comparative form of introspection, an awareness of the sinful nature of the self that is partly penitential. God and man are compared and contrasted in the most extreme of terms. Negative constructions clarify that gulf: there is no sin within God, just as mankind cannot live without sin. The language of trespass and punishment dominates the majority of the passage, as the full ramifications of Christ's unjust death are plainly expressed. There is no mention of mercy here, no forgiveness, just the horror of His torment and the agonising realisation of our own just punishment. This is given potent expression by the imagery used in the passage: a green tree, burnt and baked upon a Cross. The sinless Christ, green and vital, is roasted alive upon an instrument of torture; the reader, in contrast, is a dry stick that escapes its just punishment. Yet the nature of that just punishment is never clarified; the image is predicated upon a comparison but does not describe what ought to be done to the sinful. The line 'wat shal þenne worthe of vs dryȝe stockys' places all interpretative and imaginative work onto the reader. Much of its force, therefore, comes from implication rather than direct statement. Both dread and penance combine here in this image of comparison: the sinless and the sinful, the punished and the unpunished. They are carefully layered, each passion augmenting and extending the other. However, the text goes further, as beyond punishment lies hope – itself an emotion which resides in the irascible power. The dread inherent in compassion, and the penitential awareness it is predicated upon, are to be combined with hope: they must become 'medelid' together, which stresses their interconnectedness and combination. To consider the Passion properly, the reader must 'fille þyn affeccioun of hope in criste3 passioun' – fear of punishment and penitential reproach must be felt simultaneously with a craving for mercy (p. 36, ll. 13–14). Compassion's composite nature is constantly reinforced:

> We shul hope & triste to be saaf þorou goddis mercy, but we shul ay haue grete drede medlid with-al & þat is þat we falle not in-to presumpcioun ne in-to fals sikernesse, and we shul commende þe gret pite of oure lord & putte oure triste in his precious blood . . . and so in tristful drede lede oure life. (p. 90, ll. 6–13)

There is no single emotion here, but instead a precise blend of others. Dread, key for combating pride and presumption, now exists alongside pity for Christ's suffering: all is 'medelid' once again. The very nature of that fear is itself more complex. It is a 'tristful drede' – a state that is more than pure terror at Christ's horrific death. This emotion is of a specific order, existing as a state that eliminates pride but nevertheless evokes a core belief in the mercy of God. An element of penitential awareness exists here within the blend, a delicate sense of the magnitude of sin and the need of not presuming God's forgiveness. Here, pity mixes and merges with that specific form of dread, augmenting and magnifying its overall impact upon the soul. Within the emotive ambit of compassion for Christ, therefore, lies a world of passionate feeling and self-knowledge. Cognitively, such compassion performs considerable work, evoking a complex of emotion and relational subjectivity:

> Wenne a man þenketh deuow3tli þat ihesu crist goddis soone wolde for his sake suffere souche peyne, þenne at þe firste bi-gynneth he for to vndirstonde of wat worthynesse, and of wat dignyte and nobeleye is þe kynde of his soule, for whos resstorringe goddis sone wolde be dede þat wolde not for sauynge of alle þe worlde haue spillid oon drope of his blode, but for man he helde hit ow3te as watir al his blode for to make hym wy3te & of þis sy3t aman is reysid vp þenne for to shame of his own filþe. (p. 39, ll. 15–24)

Through pity for another we come to an awareness of ourselves. Christ's torture and suffering become the basis of a profound and deepening self-awareness. The passage is dominated by a central image: drops of Christ's blood poured out like water. The simile is of course sacramental, and alludes to the cleansing and salvific work of the waters of baptism. But beyond that sacramental register it is an image of effusion, predicated upon and coloured by horrific pain. Pity is a part of it, though that pity is used to generate a new perspective – the self viewing itself afresh, as something at once corrupted and ennobled. More precisely, the compassion evoked through Passion mediation initiates a series of states within the soul: pity shades into awe, awe into self-knowledge, self-knowledge into a hatred of sin and a sense of shame. The overall psychological impact of compassion is thus quite complex. It moves beyond a penitential sense of self-accusation, encouraging an awareness of the implications of sin that encompasses shame, as well as underscoring the inherent nobility of the soul. The self, through compassion, is at once magnified and diminished: it deepens self-awareness, fostering a relational subjectivity that brings the self into new comparative perspectives and horizons.

As the text goes on to note, through compassion for Christ the soul is 'quyckened and hertid for to lyue aungel-like', and is 'strengþid and hertid to suffree alle tribulaciouns' (p. 40, ll. 4–7). What compassion does to the soul is far more than simply evoke a sense of sorrow: it alters the soul, making it patiently endure suffering and strive to emulate the angels. The contours and horizons of the self change and expand. Through compassion, the self seeks 'to be ouerhelte with þe streme of þat blode and fulli to be þourȝe-shapen in-to crist crucified – to be saturated in blood to the point that distinctions between it and Christ no longer exist (p. 40, ll. 10–12). To be so 'þourȝe-shapen', to be so transformed into Christ, highlights not simply the potency of compassion, but also the medical effect of its constituent emotional and cognitive states. The very blood that covers and envelops the self is also the source of its treatment: the 'passioun of ihesu crist and his swete blood is my counfort & my strenþ & my hele' (p. 59, ll. 16–17). Compassion for Christ – engagement with that blood – is ultimately a form of treatment for the soul. The text is unambiguous on this point, asserting that reading and considering Christ's horrific Passion is 'þe souerayne refute & þe most soth-fast remedie aȝeynes alle synne', and works to counter pride and promote patience (p. 60, ll. 2–6). At its core, the Passion is a medical intervention:

> Criste on þe crosse visited seeke men for he bare vp-on him-self þe payne of alle oure sykenesse. We were so seke þat we myȝte not come to hym, and þer-fore he as a leche ful of pite coom to vs & heled vs with his passioun. Therefor shul we bisili visite hym aȝeyn in his lymes and haue compassioun of here sekenes se, as hit were his owne, and seie with þe apostole þus, who is seek and I am not seek. (p. 66, l. 20 to p. 67, l. 3)[58]

The cause of the Passion is reconfigured here as a universal malaise. Christ, the ultimate doctor, comes to cure the sickness of mankind. Sin and sickness become one and the same, the reason for His suffering and for mankind's own. The pain of that illness dissolves differences between mankind and Christ: there is a commonality in pain, as through that emotion we hold something in common with Christ. Yet the whole passage operates through a careful inversion. Initially it is Christ that visits sick mankind in pity, to share their pain. The roles soon switch, as mankind then visits Christ on the Cross. The point is clear: only through pain and pity can we come closer to Christ. The whole passage is a distillation of the various medical and theological aspects of compassion. The key line here is the mention of visiting Christ 'in his lymes and haue compassioun of here sekenes'. This recalls that medical definition of compassion mentioned earlier, the co-suffering of the various parts of the body due to their complex interconnection. Yet 'lymes' has a range of meanings both physical and theological, referencing both the actual body and the corporate body of the Church. In this way the passage figures a model of incorporation: through compassion for Christ we can 'visit' His limbs, become part of His body both in the historical particularity of His person and the timeless universality of His body the Church. There is, within this moment, a carefully delineated sense of intersubjectivity: through compassion we are brought to and into another, and by extension to all others.

The passage does not stop here though, and goes on to reference St Paul (2 Cor. 11:29). The mention of Paul in connection with compassion and its medical effect is a direct link to the whole theology of the *Christus Medicus*. As the text notes, 'oder medicine wole I noon but þi passioun. Oþer salue wole I noon take to my synne but þyn own blood, for seynt poule seyth withouten blood no-þynge mai be made clene' (p. 70, ll. 10–13). That blood 'shal clense oure consciences'; it is the most sovereign cure, but it is far from gentle in its operation (p. 70, ll. 16–17).[59] These references to Paul make a subtle point – Christ will heal us like He healed Paul, through the torture of compassion:

> I shal pare awey with a shelle of sharpe sorowe þe stynke of my conscience. I schal nouȝt spare my soule fro siche turmentynge tyle I may fynde my ihesu in his passioun. (p. 17, ll. 11–14)

Though brief, this passage is based upon a complex and imaginative interplay between the metaphysical and the physical. Sorrow – an intangible emotion – solidifies, becomes hard and sharp so as to cut and excise sin. It is a powerful tool of treatment, and works to surgically alter the soul in the most direct of ways. It is not an easy process, but a 'turmentynge' of the soul. Sorrow of this order and magnitude is a form of torture, and the whole passage has a relentless and merciless quality to it. This sense is reinforced by the carefully delineated imagery. The soul is gradually pared back, cut away to reveal Christ's own agony – horror within horror. To add force to the image, this process of removal is carried out by a 'shelle': not a surgical implement, but instead something fashioned from the remains of a crustacean.[60] This gives the image an unsettling brutality, the implement used lacking any pretence of professional medicine. It is used to 'pare away' the soul, a verb that means to trim or cut through scraping, and also to prepare and make ready.[61] Sorrow for Christ is, therefore, a preparation of the soul through scraping away its dead layers. The impact of this horrific image is augmented by the use of alliteration and sibilance. The 'shelle of sharpe sorowe' has a forward momentum to it, an immediacy that performs in sound what it describes in image: the sibilance makes a harsher sound much like scraping itself. The ear is made to hear what the eye could never see – the deliberate, constant scraping of the conscience. The effect enhances the image and forges connections between similar syllables. The repeated sounds in 'shal/stynke/conscience/schal/spare/soule/siche/passioun' draw force from the pattern of 'shelle of sharpe sorowe', allowing each word to echo that constant background scraping. It is a force of sound as much as sense, and it is used to convey how compassion is a 'turmentynge' of the soul.

It also allows other aspects to be shaded into the narrative. The phonetic connections between 'conscience/passioun' delicately allude to the importance of a confessional introspection in this moment. Throughout the text, the passion is often a prelude to self-examination. As it notes in a later section, Christ's blood is a remedy so powerful that 'ȝif þou be crokid ley þi soule by hit & þenne shalt þou see þyn owne crokednesse' (p. 60, ll. 23–5). More than simply sorrow, compassion can evoke a profound confessional self-awareness. The image is striking: the soul laid down beside streams of Christ's blood for the purpose of properly knowing itself. Through blood and pain come understanding. Compassion, therefore, has an aggregate quality to it; its effects are manifold and multiple. The text stresses this sense of its medically complex operation:

> A a selcouthe surryp is þis & a precious drynke, a confeccion vnprisable & a medelynge most deyntyuous for to fele a trewe inly sorwe of cristes compassioun, temperid with goostly ioie of cristes goodnesse. Þis drynke with hertili gredynesse drunken maketh a man drunken & alienyd fro hym-self like into heuenli sobernesse. Thorou considerynge of compassioun a soule is pured as gold ... compassioun clensith hit from synne. (p. 38, l. 23 to p. 39, l. 7)[62]

The effects and nature of compassion are described in precise medical terms. It is a medicinal drink that works to cleanse and purify the soul. More precisely, it is a medical compound. The 'surryp' is a mainstay of medieval medicine, usually made from a range of ingredients mixed with honey and bitter herbs. Such compounds combine ingredients designed to interact together for greater therapeutic effects; 'surryp' being a broad classification that can include other types of drinks such as electuaries.[63] The choice of metaphor is thus deliberate and telling: compassion is a blend of contrasting ingredients that work together to exert greater medical effects. The second metaphor makes this clear. Not only does compassion cleanse the soul, but it does so in the same way gold is purified. Images of metallurgy are used here to convey a sense of potency and intensity – compassion will cleanse like a burning furnace. Its composite nature is a delicate 'medelynge' of contrasting emotional states. The word has a precise semantic range and refers to a mixture of various ingredients. The composition of compassion is similarly contrasting, containing 'sorwe of cristes' and 'goostly ioie of cristes'. It is, therefore, a compound medicine, an emotional complex that incorporates multiple passions at once – comprised of 'ouer-done bitternesse' and 'ioye & vn-speckable swettenesse' (p. 38, ll. 17–19).

Its effects are strong, and the passage plays with this idea of contrast through its use of language and modulation of tone. It begins with an interjection, an expression that evokes raw feeling rather than calm exposition: this is no mere list extolling the effects of the 'surryp' of compassion, but rather a desperate cry for its medical potency. Over its course, this sense of urgency is maintained and developed, as the 'surryp' is drunk not with a cool medical detachment but with a voracious and animal-like thirst. It must be with 'hertili gredynesse drunken' – there is a sense of desperation here. Imagery of intoxication and inversion supplement this effect. The 'surryp' will make whoever drinks it drunk to the extent of being 'alienyd fro hym-self'. It is a potent mixture, able to forcibly remove the self's preoccupation with itself. In this way it generates a 'heuenli sobernesse': a 'self-less' state that is the spiritual inversion of drunkenness itself. However, while the medicine of compassion is potent, to access it can prove difficult. Compassion must be cultivated within the soul, and the text is clear that this is far from simple:

> A my herte harder þen a ston þat wole not breke with þe mynde of þis passioun, god wolde þat my herte were of ston and not of flessh. For-whi, stones al to-barsten in tyme of cristes passioun, but my herte wole not cleue neythir breke. (p. 82, l. 23 to p. 83, l. 2)

Despite the enormity of Christ's sacrifice the narrator figure is unmoved. A lack of feeling, an inanimate indifference is all that exists. The imagery used here is suggestive of the moribund nature of this state: the fleshly heart is so dense and numb that it is beyond stone in its lack of inner feeling. Instead of breaking in two, the heart remains intact. This is a damning state of being, as the whole purpose of compassion is to cut the heart, to excise sin from it, to torment it with suffering. Without that, it cannot be healed – 'I mai wel fele þat I am seek or ellis dede, þat I haue lost sauour and taste' (p. 84, ll. 5–6). Emotional insufficiency is essentially a sickness unto death. Within this short passage there is a profound awareness of a central fact – that compassion is not automatic, that its emergence within the soul must be aided and developed. The text itself aims to do precisely that, and over its course it deploys a range of devices to evoke compassion within its readers. This is, however, a gradual process. Those who seek compassion must 'suffereþ paciently dissese til þe medicyne haue wrouȝte in hym, and restored hym hele aȝeyn' (p. 122, ll. 24–5). Befitting its complexity and potency, the emotional impact of compassion builds slowly. Through the manipulation of vivid imagery, the intersubjective focus on Mary's pain, and through carefully modulated narrative moments, the text will attempt to cut even the hardest of hearts. Its length thus affords great possibilities, a vast canvas on which to display its emotive images. Yet those images are only gradually delayered; compassion does not occur all at once. Christ in his agony dominates the narrative time and again, but each aspect of his pain is carefully detailed and enumerated. The narrative develops those images of suffering, arranging and layering them in a way that maximises their impacts. This begins early on in the text, when a section that extolls the benefits of Passion meditation warps and twists into something utterly different:

> He wolde hange with crist on þe cros. And ihesu halseth him þenne ful sweteli, he wolde bowe doun his face turned into dedli palenesse and crist reysith vp his hed, with kissynge þat is swete. A þow loueli deth, a þow deth delitable, a whi ne hadde I ben þere in stede of þe cross þat crist myȝth haue ben nayled to myne hondes & to my feet. Sotheli, I shulde haue seide to Ioseph ab aramathia take him not fro me, but graue me with him for I wole neuere be departid from him. (p. 8, ll. 7–16)

The moment of Christ's death is the instant when the narrative comes truly alive. In a careful and deliberate play of time and tense, the narrative shifts from the present mention of meditation to the past time of the Passion itself. The reader, caught up in this narrative shift, moves from a consideration of Passion meditation as an activity to actually imagining taking part in a new version of the historical event. But it is the images in the passage that are truly remarkable, and the careful shifts among them. It begins with the desire to hang on the Cross with Christ. It is an image of some force, but one that is immediately blended with another to create a shocking change of tone. Hanging with Christ on the Cross is not enough, as the narrator figure turns to embrace and kiss His dead body. Violent death and decay are blended with tenderness and intimacy – the 'kissynge þat is swete' merged with the 'dedli palenesse'. Though antithetical, these images work together to create a depth to the current narrative moment, to articulate with delicacy a painful longing amidst a scene of utter horror. The repeated interjections – 'A þow loueli deth, a þow deth delitable, a whi' – are cries of compassionate intensity that express and evoke that complex depth of feeling. Alongside the clausal repetition here, they combine contrasting concepts – love with death, death with taste – elevating the force of the whole passage to new heights.

They are, however, all prologue. The next set of images move into more vividly extreme areas. The opening desire to hang upon the Cross with Christ is now transcended, blasted away by those interjections and replaced with a desire to become the Cross so 'þat crist myȝth haue ben nayled to myne hondes & to my feet'. It is a shocking moment of torturous intimacy. Much of its force is derived from the manner in which it conveys incorporation:

Christ brutally enters the soul through the torture of compassion; man and God become one in agony. As a metaphor for sin it is fascinatingly rich. The narrator figure here is made into a Cross for Christ, he becomes essentially an implement of torture for the Son of God: mankind is both the reason and the means of Christ's torment. Carefully, subtly, this metaphor conveys an almost penitential tone – the reader's sin is at the core of Christ's pain. However, the narrative does not stop at the crucifixion. Matters soon become more disturbing, moving to the burial of Christ. The narrator's request to 'graue me with him' in the tomb is a terrifying image of incorporation and enclosure: as the narrator seeks to be buried alive with the dead body of Christ, so too the reader is brought into the tomb. It is, in terms of narrative progression, a visual simulation of what compassion is – we follow the Cross and then Christ, we too are tortured with Him unto death. The overall tone resists simple classification, simultaneously horrendous yet pious. It is, therefore, the essence of compassion, the aggregate product of the emotions of fear, penance and pity.

After this visually intense moment the narrative continues with the idea of enclosure, presenting Christ's wounds of heart, hands and feet, as three tabernacles for the reader to hide in (p. 8, ll. 18–20). At its core this more fleshly sense of enclosure is an abstraction that serves as a form of narrative pause. It affords a rest from the relentless emotive intensity of the passage, and gives the reader some relief. It does not last for long:

> And nat only wole I þus be crucified with ihesu but I wole turne aʒeyn aftir þis bitternesse of his passioun to þe swetenesse of his incarnacioun. And bi-holde owre swete childe ihesu in his modres armes sowkande of hire blessid brest. & I shal fonde to sowke with him with al þe feith þat I haue & þus shal I tempore to-gidere þe swete mylke of marie þe virgine with þe blood of ihesu and make to myself a drynke þat is ful of hele. A ʒee woundes of ihesu crist þat are so ful of loue & þat mai I wel seie. For on a time as I entrid in him with myn eʒen opened, me thouʒte þat myn yʒen were filled ful of his blod & so I ʒeode in gropande til I come to þe inneerest of his herte. (p. 9, ll. 6–18)

At once tender and horrific, the images here combine in a breathtaking display of visceral force. Sense impressions jar, as language bends and twists to accommodate contrasting images with a force at once repelling and compelling. Milk merges with blood to form a medicinal drink, while the wounds of Christ become sites of entrance and immersion, enveloping the very eyes with blood: taste joins with touch, and pain with cure, in combinations that are extreme and unusual. Through structured temporal shifts in the narrative, the whole tone of the passage becomes ever more abstract and unsettling. It begins with the use of analepsis, the narrative moving its temporal focus from the 'bitternesse of his passioun to þe swetenesse of his incarnacioun'. Time past becomes part of time present. Initially, this moment of 'swetenesse' between mother and child provides a brief respite from the torture of the Passion. Yet in fact the scene works only to augment the horror. It is an emotional backdrop that re-sensitises the reader, providing a break from the torture of Christ that makes any return to it all the more forceful. All too suddenly, we move from mother's milk to child's pain, specifically His blood. The narrative focus on the 'swete childe ihesu', and the narrator figure's desire to partake of that tender moment between mother and son is immediately shot through with mention of the Passion. The effect is to generate a narrative moment of unsettling potency: powerful pity is demanded from the reader, as Christ's torture becomes the torture of an innocent child. Emotions become layered. Pity for Christ emerges from a moment of 'swete' joy at His incarnation, a moment also full of fear and horror. The central image, milk and blood merged into something that the reader must then consume, is a sublime confection of the medicinal and the horrific: the narrator figure will 'tempore to-gidere' the milk and blood, creating a medical compound – a 'drynke þat is ful of hele'. The reader must then 'drink in' the scene, with all its complex associations. The point is clear: compassion for Christ is therapeutic, a treatment that is composite and extreme.

From here, narrative time lurches forward, refocusing on Christ's violent death. This is a loose form of prolepsis, another play with time and perspective designed to maintain constant emotional engagement. The use of the interjection in 'A ȝee woundes of ihesu crist þat are do ful of loue', is tactical. It not only adds emotive force to an already charged passage, but also forges connections between the love of mother and son and the blood contained in those wounds. It attenuates the temporal progress of the narrative moment: the reader is held within an artificial present that links all those elements of tenderness and pain together in an expressive cry of desire and agony. The resonances of Christ as an innocent and vulnerable child are now brought into the realm of His Passion. Here the images are no less surreal and compelling, changing from those of mixture to those of saturation. What began as a bloody addition to breast milk now becomes the exclusive substance in the narrative. Blood is the focus, but it is focused upon in a manner that is engrossing: entry into Christ's wounds becomes a moment of reciprocal entry, as vast amounts of blood fill not simply the narrative gaze, but also the very eyes of the narrator figure. It is an image of saturation, of complete covering and admixture, that erases distinctions between narrator and Christ: now groping inside Christ's body, now covered in blood, there is little to differentiate man and God. It is a figure of connection and incorporation, and as such recalls that medical sense of compassion as intimate physical interrelationship.

The text continues to engage with such ideas. After entering the wounds, the narrator figure seeks to eat and drink from Christ's very heart (p. 9, ll. 18–20). Beyond its Eucharistic associations, such an image conveys a sense of passionate intimacy – through the torture of compassion man and God become one. Yet the text goes further still, and adds to the overall complexity of the image. After eating the bloody heart, the narrator figure notes that 'him þat I eer fonde in his modres wombe I fele now how he voucheth-saf to bere my soule as his child, with-inne his blessid sides' (p. 9, ll. 23–5). The narrative moves from wounds to womb, and in so doing the maternal imagery mentioned earlier becomes overlaid on the image of Christ's death. Such a recursive chronology charts a course from death to compassion, to tomb and then to womb, and it makes it difficult for the reader to become inured to the emotional tone of the passage. That tonal shift is precisely modulated: birth and death, tenderness and torture, infancy and agony – all held together in a pattern that magnifies the emotive impacts of each. Proximity and intimacy with Christ take on new dimensions here, with the narrator figure at once in the womb with Christ and in Christ's womb. Overall, the image is a figure of complete incorporation, at once maternal and compassionate – the reader is, at this stage, part of Christ just as Christ is part of the reader.

Such figures of incorporation continue, but soon switch to more graphically intense ones predicated upon pain and torture:

> A blessid be þat spere & blessid be þo nailes þat maden þis openyng. A þat I ne hadde be there in stede of þat spere. Sotheli I wolde neuere haue goon ouȝt fro cristes side but I schuld haue seyd þis is my reste & here shal I wone. A ȝe dulle and slowe in herte, þat þorouȝ vicious vsyng of ȝowre bodily wittes goon into likynges of al worldili vanitie & wolen not entre by þe open ȝates of þeise woundes. (p. 12, ll. 5–12)

The overall tone of the passage is densely layered and complex, at once brutal, desirous, tender and penitential. The implements of Christ's horrific torture become refigured as highly desired objects, the spear and nails now sanctified due to their brutal intimacy with Christ. They have proximity to the divine, their essential functions as implements of torture and harm now combined with their status as means of contact with God. Once again, the text blends together stark contrasts to create an aggregate image that possesses greater potency. Here injury and intimacy share the same narrative moment as well as the same conceptual space. The use of interjections in the passage reinforces and reflects this complexity of image and tone. The opening 'A blessid be þat spere' is a raw cry of passionate intensity, but one that is itself indistinct. The words which follow convey concepts that are to some extent antithetical, and so constantly modulate it. The adjective 'blessid' exerts control over that opening cry of 'A': it evokes an atmosphere of prayer, of solemnity and devotion. Yet the noun 'spere' follows almost immediately and works in the same way though to different effect: it evokes images of weapons of war, the registers of torture and harm. The emotive force of the interjection is thus composite, at once a cry of devotion and of pain. Near repetition in the next clause continues this process, making the emotive cry all the more compounded. This process continues over the course of the passage. The next interjection, 'A þat I ne hadde be there in stede of þat spere', is one of wistful longing, the expression of a fervent wish to have taken the place of that weapon within Christ. The imagery here is taken from a martial and punitive context, and applied to another contrasting one – the language of love. Subsequent lines further this, and present the wound in Christ's side as a space of repose, of restfulness. The second interjection thus continues the emotive work of the first, but moves it into new directions. Desire becomes more layered and multifaceted, the aggregate of various and often contrasting ideas and images.

The final interjection, 'A ȝe dulle and slowe in herte', signals a further change in tone and makes a subtle theological point. With it a penitential note enters the passage, as that cry is one of reproach and accusation. Its tone is different, opening a narrative moment that has different temporal dynamics to the others, moving the reader into a present moment that has more to do with penitential awareness than with Christ Himself. Here that opening desire for proximity becomes part of a wider penitential point: the place of those weapons within Christ that the narrator envies are, of course, caused by the sin of mankind. In this way the implements of the Passion are to some extent identical with the reader – the source of sin itself. Each interjection is, therefore, part of a careful pattern. They not only divide the passage into its main parts, but also take that opening cry and channel its emotive force into a penitential outpouring. Their function is one of confection: each expresses an emotional point that is merged with others to create something more. Compassion is here the aggregate of desire, reproach, penance and pain; its contours shifting with each of those expressive cries yet containing each element they articulate. Its effect upon the soul is a central concern of the text, and it makes a clear statement of its therapeutic work in a section that contains one of the most extreme images of incorporation and connection with Christ.

> For to haue mynde of cristes passioun þat we my3te þorou hit be rewled in oure affecciounys and strenþed in all vertues. Þer are foure affecciouns of a sowle: ioye and sorwe, hope & drede. Þese foure mai be filled with licour of cristes blood. For-wy the 3ettyng of þis blood is to a soule matere of endeles joye and a kuttynge a-way of all false worldely myrþis. Open now þer-fore þou cristen man with ful feiþ þe mowth of þyn herte & lete þis blood droppe in-to þe marow3e of þi soule. For wite þou wel þat cristes blood is 3itt als hote & as fresh as hit was wenne he died on good friday. (p. 35, ll. 8–19)

Thought of Christ's Passion constitutes an intensive psychological event that engages with all the soul's 'affecciouns'. Yet here the text not only shows how conversant it is with contemporary psychological knowledge, but it also makes the point that the very thought of the Passion can alter the soul in specific ways, bringing order and fortitude to it. It is through these 'affecciouns' then that the soul can be treated, healed. The key word here is 'licour'. It possesses an interesting semantic range, meaning either a fluid, communion wine, or a medicinal drink made from other fluids.[64] Each sense of the word is at play here, but the predominant meaning is medical. The 'licour' of Christ's blood is, therefore, a medical compound that treats the passions of the soul. The overall point that the text is making here is that compassion for Christ operates on the soul just like a compound medicine, its therapeutic work similarly composite and intense. Compassion for Christ will allow direct engagement with the *Christus Medicus*, enabling the passions to be 'rewled' and 'strenþed', and also constituting 'a kuttynge a-way' from the soul itself – a treatment both extreme and powerful. It begins immediately, as the passage offers a series of images of sublime force. Rather than simply note that this medical 'licour' is drunk, the narrative follows the fluid as it enters the body. The various stages of this process are rendered in vivid detail, as the reader sees first the mouth of the heart opening, followed by this medicinal blood flowing down into the very marrow of the soul. Such a procession of images is intensely physical and progressive, as the narrative perspective moves ever inwards to the utter core of the person. It begins with the first image, 'þe mowth of þyn herte', which combines sense impressions and physical body parts in arresting ways. It is itself highly concrete and defined, yet strangely abstract – the heart has its own mandibles. Ideas of sense and sensation combine within the image: taste with the physical act of consumption, ideas of the feelings of the heart with the physical organ itself.

The next image is much worse: that of blood dropping 'in-to þe marow3e of þi soule'. It is extremely graphic and, to my knowledge, without precedent in Middle English. Once again it is an image concrete and specific, yet also abstract: the immortal soul has a marrow, a fatty pulp that constitutes its innermost part. Such a physicality is visceral and unsettling, forcing the reader to conceive of the soul not as a nebulous presence, but as something tangible and, crucially, treatable. By presenting the soul in this way, the medical treatment offered by the *Christus Medicus* takes on an intensely real and disturbing dimension: Christ will cure not metaphorically but directly, cutting through to the innermost part of the soul and saturating it with His blood. Here, as elsewhere, distinctions between mankind and God degrade. The narrator's desire for physical proximity to Christ is vividly realised, as

He envelops and suffuses the soul completely. What Christ treats with His blood – the marrow of the soul – are those very emotions mentioned in the prior lines. Christ's Passion looms large; the whole scene is a carefully crafted presentation of compassion itself. The mention of 'good friday' refers to the source of that medicinal blood, and specifies a temporal frame. The past of Calvary becomes the present moment of treatment, the events of the Passion now directly affecting the reader as they did Christ Himself. Through this subtle mention, the reader is brought into the temporal moment of the Passion, aligned with it and all its horror in the most intimate of ways: the reader takes his or her position at the very foot of the Cross to drink in the scene with the 'þe mowth of þyn herte'.

Similar moments that encourage an identification and participation in the historical moment of the Passion occur over the course of the text. The most emotionally potent deal with Mary, with her pain and agony during the torture of Christ. After noting that all 'þe woundes þat ihesu sufferid in his bodi, þow sufferid in þi soule', the text asserts that she is the model of compassion response – that she was 'crucifid with hym in herthly compassioun' (p. 23, ll. 11–12; p. 23, l. 19). So great was her suffering that her very heart was 'turned in-to a lumpe of sorwe' (p. 23, l. 20). This is a fascinatingly rich image that has a clarity and force of expression. The semantic range of 'lumpe' covers the ideas of 'indistinct mass', to 'piece of clay', to 'bodily excrescence', to a fleshly growth or 'swelling'.[65] Its use here makes the metaphysical physical: pain becomes flesh, sorrow takes on physical dimensions. Its syllabic brevity gives it, in this instance, a brutally succinct force. The long vowel sound ending with a plosive allows the word to perform in sound what it describes in sense: to say this phrase requires the mouth and vocal cords to constrict and contort, to make the flesh of the throat undulate around the sorrow it expresses. In this way it functions like the earlier mention of the 'shelle of sharpe sorowe', endowing the emotional with physical dimension but doing so through sound in a manner that is evocative (p. 17, ll. 11–14). However, the text does not linger on this image, as it soon moves to present Mary as a 'vessel of peynefulnesse' (p. 23, ll. 24–5). Ever physical, Mary now moves from the bearer of Christ to the bearer of pain. The contours of her being are defined and delimited through the emotional states she endures. The precision and emotional depth of her presentation here are deliberate ways of evoking specific aspects of compassion from the reader. But the text goes further still, and offers a more vivid realisation of her pain by presenting her in the moment of the Passion:

> Þe vilehede of þat palce, þe vgly syȝt of mennis synnes, þe hydousnesse of noyse, þe wodnesse of þe Iewhes, þe feendis rabell of cristeȝ turmentouris. But to alle þese þou hadde no consideracioun for-whi þyn herte was alienid fro þe for sorwe, þou was not in þi-seelf but in affeccioun of þi sone ihesu & in the woundes of þi dere childe. (p. 24, ll. 3–9)

In an effusion of detail, the narrative presents the sights, sounds and textures of the scene of Christ's agony. So rapid is the delineation of these various sense impressions that the overall mental picture is inchoate and jarring. The effect upon the reader is dizzying, as these images rush and clash together. Yet, it lasts only for a moment. The next sentence moves away from this sensory outpouring to a narrative moment of utter fixity. All the details are cut away to leave only Mary in the narrative gaze. We assume her perspective, which is one not of sensory bombardment but one of horrific repose: she has 'no consideracioun' – sees nothing, hears nothing – as her whole heart is 'alienid fro þe for sorwe'.

This word 'alienid' has an interesting semantic range covering legal, theological and even psychological senses. Mary is, at once, surrendered to this scene, estranged from it and deranged by it. However, while she is here at a psychological remove from the physical and sensory bombardment of the scene, she is nevertheless the closest to its core and real centre. The point the text is subtly making is that Mary is utterly present to the Passion not because of her physical proximity to it, but rather due to her emotional response to it: she was 'in affeccioun of þi sone ihesu', and so in the very 'woundes of þi dere childe'. In this way she is a figure for the reader to emulate. The passage stresses this through its careful manipulation of perspective and image. That opening profusion of images of sound and sense is immediately cut away to focus only on Mary, thereby bringing her inner state of sorrow into sharper and exclusive relief. The emotive reach of the passage becomes all the greater, as it forces the reader not only to engage with those sensory details, but also to realise that her sorrow is such that it overwhelms the horror. It is through Mary that the Passion becomes all the more accessible. The visual details of Calvary and the Passion are, in a sense, incidental. What matters most here is the figuring of emotional pain based upon the relationship between mother and child. That specification of 'þi dere childe' enables universal, familial bonds to augment the emotive impact of the scene: the Passion becomes literally familiar and so more horrific through this relationship.

Beyond its emotive impact, the use of this familial relationship has wider and more nuanced implications. Specifically, it allows the intersubjective aspects to compassion to come to the fore. Such aspects are subtly evoked. It begins with the line 'þe vgly sy3t of mennis synnes'. Here the presence and role of sin within the Passion are given deliberate attention. This serves to not only remind the reader of the essential purpose of Christ's Passion – to remedy Original Sin – but also to allow a penitential aspect to enter the passage. Sin is the cause of this horror and suffering, both universally in the sin of mankind and particularly in the sins of the reader. The narrative aligns the reader with 'criste3 turmentouris'. This initial presentation of the consequences of sin is soon enhanced by the focus on Mary's pain and suffering at the torture of her child. It enhances our sense of culpability in the Passion, as it focuses on the pain of others: mother and son suffer because of our misdeeds. Compassion becomes more layered and complex, aware not only of the pain of Christ but also His mother. The process does not end here, however, as the narrative beings to rapidly increase its rhetorical and emotive force:

> Turne a3eyn good ladi to þi firste place last þat we lose þe also with oure goode shepherde & so in o tyme we for-bere þe rewlynge of 3ow bothe. Hit is not custummable ladi þat we punishe wymmen wit siche maner deþ, but I hope þou may not here me for þi herte is so ful of sorwe – A a selcou3t þynge is þis, þou art al turned into þe woundes of crist & al cryist is crucified with-inne þe sides of þi herte. A þou wounded ladi, wounde thow oure hertis & renewe in oure soulis þe passion of þi sone ihesu. Ioyne þi herte in-to ourys þat we mai be woundid with þe. A lady 3if þow wolt not 3eue me þi sone crucified, neþer þi-self woundede, I praie þe 3eue me þe despites & þe repreues of þi sone. (p. 24, ll. 9–22)

So vivid is the narrator's meditation on Mary, that the boundaries between thought and historical reality break down and become porous. Instead of watching this scene, we become part of it, and attempt to stop Mary following Christ to her own death. It is an interesting moment of participation with the biblical scene, with the narrative voice breaking into the passage and addressing the Virgin directly. The mention here of the execution of women – that it is 'not custummable' – forces the emotive parameters of the Passion narrative to expand and envelop other, more shocking, associations. It therefore makes the reader more sensitive to the whole event, and thereby aligns the reader more closely with Mary in her pain. Yet, while this would be the perfect moment for Mary to offer a reply, she remains impassive. Instead of words and explication, we get emotion, a lingering insight into her inner state. As soon as we apprehend that her 'herte is so ful of sorwe', the passage abruptly launches into an impassioned and almost rhapsodic register. The line breaks off, followed immediately with 'A a selcouʒt þynge is þis'. Language and imagery now become more intense. It begins with that interjection 'A', a cry of emotive force that endows the words that follow it with further intensity. That cry is immediately modulated by the adjective 'selcouʒt', a word with meanings that range from 'marvellous' to 'strange', 'shocking', 'outrageous' and 'monstrous'. All of these senses are at play here, that opening cry one of shock and horror as it is of wonder. The narrative breaks down under her grief, the reader crying out to her and becoming one with her in agony.

The images which follow make this clear, as Mary and Christ morph into one. They are images of reciprocal agony, predicated upon the bonds of family. Mary's body becomes the locus for physical pain, her heart a source not of tender feeling but of torture, of inescapable agony. Just as the full weight of these images begins to take hold, the narrative breaks off again with another interjection. The 'A þou wounded ladi, wounde thow oure hertis' maintains that emotive force, but channels it into a cry of prayer. Its chiastic structure performs a number of functions. Initially it extends the expressive force of the interjection for as long as possible: the impassioned note it strikes is effectively held through a form of echoing. Beyond that, it generates a mode of intersubjectivity: it aligns the reader with Mary again, blurring them together in a moment of shared injury, idealising her compassionate response and making her a role model. The next sentence furthers this with the specific request to 'Ioyne þi herte in-to ourys þat we mai be woundid with þe'. It is a delicate image, but nevertheless one of strangeness and unsettling force: it combines emotions with bodily organs, and relocates the centre of Christ's torture within the reader. The emotive charge of this image is not allowed to dissipate, as the passage deploys yet another interjection. The cry itself, 'A lady', begins more formally and is more prayer-like in terms of structure. What it asks for – 'I praie þe ʒeue me þe despites & þe repreues of þi sone' – articulates the essence of compassion: the desire to be tortured with Christ. Yet this request rests upon highly crafted and cultivated intersubjective dynamics. Mother and son are in agony, but the reader is amongst them, the cause and reason for it all. The point the text is making is clear – the soul can be tortured most effectively through considering the torture of Christ's Mother. Further detail soon emerges:

> And ʒit more hit agreggid his bittirnesse, oure caytif vn-kyndenesse, þenne al his bodili peyne þat we are so vnkynde to hym, and so litel deynte haue of þat dede þat he hym-self most chargeth, þat is his passioun. ʒehe & ʒit was his pyne moche more for compassioun of his modir. For-wy he saw hir swowne for sorwe and þat was his sorwe, for þe mykel loue and þe grete compassioun þat was by-twenehem bothe, þei were crucified togedere. His modir knewe wel þat ihesu suffred deth for hire als he dide for odre, and ihesu al-so knewe wel þat þe sword of compassioun percyd

his modris herte. A þou cristen man þenke ofte of þis passioun & turne þe to þi herte & fille hit ful of sorwe & peynes, wenne þow seest þi god and þi maker suffre þus for þe. (p. 29, ll. 12–15)

The constant shifts in narrative perspective between the narrator, Christ, His Mother and the reader encourage an awareness of the intersubjective dynamics of the Passion. Detail is directed towards His emotional pain. His 'bodili peyne' is only briefly mentioned, used by the narrative to serve as a contrast to the real suffering He endures: the agony of our indifference. Here the passage focuses on the reader, at once assuming and castigating their apathetic perspective. The careful use of the possessives and repetition in 'oure caytif vn-kyndenesse' and 'we are so vnkynde', simultaneously describe and ascribe an abnormal emotional state to the reader, aligning him or her fully with the narrative moment. It is a technique that enables highly choreographed self-reflection: permitting both proximity and distance, the reader comes to see his or her self in a certain way, as an 'other' and unnatural self within the confines of the narrative. There is an unmistakable penitential tone here, as the reader is made to feel guilty through the simple act of viewing the Passion. Yet the passage does not linger with the reader, but instead shifts to the perspective of Christ. From here the text begins to articulate a model of compassionate response and psychology: the co-torturing of both mother and son. Beyond the pain of the reader's indifference lies the torment of His Mother, and to convey that intensity the passage becomes more rhetorically and structurally sophisticated. A form of parallelism between the two is created through conceptual and linguistic means. The sibilance of the line 'he saw hir swowne for sorwe, and þat was his sorwe' merges the suffering and person of Mary with the suffering and person of Christ. Sharp contrasts between the two are broken down through sound. This is given visual force through the shocking image of co-crucifixion: their compassion for each other, their shared feelings, enable them to be 'crucified togedere'. Distinctions between mother and son dissolve in pain, as both coalesce through compassion.

The impact of this compelling image is maintained through a loosely chiastic clause structure. The line 'his modir knewe wel þat ihesu suffred deth for hire als he dide for odre, and ihesu al-so knewe wel þat þe swerd of compassioun percyd his modris herte' places both perspectives in parallel, allowing the narrative to rapidly shift between them, further blurring them together. The overall result is to generate a moment of mirrored torment, designed to amplify the emotive force of the text. The narrative carefully moves the reader from Christ and the extent of His wounds, to a moment where He thinks only of another. That narrative space allows the reader to occupy a different position: to see that Christ 'dide for odre' and that Mary suffered 'þe swerd of compassioun'. That image of the sword recalls Christ's own infancy narrative, and thus adds a sudden gravity to the passage, as the reader is forced to see a woman grieving for the death of her innocent child. Thus, a focus on the intersubjective dynamics of the Passion forces the reader to apprehend the wider impacts of sin – that it wounds His Mother as well as His own person. This penitential aspect is confirmed in the next line, as the passage moves to a more impassioned register. The opening interjection in 'A þou cristen man þenke ofte of þis passioun', heightens the emotive force of those images, their heavy awareness of sin, and channels it into a new narrative moment of self-accusation. Narrative perspective moves now to the narrator figure, who directly addresses the reader with the succinct charge that all the pain and agony between Christ and His Mother was suffered 'for þe'. It is a moment of layered emotion, and of nuanced self-awareness. Intersubjectivity is thus a key part of compassionate response, one that allows the full intensity of this emotional complex to come to the fore. However, heightened compassion is simply the means; the end is the treatment of the soul.

The text is assiduous in ensuring that the reader can cultivate the emotional medicines within compassion. Pity and patience are the most overt. Over the course of the text the reader must patiently endure the often luxurious and languorous descriptions of Christ's agony; and with the additional mention of Mary and her sorrow, a pervading sense of pity is evoked. All of the images and scenes looked at thus far are clearly aimed at evoking both. Yet, there is another emotional state that is part of the treatment offered by the *Christus Medicus* – humility. As with Paul, the reader must be tortured by compassion, must suffer it so that humility can be generated within the soul. This is a complex state, and it is only begun through compassionate response to Christ. In various passages throughout the text there is evident a deliberate attempt to encourage the beginnings of humility, to make the reader 'mykel holdande hym-self' (p. 75, l. 13). At times this is quite overt, with some sections offering little else than a series of extreme comparisons designed to encourage self-hatred and contempt, to make the reader feel ever more humble. These sections directly address the reader as 'so vnconnande a wrecche', as 'vile & lewd' and as 'vilese of all oþer' (p. 74, ll. 5–16). Other sections operate more subtly, generating a sense of humility gradually over their course, through lines that are ostensibly directed towards evoking compassion. In chapter nine, entitled 'a preier to oure lord a-boute his passioun', initial details of the ignominies Christ suffered soon give way to something rather more complex:

> A lord ihesu hit is wondir to **me** þat þou woldest suffre deth for **me**. Whi dedest þou so lord, whi louediste þoue **me** so mikel? Goode ihesu, what art þou and what am I? Thou are goddis sone and I am a vile stynkande wrecche, a feendis felaw and a bestli man. What nede haddiste þou of **me**, þat þou was so tendirli bisye a-bouȝte for to seke **me**, and to biȝe **me** with þi blood? I loued not **þe** but þou loued **me** & I hated **þe**. I chese not **þe** but þou chese **me**, not for any þyng þat þou sawe in **me**. For-whi what seyȝe þou in **me** but synne? (p. 67, l. 25 to p. 68, ll. 1–10, emphasis mine)

The opening interjection and address to Jesus signals an important tonal shift away from the horrors of the Passion to the mystery of it – the 'wondir' of why Christ would bother to die for someone who clearly despised Him. It is, in essence, a cry of prayer, but one of considerable nuance. It is precisely modulated, beginning as an effusive expression of wonder, before swiftly shading into a form of self-analysis and eventually self-reproach. Gradually, the magnitude of Christ's sacrifice is brought to bear upon the reader through lines that constantly and recursively articulate his or her unworthiness. Rhetorically, the passage is quite sophisticated, deploying tactical mention of the Passion alongside rhythmically expressed comparisons. The lines 'þou woldest suffre deth for me' and 'biȝe me with þi blood' refer to the Passion, but with none of the expressive visual force of earlier passages. Any and all visual complexity is reserved for describing the reader – who is variously a 'vile stynkande wrecche, a feendis felaw and a bestli man'. The function of the Passion here, therefore, is different. Instead of overwhelming the reader with disturbing visuals, these mentions channel the emotive force of the opening interjection into a different context: they articulate not horror and fear at the Passion but the contours of a relationship, reminding the reader at key moments in the passage that Christ suffered death 'for me'. Personal pronouns are given the most rhetorically sophisticated treatment. Rhythmically, they structure the entire passage, marking not only separation between clauses but also forms of emphasis. This is evident from the very first line. The repetition at the end of the clauses in 'wondir to me/suffre deth for me/whi louediste þoue me' carries forward the force of the opening interjection throughout the passage: the repeated 'me' generates a loose form of epiphora, at once echoing and emphasising that opening cry.

Later use of this technique operates in similar ways. The repetition of 'me' at the end of the clause in the last few lines enables them to connect directly back into the opening cry. Yet the text goes further still (p. 68, ll. 5–9). There is a subtle prose rhythm generated through the rhyme between 'me' and 'þe'. This is an integral part of the function of the passage, as the rhyme articulates a relationship: it constantly compares and contrasts Christ and the reader. Through such patterns of sound, the reader is brought into a specific relational context with Christ – one of utter contrast to His selfless acts of suffering and death. Humility is the result, as the reader moves closer to the realisation that all this pain was only ever for them. Here, self-awareness soon becomes self-accusation. The rapid oscillation between 'me' and 'þe' ends with a focus on the self, with the question 'what seyȝe þou in me but synne?'. The penitential aspect in this passage moves to the fore, adding a further affective charge to the general sense of the reader's unworthiness. It is a highly tactical use of penitential feeling that the text often employs to evoke humility. As it notes most clearly towards its end, no one may approach God unless 'he a-counte hym-self as a wrecche and as nouȝte' (p. 166, ll. 9–10). The emphasis is clear: the reader must 'come first to god mekeli with shame of his owne synnes and wiþ greet reuerence and drede . . . and þat he knowleche þanne goddis gretnesse & his worþynesse, and his owne litilnesse, and his wrecchidnesse' (p. 166, ll. 10–16). Penance is an integral part of self-knowledge, the essential prerequisite to a deep and abiding sense of humility for the presence of sin and the consequent death of Christ:

> But gode lord ihesu, what disseruyd I for to resseyue of þe ony gracious ȝifte? Soþeli no þynge, but þou ȝeldest gode for yuel & þat wel bi-cometh þe. I haue pursewed þe and þou hast turned me to þe. I haue spitted in þi face and þou wolt kisse me. I haue wounded þe with iren & þou woundest me with þi loue. I filled þe ful of sorwe of my synne & þou ȝettist me ful of coynfort of þi grace, I shlow þe and þou hast quykened me & ȝeuen to me lyȝf endeles. A þis is a selcouȝt chaunge. (p. 109, ll. 16–25)

This is a meditation on merit as much as the Passion itself, on what is truly 'disseruyd' by actions of the narrative voice. Constant comparison with the actions of Christ fuels the entire passage, and brings it into a vividly realised and personalised re-enactment of the Passion. The Biblical account is immediate, its events indistinguishable from the actions of the narrator figure. Time past and time present merge into one, as the lines relocate the reader's awareness of the presence of sin onto an awareness of his or her culpability in the Passion narrative itself. Constant use of exegematic narration is part of this, and it is augmented by the switching in tense when describing action. The narrative voice acts always within the past tense, while Christ is in the present tense. This subtle difference has the effect of placing the horrific details of the Passion in the background, and the selfless love of Christ in the foreground. A penitential mood is established: the past sins and atrocious deeds of the reader are constantly contrasted with the ever-present generosities and mercies of Christ – His inexhaustible 'gracious ȝifte'. However, this mood is strictly controlled. Penance is not permitted to spill over into self-accusation and reproach. Instead, the mood builds to a moment of profound and humble self-awareness. The final line – 'A þis is a selcouȝt chaunge' – begins with an interjection that elevates the entire passage into a cry of wonder rather than alarm. Those constant contrasts between Christ and narrator establish a rapid narrative pace, a forward momentum that is focused and expressed by that interjection. It articulates best the humble awe created by Christ's death. The wide semantic range of the adjective used to describe it – 'selcouȝt' – only adds to this. Through that ending cry of emotion, the narrative can relocate the wonder, horror, marvellousness and unnaturalness of the Passion onto the reader – expressing, in a moment of intensity, words which convey how low and humble the reader is in the presence of Christ's pain, and how wonderful it is that He would deign to endure it.

Compassion for Christ, that complex blend of emotions, has treated the soul in the most direct and intense of ways, bringing the reader into far closer contact with God than through fear or penance alone. It truly is a compound medicine, one that requires the sophisticated deployment of rhetorical and poetic effects to evoke and layer its many parts. Yet, it is nevertheless a preparatory treatment. As Julian notes, 'be compassion we arn made redy': it does not completely heal the soul through its painful intensity, but instead acts as a prologue to something more profound.[66] As the text notes, 'no man may parfiteli fynde god til he kon parfitely first lesse hym-self' (p. 85, ll. 13–14). Kenosis, the loss of the self, is an essential condition for coming close to God – to sowle-hele. Achieving this requires more than an initial sense of humility, it must be developed further and go beyond humility into something more complete: a 'meekness' that will utterly change the soul for the better. To achieve that will require the emotional capacities of the soul to be pushed to their limits; to make the soul not simply desire Christ, but to cry out in agony for Him. It is to that most complex emotional state, the painful 'longynge' for God, that the next chapter turns.

4

Longing for Health

Take good gracyous God as he is, plat & pleyn as a plastre, & legge it to þi seek self as þou arte. Or ȝif I oþer-wise schal sey, bere up þi seek self as þou arte & fonde for to touche bi desire good gracious God as he is, þe touching of whome is eendless helþe by witnes of þe womman in þe gospel: Si tetigero vel fimbriam vestimenti eius, salua ero.[1]

Contemplation is ultimately a medical intervention. For this text, the most sophisticated of its type in Middle English, it is contact with the divine that offers the most effective healing touch. Yet this 'touch' is itself a complex of emotional states, of self-emptying abnegation, and of a relentless focus on God. The reader is encouraged to 'touche bi desire good gracious God', to 'bere up þi seek self', and to ignore anything that pertains to 'þe beyng of þi-self or of God' (p. 139, ll. 5–10). The reference here to the healing of the bleeding woman by Jesus serves as an instructive paradigm: one must contemplate God not casually or curiously, but with all the urgency and intensity of someone desperately seeking a cure.

Suffering, though painful, offers a clarity of perception. Contemplative aspiration is far from gentle, and is instead full of intense, painful, longing. When this text speaks of desire for God, it is a desire that is best understood within that medical context of the desire for health. This central claim regarding the health of the soul is conveyed with emphasis. The heavy use of alliteration in the first line builds a sense of forward momentum that compels the reader into accepting the main points of the following lines. Through alliteration, the opening line of the passage performs what it describes. The rapid succession of velar plosives forge connections between the various concepts each word expresses, merging them together in a pattern of sound and sense that encourages the reader to understand God as a medical treatment. The phrase 'plat and pleyn', a Middle English idiomatic expression meaning 'exactly like', allows metaphor to give way to a functional equivalency between God and medicine.[2] Yet this cure has certain requirements. The contemplative must 'touche bi desire' – must be in a state of wanting and longing before any healing can take place. The last medicine of the soul is, therefore, a profound desire for God; a desire that is as complex as it is acute. As Julian notes in her *Revelations*, a 'trew longyng to God' completes the soul's programmatic treatment. Julian's term, 'longyng' has an interesting semantic range that signals its intricacy. It primarily means 'to languish or pine in erotic or spiritual love'.³ Pain is a key part of this desire, as it is so intense, is felt so keenly that it hurts and enfeebles the soul. *The Cloud of Unknowing* provides some additional detail:

> sorow, when it is had, clensiþ þe soule, not only of synne, bot also of peyne þat he haþ deseruid for synne. & þerto it makiþ a soule abil to resseiue þat ioye, þe whiche reuiþ fro a man alle wetyng & felyng of his beyng. Þis sorow, ȝif it be trewly conseyuid, is ful of *holy desire.*⁴

True sorrow for sin contains a form of desire for God. In the same way, true desire for God contains a profound sorrow for sin. Desire is, therefore, not an emotion per se, but rather an emotional complex, a layering of intensive and contrasting emotions that are all directed towards a single goal. True longyng for God demands the utmost from the soul and its passions. It is not a shallow enthusiasm for God, but instead a specific state of the whole soul that requires the cultivation and emergence of cognition, of specific modes of self-awareness and self-emptying, and of intersubjective relations. In this sense it is like compassion – an aggregate of various other emotions directed to both the self and God that are used to move the soul closer to God. Yet it is also much more. Longyng is the perfection of the soul's prior emotional treatments, and moves it into a new reformed state. This chapter deals with longyng as the last and most complex medicine of the soul. It begins by exploring what longyng essentially is, how it is understood medically, and ends with a consideration of a text within the Vernon manuscript that seeks to evoke it within the soul: *A Talking of the Love of God.*

A Desire to be Healed

> Sothly bot a perfit man or womman, that has gedird to gedire all the desires of thair saule, and with the naile of luf festid thaim in ihu crist, swa that thaim thynke an oure of the day ware ouere lange to dwell fra him, for thaim langis ay til him, bot an that lufis noght swa has na langynge that he come, for thaire consciens says thaim that thai haf noght lufid him as thai sould doe.⁵

For Rolle, 'langynge' is far from easy or gentle. Glossing Psalm 12 in a way that puns on long (duration) and to long (to yearn), he speaks here of those who truly desire God and are impatient to be near Him. The central image he uses to convey the nature and extent of this desire is both sinister and sublime: 'the naile of luf'. It is arresting in its potency and strangeness, as it takes any sense of love as something mild or welcoming and reconfigures it as a sharp tool or implement. Love penetrates, but it is whom it penetrates that gives the image imposing force. The contemplative must pierce both his or her own soul and God with this nail: the desire for God becomes here a form of personal crucifixion that participates in Christ's own. Love, and any pre-existent sense one has of it, warps and changes here into something strange and almost horrific. This image allows aspects of the Passion to enter into the contemplative desire for God in a way that shocks.

It is not enough to love God, nor to have pity for his Passion; we must instead participate in that process and nail ourselves to Christ as He was nailed to the Cross. Desire for God becomes an act that manifests itself as a shocking double crucifixion. But of course therein lies the point – 'longyng' is not something pleasant but is inherently painful and intimately connected with sorrow and suffering as it is predicated upon an absence and a lack. Moreover, it also contains a penitential reproach. As Rolle notes of these contemplatives, 'thaire consciens says thaim that thai haf noght lufid him as thai sould doe': despite sharing Christ's Passion in this highly literal way, it is still not enough. Conscience, and that penitential state of awareness it requires, is never left behind even in the heights of contemplation. While this longyng is the utmost expression of desire, it is a desire that is itself a combination of all the other emotional medicines of fear, penance and compassion. True longyng will be so intense that it will be painful, will contain as much fear of God and sorrow for sin as it does compassion and ardent love for the Divine.

A key theological treatise that deals with this type of emotional complex is the *De quatuor gradibus violentae caritatis (Four Degrees of Violent Love)* by Richard of St Victor.[6] In many respects it is a religious analogue to the medical interest in love-sickness during the twelfth century. It delineates four levels of love for God, each one superseding the last in terms of intensity and potency. None of them is gentle. The first is presented as a wounding of the soul through love: the 'fiery dart of this love penetrates the inmost mind of man, pierces his affections'.[7] Such an affective injury increases in the second degree, a 'binding love' that 'burns up the soul in a continual heat as in a state of fever'.[8] The use of a medical register is not accidental: this love operates like a disease. The third stage 'excludes every other love' and makes 'hand and feet nerveless as in illness'.[9] Once again, medicine serves as a way of understanding the nature and form of this kind of love – it enfeebles the soul. The fourth and final love is the most terrible, as it exceeds all the prior degrees and is 'unlimited in its expansion'.[10] It is presented as a form of torture: Richard notes that no form of love can 'crucify [the heart] more cruelly' than the fourth.[11] So great is it that the medical metaphor he has been using is tested to the limits. This love is,

> morbus irremediabilis et omnio desperabilis ubi semper et remedium quaeritur, et nusquam invenitur, imo quidquid praesumitur ad remedium salutis, vertitur in augmentum furoris.
>
> (An incurable and wholly desperate sickness, in which a remedy is forever being sought and never found, in which indeed, whatever is considered remedial to health turns into an increase of the raging sickness.)[12]

Beyond treatment, beyond relief, this love destroys everything it touches. But that is how it should be: in its purest and highest form the love for God is a state of painful intensity. Moreover, it also contains within it a specific form of self-awareness. Speaking of its effects upon the soul, he notes that 'in the first she goes forth on her own behalf, in the fourth she goes forth because of her neighbour . . . in the fourth she goes out in compassion.[13] So strong is this love that it not only ravishes the soul like an illness, but it also fosters within it a profound sense of intersubjective awareness – this love extends from the self to God, and then to everyone else. The text underpins Rolle's own understanding of the love of God, though he only speaks of the first three degrees. Nevertheless, for other texts of Middle English mysticism, such an apprehension of love's complex extremity is very much foregrounded. As the *Cloud* author notes in his *A Pistle of Preier*, desire for God is a complex state:

þe goostliche experience of þe profe of þis worching, it stondeþ al in a reuerent affeccioun þat a man haþ to God in þe tyme of his preier, causid of þis drede in þe grounde of þis werk and of þis stering of loue, þe whiche is brouȝt in bi þe goostly steppis of þis staf hope touchid before. For whi reuerence is not elles bot drede and loue medelid togeders wiþ a staf of certein hope.[14]

The 'reuerent affeccioun' so crucial for effective prayer is itself a combination of specific emotional states. While fear and love are distinct emotions, they nevertheless function in a complementary manner at this stage in contemplative activity. The key word in this passage is the verb 'medelid'.[15] It is a word with a range of connotations, some even sexual, but all of which convey a sense of complete combination and admixture. As a result the passage is not advocating the experience of fear and then love at this stage in contemplation; emotional combination is much more fundamental than that. Instead, the text insists that both love and fear are experienced together and at once in this 'reuerent affeccioun' for God. Such an insistence makes a subtle but significant point. Fear and love, though not antithetical emotions, do contrast to some extent with each other. In terms of medieval psychology, these specific passions were held to emerge from distinct powers or appetites within the soul. Fear is located within the irascible power of the soul; love, in contrast, resides in the concupiscible power. By feeling a true 'reuerent affeccioun', both powers of the soul are engaged and united in contemplative activity. A 'medelid' affection thus fosters a similar unity within the soul, focusing all powers upon God.[16] Such an emotional complex results in more complete forms of contemplation, and is wholly based on the medieval understanding of the theology of fear. As mentioned in Chapter 1, *timor servilis* must grow and develop into *timor filialis* – a form of fear that is itself based upon a form of love. This movement from an initial to a more complex form of fear is emphasised in religious texts aimed at all levels of spiritual development. The *Prick of Conscience* notes from its outset that 'drede may a lofe bygyn'.[17] Emotional states move and shade into others, combining in a manner that permits both to operate upon the soul:

> For if drede stand by itself anely,
> Na mede of God it es þan worthy.
> Þarfor drede suld be lufes brother
> And ayther of þam stand with other,
> For whaswa lufes God on ryght manere
> He has grete drede to wrethe hym here.
> Þan lufes he his bydynges to fulfille
> And dredes to do oght ogayne his wille.[18]

The relationship between dread and love is precisely expressed: they are not opposites but rather siblings. Such a metaphorical rendering is immediately intelligible and accessible, and expresses a complicated point with clarity and force. Dread and love are not abstract concepts expressed through abstract language, but instead brothers who stand together before God. The text reimagines and reworks the theology of fear into a more expansive familial setting that the reader can easily interpret. *Timor filialis* is here less a theological abstraction and more a domestic drama, as the two brothers Fear and Love work ceaselessly to please God.[19] The metaphor conveys the deep interconnection between these two emotions – they are blood relatives – yet it is also flexible enough to accommodate a sense of distinction within such unity. Subsequent couplets exemplify this idea. The lines 'þan lufes he his bydynges to fulfille / And dredes to do ouht ogayne his wille' and 'He lufes to be with God ay / And dredes to be put fra hym oway' convey not only the unified action of love and drede but also their distinctive qualities: both emotions act as the main verbs in each couplet, but they carry out activities that are inversions of each other.[20] Such inversion generates a sense of complementarity and simultaneity. Each 'brother' works ceaselessly in a manner that complements the other, and that is carried out at the same time as the other: they are truly 'medelid' together, as their actions upon and within the soul occur at the same time and are directed towards the same goal. Emotions become here aggregated and intertwined. That initial dread of punishment gradually changes into the dread of sons – a state characterised by love as much as fear: the soul desires only to please God, to be near Him, and to do his bidding; but at the same time it also fears failing to do so. The object of focus subtly shifts from the self to God.

In the initial stages of fear there is an exclusive preoccupation with the self, as the fear of punishment is in part based upon a form of self-regard. In the advanced filial fear there is instead a preoccupation with God, a fear of failing Him and His requirements; a state that is essentially selfless. The last two lines of the passage articulate this, as emphasis falls on God, His commands and His will, while all mention of the reader fades into the background. The focus is, by the end, only on God; not the self. Through this combined emotional complex there emerges a more sophisticated sense of intersubjective relations. As the *Epistle of Prayer* notes, this 'medelid' affection contains hope as well as love and fear. Hope is also understood as a passion of the soul that resides in the irascible power. However, it has a specific temporal aspect – one that is directed towards the future and the apprehension of a good.[21] In this text it is the hope of God's mercy, an emotional state that is predicated upon an intersubjective relationship and that requires the development of specific attitudinal frameworks. It is not enough to simply feel; rather, the contemplative must feel a certain way regarding the unknown agency of another – here God. Hope of God's mercy, by its very nature, fosters a relational context that delimits the agency of the contemplative by emphasising that of God's. Through hope the self is placed in a subordinate position characterised by possibility not certainty. There is the expectation of God's mercy, not the sure knowledge of it.

The 'reuerent affeccioun' that the texts extolls is an emotional complex that places those who cultivate it into a specific attitudinal and intersubjective state that fosters an active passivity and humility. Through this 'reuerent affeccioun' the contemplative becomes utterly focused on God and utterly submissive – in essence, meek. This state of selflessness is seen as a crucial aspect of the longyng for God:

> He suld luf him and drede in thoght
> Mare þan anythynge þat es wroght;
> And luf and drede in alle thinge
> May sonest a man to Mekenes bringe.[22]

Though the *Speculum Vitae* is not concerned principally with matters of high contemplation, it nevertheless displays the general understanding of what fear and love cultivate within the soul. The idea of aggregate emotions is as much a part of the era's pastoral materials as it is of its contemplative materials. Here the emotional complex of 'reuerent affeccioun' leads to the virtue of meekness, without which man cannot approach the Divine. It is not presented as something additional to drede and love, but rather as something predicated upon them: 'Of swilk thoght comes luf and drede / þat may a man to Mekenes lede'.[23] 'Mekenes' can only exist if the fear and love of God are truly felt, in combination, within the soul. The 'longyng' for God is thus much more complex and layered than simple enthusiasm. Its various constituent parts are given much more sustained elaboration in Julian's *Revelation*. For her there are four kinds of drede, 'drede of afray', 'drede of peyne', 'doutfull drede' and 'reverent drede', each of which increases in intensity and merit before God; the fourth being the most important and useful.[24] The higher forms do not displace the prior, but rather incorporate them, and they chart a course from the purgation of the soul, to an almost penitential awareness of sin. Referring to the last, she notes that:

> Love and drede are brethren; and thei arn rotid in us be the goodness of our maker and thei shall never be taken fro us without end. We have of kinde to loven and we have of grace to loven, and we have of kinde to dreden and we have of grace to dreden ... And thow this reverent drede and love be not partid asunder, yet thei arn not both one, but thei arn ii in properte and in werking and neither of them may be had without other.[25]

Once again, the idea of dread and love as brothers is used here to great effect. As with the *PoC*, this analogy allows the theological concept of *timor filialis* to be given a more direct articulation. Yet here it is also augmented with the use of a physiological metaphor: dread and love are rooted within the soul. Such a rendering of each endows them both with a sense of naturalness and of purpose. Both are placed within the soul by God, and both ought to work towards Him. Ideas of biology and family, of nature and nurture combine here in Julian's presentation of reverent drede. The repetition of 'kinde' and 'grace' reinforces this combination of naturalness with Divine purpose. Through analogy and metaphor she is able to convey the sense of their complete interconnection and distinctive operation: while they share blood ties, they nevertheless work upon and within the soul in different ways. The specification that they 'arn ii in properte and in werking', conveys the sense of their aggregate function. While conceptually distinct in terms of their nature and operation, dread and love work together towards a common, divine, goal. Crucially, their focus is wholly upon God, and permits no room for self-regard. Within this specific emotional complex lies an inherent selflessness:

> This reverens that I mene is a holy, curtes drede of our lord, to which mekeness is knitt: and that is, that a creture seith the lord mervelous grete, and the selfe marvelous litil; for these vertues arn had endlessly to the lovid of God.[26]

Far from being an accidental by-product of reverent drede, the virtue of meekness is so closely connected to it as to be almost indistinguishable. The word 'knitt' has a range of meanings such as 'conjoined' and 'interlaced', and so meekness is itself an integral part of dread. Its use conveys the sense of intimate and fundamental union between reverent dread and meekness. The text does provide some clarification, and carefully notes how reverent dread generates particular forms of self-awareness and intersubjectivity. By necessity, this emotional complex places those who experience it within a relational context to God. It ensures forms of comparison and discrimination: through dread God is not only perceived as 'mervelous grete', but the self is also seen as 'marvelous litil'. It is this intersubjective form of self-assessment that meekness is predicated upon, as the nature of the self is only mentioned insofar as it pertains to God. Dread at this level ensures that the contemplative's focus is no longer on the self but rather on Divinity. Such selflessness is subtly figured in Julian's idea of the medicines of the soul. She notes that through 'trew longyng to God we arn made worthy': the result of this emotional complex is directed towards another, as longyng results in worthiness – in making the soul worthy for God, worthy to receive Him; not for itself.[27] The contemplative longyng for God treats the soul, therefore, through the meekness it generates. While the other emotions that comprise longyng also have an effect, meekness is the distinctive therapeutic potential that longyng possesses.

Julian is not the only writer to note the medicinal effects of meekness. It is a recurrent topic in several influential texts of spiritual guidance. The *Pore Catiff*, for instance, contains a whole section on the topic. It offers a highly figurative rendering of meekness as the mother of Christ, and stipulates not only how essential it is in loving God, but also how it is a form of medicine. 'Þerfor if þou wolt conseyue ihesu, þat is saluacion eþir helþe of soule, bicome þou meke.'[28] While this makes a standard point, that to get as close to Christ as Mary did one must become utterly selfless, it also makes a connection between meekness and sowle-hele: Jesus is the health of the soul, and to conceive Him one must be meek. Later in this section of the text, it asserts how meekness is a form of medicine: 'meke suffryng of siiknesse, it purgiþ þe soule fro synne'.[29] Meekness operates in the manner of a purgative cure, targeting and removing sin from the soul. Other texts of spiritual guidance make similar claims. In the *Chastising of God's Children*, the therapeutic work of meekness is clarified. Initially the text uses analogy to explain its function: 'Also we fynden wele þat fier purgieþ goold and siluer, but man is preued bi mekenesse in chastisynge' – meekness is a purgative for the soul.[30] Later in the text it makes a more precise claim, asserting that meekness is essentially 'a special remedie aȝens pride'.[31] Such accounts of meekness are sparse, and offer more summary information rather than a sustained elaboration of this virtue and its specific effects upon the soul. Other texts, however, go into much greater detail regarding the nature and operation of meekness. Hilton's *Scale of Perfection* is one such text. Although it does not offer a profusion of medical metaphors or statements regarding meekness as a medicine, it does view meekness as a treatment for the soul that enables its overall reformation:

> The lasse thou felist that thou art or that thu hast of thisilf thorugh mekenesse, the more thou coveiteste for to have of Jhesu in desire of love. I mene not oonli of that mekenesse, the whiche a soule feelith in sight of his owen synne or frieltees or wrecchidnesse of this liyf, or of the worthinesse of his evene Cristene. For though this mekenes be soothfast and medicynable, nevertheless it is boistous and fleschli as in regard, not clene ne softe ne loveli. But I mene also this mekenesse that the soule feeleth thorugh grace, in sight and biholdinge of the endeless beynge and the wondirful goodnesse of Jhesu. (2, ll. 1147–54)

Meekness consists of two levels, both of which are presented here as therapeutic. The first is penitential, arising from a confessional self-awareness, and the acknowledgement of sin it entails. In it 'a man feelith of bihaldynge of his owen synnes and of his owen wrecchidnesse, thorugh which biholdynge he thenketh himsilf unworthi for to have ony gifte or grace or ony meede of God' (2, ll. 2573–5). The second is, though related, vastly different. It incorporates the first form but then transcends it, and consists of the contemplation of God. Such meekness 'setteth at nought itsilf with alle the synnes and alle the good deedis that evere he dide, as yif there were nothinge but Jhesu': it is wholly intersubjective, based upon a comparative awareness of one's limitations in the face of the Divine (2, ll. 2593–4). This higher form of meekness alters the soul, reforming it and its emotional capacities. Despite their differences in degree both share key similarities: they are not only therapeutic, but also reciprocally connected to the desire for God. Meekness, in any form, is essentially a 'medicynable' manifestation of a Divine desire – of longynge. It is this desire for God inherent in longynge that is given a sustained medical rendering. Initially, Hilton begins by asserting that 'For this name Jhesu is not ellis for to seie upon Ynglisch but heelere or hele' (1, ll. 1224–5). A few lines later, this instance of translation is amplified and elaborated into a complex metaphorical construction where the desire for Jesus is equated with the desire for spiritual health:

> But this gostli heele mai noo man have that hath use of resoun but yif he desire it and love it and have delite thereinne, in as michel as he hopith for to gete it . . . Nothinge is so dere, ne so nedeful, ne so mykil coveited of hym, as is goostli heele; and that is Jhesu, withouten which alle the joies of hevene mai not like hym. (1, ll. 1231–42)

Once again a medical metaphor is used to understand the necessary intensity required by contemplative activity. Desire is an urgent need that excludes all others, not a shallow enthusiasm. Yet the text is also making a subtler point: the desire for God enables the healing of the soul. To desire God with such urgency is to be healed by Him, specifically through the meekness such desire naturally generates. As Hilton asserts in the second book of the *Scale*, who 'hath the gifte of perfite mekenesse . . . hath the gifte of perfighte love' (2, ll. 2675–6). As the highest desire for God constitutes the highest level of meekness, perfect meekness is the most potent treatment for the soul – it will reform it utterly.

Its impacts upon the soul are given considerable attention. Initially, perfect meekness counters pride and makes the soul wholly focused on God (2, l. 2568). Following on from this, it then performs additional reforming work as a manifestation of perfect love:

> Love wirketh wiseli and softeli in a soule there he wole, for he sleeth myghtili ire and envie and alle passions of angrinesse and malincolie in it, and brengeth into a soule vertues of pacience and myldenesse, pesiblité and lovereden to his even Cristene . . . for whi love feighteth for him, and sleeth wondir softeli siche risynges of wraththe and al malencolie, and maketh his soule so esi, so pesible, so suffrande, and so goodli thorugh the goostli sight of Jhesu, with the feelynge of His blissid love, that though he be dispiced or reproved of othere men, or take wronge or harm, or schame or velany, he chargeth it not. (2, ll. 2680–98)

Though this perfect love is 'softeli' it is nevertheless forceful, and is endowed here with a martial power and potency. Its operation upon and within the soul consists of two forms. The first is one of elimination. Love is the ultimate combatant: it 'sleeth' sins and undesirable affective states from the soul in the most direct of ways. Reformation in 'feelyng' is not a gentle process, but instead a violent crushing achieved with remarkable ease. The words used to describe this operation – 'sleeth wondir softeli' – construct an arresting image of effortless slaughter. Their alliteration and sibilance at once convey a sense of speed but also of almost sinister ease as several of the seven deadly sins are themselves killed. Love 'feighteth' the sin in the soul and eliminates it: there is no accord made with sin, only its utter vanquishment. In this way love is almost personified, rendered not as an emotion but rather as an heroic champion who protects the soul by conquering it.

Such a presentation of love is reinforced by the second operation it performs on the soul. After crushing sin, Love 'brengeth into a soule vertues', liberating it from the bondage of sin. Building upon the presentation of contemplation as the Heavenly City in Chapter 21, Hilton here presents Love as the ultimate hero who frees the soul from sin and installs a new order within it. Though implicit, there is nevertheless the sense that Love is a protector and steward of the soul as much as its prize fighter. In addition to this, perfect love also enables further changes within the soul that are more directly associated with its dual aspect of perfect meekness. Specifically, it reconfigures any idea of sociality within the soul. The 'he goostli sight of Jhesu' is an exclusive one that precludes any other form of social awareness. Through it all normal modes of social life are removed, as the soul becomes unconscious of the evaluative judgements and behaviours of others. Irrespective of the negative actions marshalled against the soul, perfect love will ensure that it 'chargeth it not': the exclusive focus on God reforms the soul in the most direct of ways.

Love's ability to slay sin and specific emotions does not end with anger and envy. Love 'sleeth coveitise, leccherie, glotonye, and accidie, and the fleschli savour and delite in alle the fyve bodili wittes' (2, ll. 2745–7). Taking each sin in turn, the text notes how and in what manner Love slays it. Once again the martial force of Love is made clear. Love becomes a weapon – the 'swerde of goostli love' that kills each deadly sin with ease (2, l. 2768). So powerful is Love that it transforms vice into virtue. When the text discusses covetousness, it asserts that 'Coveitise also is slayn in a soule bi the wirkynge of love, for it maketh the soule so covetous of goostli good and to heveneli richesse so ardant' (2, ll. 2748–9). As Hilton notes in his text sin is essentially disordered desire, and so when love is properly directed towards God, all sins cease to be (1, ll. 1556–8). Through perfect Love and the exclusive focus on God it generates, the soul covets what it properly should; in so doing it acts virtuously. This emotional alteration constitutes the essential part of the soul's reformation in 'feelynge' – the second stage of its programmatic treatment when it is 'firste heeled of goostli sikenesse', when 'alle bittir passions and fleschli lustis and othere oolde feelynges aren brente oute of the herte with fier of desire' (2, ll. 859–65).

Sin, the soul's chief sickness, can only be healed through intensive emotions. Here it is burnt out of the soul through the 'fier of desire' and a 'brennynge love'. Medically, the soul must be cauterised of its sickness: the imagery of fire and burning conveys a sense of potency and intensity. The Holy desire for God is not an easy or gentle state, but instead a purgative process that sanitises the soul by setting it aflame. Sin, itself an emotional disorder, is destroyed by an even greater emotional state. The complexity of this desire is also noted, as the cleaning fire brings 'newe gracious feelynges' into the soul: the specific use of the plural makes the point that longyng for God is not one emotion, but an aggregate of confected emotions and intersubjective states. As a treatment for the soul, it works as a compound medicine: longyng, through the painful desire it contains, the filial fear it evokes, the meekness it generates, and the penitential and intersubjective modes of awareness it fosters, will alter the soul and its emotional and cognitive capacities to enable sowle-hele. Though it is the most complex medicine of the soul and requires some element of Divine Grace, it is a treatment begun with specific forms of reading. Certain contemplative lyrics, forms of prayer, and even prose treatises can all be seen as aiding the soul in evoking this complex state, in igniting this cleansing fire. As this Holy Desire for God pushes the soul to its utmost, so too the texts that evoke it take language to its limits.

Texts of Longynge

To 'taast of þat triacle' and achieve sowle-hele, is a process that requires both patience and practice. For Hilton, this idea of contemplative progress and its iterative and reiterative stages is the subject of extensive investigation. Over the course of the *Scale*, he systematically breaks down contemplation into various shades of advancement in spiritual development. Its heights cannot be scaled all at once; there are stages to pass through, skills to practise, and there is always the necessity for Divine Grace:

> For a man schal not come to goostli delite in contemplacioun of His Godhede, but yif he come first in ymaginacion bi bitirnesse and compassioun and bi stable trouthe and stidefaste mynde of His manhede. (1, ll. 922–4)

Passion meditation is a key practice in furthering spiritual development and achieving sowle-hele. Yet, while its benefits are extolled, so too are its emotive impacts mentioned. Neither sweetness nor savour characterises this activity – only 'bitirnesse' and 'compassioun'. To come to contemplative union with God, to reach sowle-hele in its purest form, requires pain and unpleasantness, the harrowing agony of compassion for Christ. The 'triacle' of longyng is as much a drawn-out ordeal as it is a medicine: greater proximity to God requires ever more potent and demanding emotional states. Hilton pays considerable attention to each gradation, and specifies three manners of prayer that encapsulate this process. The first is the 'comon praier of the ordenaunce of Holi Chirche', consisting of the *Pater Noster* and 'matynes and evesonge' (1, l. 715; l. 683). It requires attention and practice, and specific forms of reading: those who engage in it must 'seie his Pater Noster and his Ave Marie and rede upon his sautier and sich othere' (1, ll. 704–5). While the Psalter is specified, the importance of additional religious texts is also made apparent, and left generally open. Such prayer and reading are controlled, and do not test the emotional capacities of the person, nor encourage meditations or visions. The second and third forms are completely different, characterised by diminished degrees of textuality and increasing degrees of emotional intensity. In the second stage, the speaker focuses on 'rehersynge hise synnes and his wrecchidnesse or the malice and the sleightes of the enemye, or ellis the godenesse and the merci of God' (1, ll. 739–40). Such penitential states of awareness culminate in an outpouring:

> And with that he crieth with desire of herte and with speche of his mouth to oure Lord for socour and help, as a man that were in peril amonge his enemyes or as a man in sikenesse, schewynge

his sooris to God as to a leche, seiynge thus: Eripe me de inimicis meis, deus meus (Psalms 58:2) Lord, delyvere me fro myn enemyes, or ellis thus: Sana, domine, animam meam, quia peccavi tibi (Psalms 40:5). A, Lord, heele my soule, for I have synned agenys Thee, or sich othere that come to mynde. And also hym thenketh so mykil godenesse, grace, and mercy in God, that hym liketh with grete affeccioun of the herte for to love Hym and thanke Hym by siche wordes and psalmys as acorden to the lovynge and preisynge of God. (1, ll. 740–9)

Speaking to God as if he were bodily present, prayer here is caught up in an effusion of emotion and its scripted articulation. Desire is the key state here, a heartfelt cry to God with all the urgency and force the soul can muster. It is that precise word – 'crieth' – that marks the central distinction of this stage of prayer. It is full of anguish and force, not tranquility or calm. So potent is it that it tests the limits of language: this is more a shout than a speech, raw and powerful and almost inarticulate. It is a heartfelt wail of desire for God that at once is consumed with and expresses urgency and intensity. Yet it is connected with reading the Psalter aloud and in a precise manner. The Psalms are used in a way that goes beyond mere repetition and moves into the area of immediate and personal intensity. They become not a prompt for feeling, but the actual expression of it. Once again it is medicine, and the language of healing, that characterise such intensity. The speaker must cry to God 'as to a leche' – as if desperately seeking a cure. This sense of urgency is reinforced through Hilton's translation of the second Psalm. The line 'A, Lord, heele my soule', begins with an interjection – that part of speech which signifies *per modum affectus*. Its position in the translation underscores the importance of emotional intensity: the Psalm begins, first and foremost, with a raw expression of emotional force and potency. So too the speaker's cry to God must begin with similar intensity. Reading, particularly at this stage of prayer, is a key means of enhancing emotions. While its importance diminishes in the third stage of prayer, a stage that is 'oonli in herte withouten speeche' and in which these raw expressions of emotion alter the soul and transform into 'goostli savoure', its overall importance in enabling sowle-hele cannot be overstated (1, l. 789; l. 794). The cries of prayer that the Psalms enable the reader to make are understood here as cries for health: reading possesses a key and instrumental function in treating the soul.

As discussed in Chapter Two, the Psalms ought to be understood as vessels of emotive force, as the metrical and rhythmical means of engaging the soul at the utmost of its emotional range. Their use here, though not penitential, is all about intensity. It is desire they help evoke, a longyng for God that is as painful and demanding as it is therapeutic. However, they are far from the only texts to enable and provoke emotion at this level. For instance, *A Talking of the Love of God*, is a text similarly concerned with the health of the soul, and with evoking longyng in its readers. From its outset it stipulates that it is 'mad for to sturen hem þat it reden, to louen him þe more. And to fynde lykyng and tast in his loue' (p. 2, ll. 1–3). It is designed to augment, enhance and extend emotional states. Such a goal is dependent upon specific modes of usage:

Hit falleþ for to reden hit esyliche and softe. So as men may mest in Inward felyng, and deplich þenkyng, sauour fynden. And þat not beo dene, but bi ginnen and leten in what paas so men seoþ þat may for þe tyme ȝiuen mest lykynge. (p. 2, ll. 3–6)

Reading is here not a linear and functional process, but instead a personal and intimate engagement. The text offers itself as a tool of emotional focusing and expansion, as a means of deepening the desire for God. The reader does not race through the text in a careless manner, but instead reads 'esyliche and softe' – with careful deliberation. It is not necessary to read the whole thing in one go, but only to engage with those sections that are most beneficial to the reader at a given instance. Reading is an act governed as much by the reader's emotional disposition as it is by the injunction to read 'esyliche and softe': it is an act tailored to the individual, by the individual, and depends upon an honest assessment of his or her own interior state. It is a form of personalised medicine, and as such pace is key. The reading process has to be carried out within some more general structures than the reader's own feelings, and so the text is composed within a certain rhythmical pattern: 'men schal fynden lihtliche þis tretys in Cadence . . . rymed in sum stude, to beo more louesum' (p. 2, ll. 17–19). This specific metrical style combines form and function, as it serves to regulate the reader's passage through the text and to endow its contents with an additional emotive charge. Style is thus central, as it allows the text's often repetitive comments and contents to take on lyrical potency and force:

> Ihesu soþ God, Godes sone, Ihesu soþ God, soþ mon. Mon Maydenes child. Ihesu myn holy loue. Mi siker swetnesse. Ihesu myn herte, my sele. My soule hele. Ihesu, swete Ihesu. Ihesu, deore Ihesu, Ihesu, Alimihti Ihesu. Ihesu mi lord, my leof, my lyf, myn holy wey, myn hony ter, Ihesu al weldinde Ihesu. Ihesu þou art al þat I hope. Ihesu mi makere þat me madest of nouȝt, and al þat is in heuene, and in eorþe. Ihesu my Buggere, þou bouȝtest me so deore, wiþ þi stronge passion, wiþ þi precious blod and wiþ þi pyneful deþ on Roode. (p. 2, l. 21 to p. 3, l. 4)

The text really begins here with its central preoccupation: Jesus. This opening is compelling in its lyrical and meditative potency, as the constant repetition of the Holy name and the careful use of alliteration generate a familiar and recursive pattern of sound and sense that is as hypnotic as it is rhetorically exuberant. Jesus is all, presented as God, as 'Godes sone', as a 'Maydenes child', and as 'Alimihti'. He is at once the Christ-child, and the Heavenly King, the obedient son and the omnipotent God. Each repetition of the Holy Name is followed by a qualification or description of one of His many roles, and each builds upon and connects to the prior one. The cascade of repetition builds up an emotive charge, a breathless yearning for Jesus that is made manifest through His associative range. Jesus is everywhere and everything, beyond yet also a part of creation – 'soþ God, soþ mon'. The sudden delineation of what Jesus actually means to the speaker augments this further: a profusion of possessives adds personal and tender meanings, as Jesus becomes 'Mi siker swetnesse', 'myn herte, my sele. My soule hele'. This technique is repeated again with greater force, with the more tightly repetitive and climactic 'Ihesu, swete Ihesu, Ihesu, deore Ihesu. Ihesu, Alimihti Ihesu' being immediately followed by the heavily alliterative 'mi lord, my leof, my lyf, myn holy wey, myn hony ter'. The speaker is overcome by Jesus as, in all His meanings, He overwhelms any simplistic categorisation. The pace of this opening is key, and it consists of patterns of identification and interpretation. Initially there are only statements of what Jesus is, glimpses of Him as Lord or Son; the personal relevance and meaning of those images is purposefully delayed only to be released in a sudden profusion of what Jesus means to the speaker.

Images of Jesus, and their interpretations, occur only in concentrated bursts. Such a structure works to deepen and intensify.

Through this opening, the reader is compelled to adopt a specific cognitive and emotional outlook that places Jesus at the centre of all things, and that glorifies His nature first and foremost. Yet desire is never simplistic. While the initial lines offer an exuberant presentation of Jesus' divine and human nature, subsequent lines add darker tones. The mention of His role as Redeemer casts the shadow of the crucifixion over the passage. The reader moves from Jesus as 'Myn hony ter' to the 'þi stronge passion' and 'þi pyneful deþ on Roode'. Emotions become layered, as the jubilant and ecstatic aspects of the first few lines are mixed with compassion and pain. The yearning for Jesus begins to reach a painful level of intensity, as the images in the passage combine in jarring and shocking ways. Within the space of a few lines, the 'swete Ihesu', who is the therapeutic balm or 'holy wey' that ensures 'soule hele', morphs into the broken and tortured body of Christ on the Cross covered in blood. These strange images of blood and honey, of health and harm, are held together structurally by the 'cadeance' of the passage: the use of alliteration, and the repetition of 'Ihesu', binds this bricolage of images together into a unified whole. The emotive impact of the passage is thus similarly composite: the 'Ihesu' the reader speaks to cannot now be viewed as the object of desire without the emotive overlay of the Passion. Jesus is made here the locus of longyng – the object of that unique blend of love and pain. Such a layering of emotion occurs at key moments throughout the text, and is supplemented by sections that seek to evoke specific forms of self-awareness. Shortly after the opening impassioned address to Christ, the text moves the reader into crafted postures of self-reflexivity:

> A Ihesu þin ore, whi have I likyng in oþer þing þen in þe þat bouȝtest me so deore. Whi ne be holde I algates wiþ eȝe of my herte hou þou henge for my loue streyned on Roode. Þin Armes wyde I spradde þi derling to cluppe, wiþ toknyng of trewe loue þat sprong out of þi syde. Whi nul I beo þi derling and loue þe ouer alle þing, and comen to þi clupping to cleuen in þin armes and cluppen þe swete. A derworþe Lord. (p. 6, ll. 5–11)

Lack, that inability to feel a desire for Christ, is the central focus here. Through the careful use of rhetorical questions, the narrative engages with the issue in a manner that compels the reader into occupying that specific position. The reader must confront their own emotional deficiencies, must understand that they themselves represent the biggest obstacle in moving closer to God. The interior, the psychological landscape, is the central focus here as the reader's own self is investigated and explored through the same visual and stylistic techniques found in the opening. Images of Christ still predominate, but they are focused upon in a manner that interrogates the self, that fosters a specific modality of self-awareness.

None of this is gentle or easy – there is a similar emotional intensity and exuberance. It all begins with the opening cry of 'A Ihesu' – the careful use of the interjection to set a specific emotional tone. The narrator, and by extension the reader, cries to God in anguish at their own emotional malaise. This initial outburst, and the emotive potency it contains, is sustained and carried through the rest of the passage by being constantly connected and re-connected to the Passion. The opening 'A Ihesu þin ore', with its subsequent rhetorical question, is rhythmically connected to 'þat bouȝtest me so deore': the Passion and its work are metrically and conceptually fused to this form of self-awareness. Introspection becomes self-reproach at the foot of the Cross as further rhetorical questions reinforce this connection. Yet the affective potency of the passage is sustained by the increasing use of romance tropes and love language. Christ is not just the Saviour, but the tortured 'derling' of the reader. Such language allows for compelling and vivid imagery. The blood and water that burst forth from His sides are now 'toknyng of trewe loue'; the physical contortions caused by the crucifixion – Christ's 'Armes wyde' – are now an invitation to a tender embrace. The use of alliteration and near repetition in the last line generates a mounting urgency to the passage, fusing Christ's death agonies with a jarring sense of lovers clasping and clutching at each other. Such energy builds up to the climax 'A derworþe Lord', another interjection that frames the passage, echoing and extending the emotive force of the opening line. This is a language of extremes – the extreme pain of Christ on the Cross becomes connected to and surpassed by the extreme cruelty of the reader's ultimate indifference to Him. Through such language the reader is guided into a posture of charged and profound self-analysis:

> Whi ne fele I þe lord in my brest roote. Whi art þou me so fremde, þow þat art so swete. Whi ne con I loue þe and loueueliche wouwe þe wiþ sweete loue wordes and lykynge þouȝtes. Aller þing swettest. Aller þing louelokest. (p. 8, ll. 8–12)

The 'brest roote' is a powerful metaphor, at once visceral and abstract. As a way of describing the heart, it conveys a sense of depth and centrality: the 'root' within the breast is in effect the very core of the person, something hidden and buried, but alive and internally vital. There is an almost uncomfortable medical quality to the image of the root within the breast, as it conveys more forcefully a sense of introspection. But of course that is the point. Its use signals difference, articulates that what will follow is not the familiar clichés of the 'heart' as a trope of interiority but something altogether more intense. The metaphor indicates that the depths of self-analysis that the text is moving towards are of a different order and magnitude, that they move beyond confessional modes of self-awareness, and into something more profound.

Sin is mentioned only very generally and only of its ability to get between the soul and God (p. 8, ll. 16–18). In this respect the text is much like the *Cloud's* advice on the subject, detailing only the general impact of sin upon the soul while eschewing all categorising frameworks and taxonomies.[32] The focus, therefore, lies elsewhere: the text is not concerned with addressing sin per se, but rather the inability of the reader to feel desire for Christ. The repeated questions deal with the incapability to feel properly, and interrogate the dispositions and actions of the soul at its most fundamental level. It is this indifference that the text seeks to address. It wishes to treat this emotional malaise, and specifies Christ's Passion as a key means. He is the 'bote' or remedy, 'of alle Medicine fruit and Roote', and it is His Passion that delivers this medicine to the reader: 'let þy woundes hele þe woundes of my soule' (p. 8, l. 32; p. 10, l. 6). Only through them, through this treatment, can a kenotic self-emptying be achieved – 'In liue not in lyue þat I liuede, but crist liueþ in me þrow wonyinde grace' (p. 10, ll. 12–13). As the text makes clear, 'wiþ pouert & wiþ wo schal me wele buggen' (p. 42, l. 33). Sowle-hele comes from the Passion, and so the text soon moves into a highly crafted meditation sequence designed to remedy indifference and push the soul to its emotional limits. After carefully describing the events leading up to the Passion, the scourging and crowning with thorns, and the insults suffered by Jesus, the narrative turns towards Calvary:

> A derworþe lord what schal I nou dou. Nou mai I liue no more for serwe and forsore, now my dere lemmon schal vnderfonge deþ. Nou mai I Murne strongley, nou mai I wepe bitterli nou mai I syke sore & serwen euer more. A now me leden him forþ to mount of caluarie, to þe qualstouwe to don him þere o dawe. A my deore lemmon, he bereþ þe Roode tre on his bare scholdre for þe loue of me. His bodi is so tendre, his bones longe and lene, al stoupynde he goþ þat del hit is to seone. A Mi swete lemmon, þe duntes þat þei smyte þe, þe serwe þat þei don þe. (p. 48, ll. 23–33)

Unlike prior passages in the narrative, this one deploys a range of techniques to enhance the reader's emotional reactions to the events it describes. It begins with the impassioned interjectional cry to Jesus that recalls the self-reflexive sections earlier in the text. This emotional cry sets a tone for the rest of the passage, carefully sustained through repetition and additional interjections. Initially, the urgency and force of the opening question what 'schal I nou dou', is sustained through subsequent clauses by the repetition of its immediate answer 'Nou mai I'. Through this repetition, each clause is connected back to that forceful opening in a manner that directly recalls its emotive energy. The reader is thus constantly brought back to that cry throughout the whole section, its force and potency endowing each clause and the details each contains with added emphasis. Additional interjections break up the passage into dominant sense units and mark progress in the narrative, but they all work in the same manner to express and evoke raw emotion. The result is that each stage in Christ's crucifixion is marked not by detail but rather by the emotive reaction to it. The whole passage thus plays with ideas of action and reaction. Until this moment all events in Christ's Passion have occurred in the distant past, but now the present tense is used exclusively: the past of Calvary merges with the moment of narration, and by extension the moment of reading.

Such careful manipulation of narrative time in the passage allows the reader to be both within and outside the events it describes. The reader is at once present but also helpless, unable to act – only to react to Christ's torture. While prior portions of this text have concentrated on the reader's inability to feel for Christ, this section functions to make feeling and reaction the only possible option. A careful pattern is established, with the interjectional cry beginning a sentence and framing the scene, and subsequent clauses articulating an increasingly nuanced emotive reaction. The narrative then immediately moves on – the reader cannot act, nor look away, only react to the scene and its events. Emotional intensity is maintained through concentrated bursts of detail that shade into self-description and introspection. The I-voice observes, and provides detail, but then reflects on that detail, becoming increasingly articulate of its inner state. The narrative voice feels 'serwe and forsore', can 'Murne strongley' and 'wepe bitterli', when it views how Christ 'bereþ þe Roode tre on his bare scholdre for þe loue of me.' While the rhyme between 'tre' and 'me' works to rhythmically connect the reader to the Cross, it is the use of exegematic narrative that further embeds the reader in the scenes described. Through its use, the movement of the narrative becomes the reader's own. Yet narrative control persists beyond this point. After several more repeated instances of this pattern of description and reflection, the narrative landscape suddenly shifts from Calvary to the immediate present of the reader. Instead of reflection, the reader is moved to action, into a position of heartfelt prayer: 'Lord þat art Almihti, ȝif me for þi merci muynde of þat vileny, and felyng at myn herte þi peynes hou þei smerte' (p. 50, ll. 2–4). The emotive energy of the prior lines has been carefully increased and controlled, directed towards a moment of prayer. This shift in the narrative interposes a different kind of emotional impulse. The prayer is essentially penitential, a request for mercy and constant recollection of the Passion. It inserts a sense of sorrow, of personal pain and culpability, to the overall presentation of pity and compassionate response. Such emotional layering reaches its climax at the actual crucifixion:

> Allas my deore lemmon, hou may men for reuþe a ȝeyn so muchel fordede, do þe al þat wo. To þe þat art so loueli, so feir and so freoly, and þoledest so mekeli al þat þei wolde do. A Ihesu now þei driuen, þe blunte vnruide nayles, þorw þi feire hondes and þi frely feet. Nou bersteþ þi skin, þi senwes and þi bones. Min herte cleueþ in my brest for reuþe of þi mones. A Ihesu swetyng wher is eny wepyng, wher is welle of teres, to lauen on my leores þat I neuere bi day stunte no be nihte nou I seo þi feire lymes, so reuþli I dihte. (p. 50, ll. 11–19)

Both narrative progress and perspective are tightly controlled over the course of the passage. It begins with a cry of woe, an expression constantly augmented and reiterated through the repeated interjections and supplementary detail. At this stage detail is rather lacking; all that is mentioned is a series of comparatives regarding Christ's beauty and patience – nothing visually concrete. The next sentence differs. Here, the reader's perspective is carefully modulated, with specific details dominating the gaze at any given moment. The narrative holds focus on compelling images: 'þe blunte vnruide nayles, þorw þi feire hondes and þi frely feet'. We move from the general scene of the Passion to an extreme focus on the crucifixion nails. This sudden shift in perspective is disorientating, and is supported by the very structure of the clause. The first adjectives used to describe the nails, 'blunte' and 'vnruide', generate a slow and lingering pace. The monosyllabic bilabial plosive 'blunte' is slow, and is further drawn out by the trisyllabic 'vnruide': the pace of the clause becomes heavy, the reader forced to linger over those nails in an elongated moment. Yet, this contrasts sharply with the alliteration of 'feire/frely/feet', which endows the end of the clause with a fast pace, the fricatives offering a phonic softness that is at once sinister and gentle: the nails, suddenly, sink into the flesh. Imagistically, the narrative starts at the edges of the Passion. The reader is shown here only the top and bottom of the Cross, the hands and the feet. The narrative then progresses from this fragmentary image. The fast pace set by alliteration moves into an animated moment – 'Nou bersteþ þi skin, þi senwes and þi bones'. The images described suddenly move and morph into another, as the narrative progresses internally, exposing the actual penetration of Christ's body by those nails. The impact, the ripping and the horror, become articulated rather than implied. As narrative focus deepens on Christ's body, narrative time becomes attenuated: the moment of torture is drawn out as the agony continues beyond expectation, impressing the event more firmly upon the reader and forcing him or her to view it afresh.

The sense impressions the text evokes immediately switch from arresting visuals to sound. Until this point, all has been carried out in silence, a silence now rent asunder by Christ's powerful 'mones'. Verbal patterning and rhythm in the last lines of the passage support this, with 'bones' and 'mones' merging together through rhyme – fusing agonised body and breath into one. These reported cries, and the effects they have upon the narrative voice, generate a powerful though subtle sense of parallelism. Such is their force that the narrator's own 'herte cleueþ in my brest'. The choice of words not only recalls the 'brest roote' mentioned in an earlier passage of self-analysis, but also places Christ and the narrator into a form of harmony: just as Christ is punctured by these blunt nails, so too is the narrator pierced internally by His cries. Such techniques layer emotions within the reader. Initially these images of torture generate a sense of horror and fear. Yet they are carefully manipulated to generate compassion – 'reuþe' – for the broken Christ, before morphing into almost penitential self-awareness. After this scene of mirrored torment, and its emotive exuberance, the narrative is propelled into a self-reflexive mode: the narrator, and by extension the reader, asks 'wher is eny wepyng, wher is welle of teres to lauen on my leores'. The question has the tone of self-reproach to it, an open address to God that confesses a deep lack of adequate feeling. This is supported by the loose rhyme between 'teres/leores', that connect the well of sorrow with the narrator's dry cheeks. An emotional complex is generated, along with a particular modality of relational self-awareness. As with earlier portions of the text, the reader is placed within a particular pattern of affect, its articulation, and guided self-examination. The effect is hypnotic. We are brought into ever more carefully delineated visual and kinetic moments, forced to linger over them, with our responses partly suggested and similarly drawn out. The next section focuses more on images that act to augment and intensify these pre-existent emotional postures:

> Þe blood of þi woundes springes do breme, and stremeþ on þi white skin, so reuþe to sene. Þy Moder lokeþ þeron, þat virgyne clene, hir serwe sit þe sarre, þen þin as ich wene. A now þei setten vp þe cros & setten vp þe Roode treo, & þi bodi al be bled, hongeþ þer onne. A Ihesu now þei setten þe cros in to þe morteis, þi Ioyntes sturten out of liþ, þi bones al to scateren, þi woundes ritten a brod for foled so wyde. Lord þat þe was wo bi gon in þat ilke tyde. (p. 50, ll. 19–26)

While the last passage interposes moments of self-reflection and the language of love and romance amid arresting visuals, this passage focuses much more on the visual spectacle of the Passion. It focuses tightly upon specific details, not the entire scene. Unlike a painting, the reader cannot take in the whole Passion in one visual moment: we cannot compass the torture of Christ, but instead are led through it instance by instance. The narrative perspective alights only upon specific details of specific moments in the Passion, and then animates them. Instead of static tableaux, the images the narrative describes are kinetic and alive, moving within their invariable confines. The blood of Christ's wounds 'springes do breme' and 'stremeþ on þi white skin': it is described and presented in motion, as a dynamic presence in and of itself. In contrast, Christ's body remains static and diffuse; 'þi white skin' can refer to any part of it. Blood is the focus of the narrative perspective, not the overall bloody spectacle of Jesus' body. The reader sees very little – just gushing blood running down white skin. Such an image is almost disconnected from the Passion, yet it has a sinister menace, forcing the reader to view up-close the consequences of sin. As this is an image in motion, it has a dynamism and force that are extremely compelling. It is enhanced by the careful use of rhyme to generate a cascading effect: 'breme' rhymes with the first part of 'stremeþ', while the end rhyme between 'stremeþ' and 'reuþe' pushes the narrative forward with greater force. Yet, the background image of the static saviour contrasts sharply with the image of running blood. As a result, the reader views not a picture of the Passion, but a textual simulation of a moment in time that has been captured and conveyed with great care. The focus on a fragment of the Passion allows the images it is comprised of to gain far greater concentration and potency. It is a technique repeated and extended when the narrative details the raising of the Cross.

Once the Cross is placed upright, the narrative focus moves to Christ's body. The reader is once again confronted with these animated imagistic fragments, all of which are overlaid upon the static background image of Christ on the Cross: Jesus' 'Ioyntes sturten out of liþ', His 'bones al to scateren', His 'woundes ritten a brod for foled so wyde'. Each encapsulates and conveys a simulated moment of horrific torture and pain, and each holds the reader's attention upon a focused point. Collectively they manipulate narrative time, forcing the reader to view the physical consequences of the raising of the Cross as if in real time. The Passion, in all its horrors, is made fresh and vividly real.

To add extra emotional intensity to these fragments, the narrative deploys broader shifts in perspective. When Mary is mentioned, she is referred to as 'Moder' – her relationship to Jesus is foregrounded. From this point the narrative moves into the psychological interior of Christ: when He sees her watching Him suffer 'hir serwe sit þe sarre, þen þin'. This moment of introspective comparison is made accessible to the reader, as we move from the contours of Jesus' body covered with blood, to the contours of His thought. It is a pattern of self-reflection that the reader is being encouraged to follow. The rhyme between 'clene' and 'wene' interposes the reader among the reflected 'serwe' and 'sarre' of Christ and Mary. Yet this moment of intersubjective torment, of emotional pain, does not last long. Rapid narrative shifts immediately occur, as the perspective moves outside again to Christ mounting the Cross and the Cross being raised. Once it is raised the narrative moves back inside, to the interior of Christ's body, to the damage done by the crucifixion.

Such dizzying oscillation in perspective is done with great intention. The reader cannot become inured to an image or scene, as it keeps shifting and morphing into something quite different, though ultimately related. The Passion thus becomes not a static tableaux but a partial simulation, a sequenced parade of Christ's sufferings. Emotions become layered and mixed: fear comes from the horror of these images, but so too feelings of pity and penance. The narrative shifts in perspective allow the images and the emotions they initiate to fold back upon themselves. The reader moves from one instance to another, to an interior state, then back again to the visual agonies. The interjections that punctuate this passage not only signal new torments for Christ, but also amplify those emotions: the reader, made a witness to the scene described, also cries out in anguish for Christ. Each interjection evokes and expresses this kind of high-level emotion, one carried through the rest of the clause. They build up an emotive charge throughout the passage, echoing each other in similar patterns of sound and visual horror. Interjections are a constant presence throughout the entire Passion sequence of the text. As such they generate a loose form of anaphora, tying each instance of the Passion together, and establishing a rhythmical parallelism in prose form that is hypnotic and evocative. Through them, the reader is led not simply into the Passion but also into specific instances of self-reflection:

> Weo, lord, vre loue it luitel worþ þat costen þe so deore. And ȝit vnne we hit nouȝt þat þou hit haue here, but folewn vr lustes in þe deueles fere as þauȝ he be beter þen þou, and more worþ

were. Allas Allas for reuþe þat I schal þe my lemmon, so foule seo demeynt, and myn is al þe gult. Al for drawen and for rent, bi spit & schomeliche schent, to sauen vs þer we weore for þat was al þi cause. A Ihesu swete lemmon, hou mai I nou libben. Nou I seo þe leoue lyf, þe loue of myn herte. Mi derling, my longyng, Mi blesset lord my swetyng, wiþ armes white and louely streyned so streytly wiþouten eny merci. (p. 50, l. 35 to p. 52, l. 9)

The opening interjection of 'weo' follows the pattern established in the preceding passages of the text. Yet its use here enables a significant change in the narrative. Its emotive intensity is the same as 'allas' or 'A Ihesu', and it is that similarity that allows it to merge the prior Passion narration into self-narration. The reader moves seamlessly from observing the Passion directly, to personal observations in a moment of meditative self-scrutiny. All those scenes of horror and pain described in the present tense, now move into the reader's own present tense sorrow and compassion, and his or her sense of personal culpability. The use of internal rhyme 'deore/here/fere/were' accentuates this movement, and through careful use of the interjection, a form of emotional transposition and layering occurs. Emotions evoked in prior sections now are used to generate a specific mode of self-awareness: fear, sorrow and pity now fuel an analysis of the self.

The following sentence begins with the repeated 'allas' – another interjection that signals a change in perspective back to the crucifixion and shaming of Jesus. Persons and tenses, passions and perspectives, become mixed and merged together. Emotions, and a specific modality of self-awareness, are overlaid upon another moment of Passion narration. This has the effect of deepening engagement with the scene described, with making the sufferings of Jesus become intensely personal. Language shifts from the sinister rhyme of 'rent/schent' to a highly charged register of love longing: Jesus is no longer addressed as 'lord' but as 'swete lemmon', as 'Mi derling, my longyng, Mi blesset lord my swetyng'. The narrative voice reflects not on specific sins, but on a general sense of 'gult' at the Passion. This reflection soon changes into the more impassioned 'A Ihesu swete lemmon, hou mai I nou libben': penance and self-accusation deepen and intensify into a profound regret towards a lover.

It is 'longyng' that now emerges, that blend of fear and love, of meekness and humility. The narrative voice is humbled by the nature of Christ's sacrifice, as emphasis rests not upon the presence or nature of sin per se, but rather upon the deep sense of humility at being the cause of all this. The rhetorical question that opens with an interjection is the key to the whole passage: it aims to make the reader humble, by forcing them to confront the extreme lengths God will go to for 'ure loue'. Language changes as a result. The image of Christ on the Cross now becomes the image of 'Mi derling, my longyng, Mi blesset lord' upon the Cross: this breathless series of possessives gives the image an added depth, endows it with a more complex emotional resonance. He is described as having 'armes white and louely streyned so streytly': Christ is in utter torment, but also in a position of open embrace. It at once recalls that earlier image of blood running down white skin, with all its emotive associations. The reader is also thus positioned to engage with that embrace, with the horror of the passion and the longyng for Christ. 'Longyng' for Him is being carefully encouraged, as the reader is ultimately held by the construction of the narrative in an emotive embrace that evokes fear, love and meekness.

From here onwards the focus of the text begins to change. Passion sections start to recede into the background, and the text considers Mary and her pain before taking up a quasi-lyrical preoccupation with the longyng for Jesus. These sections function like lyrics, amplifying and extending the prior emotional complexes the text has evoked:

> A swete Ihesu sweete leof, my lemmon my deore lord, swettest of alle þing, my leue lyf, my lyues loue, þou me hast defendet a ȝeyn myn enemys þreo wiþ al þi lyf, wiþ þi deþ. And madest of me vnworþi, þi lemmon and þi spous. And brouȝtest me so seliliche out of þe false word as þin owen derling to þin owne boure. And as I weore þin owne bird here in to þi cage, to wone wiþ þi self in þis holy place. (p. 58, ll. 7–13)

The narrative voice cries in rapture towards Jesus, the 'sweete leof' and 'lemmon'. This interjectional cry is full of emotional potency, of love-longynge and desire. The use of alliteration and repetition in the first line builds a sense of forward momentum and interconnection between the key concepts it describes: 'leof', 'lyf' and 'lemmon' all join together in the presentation of Jesus, just as the chiasmus of 'my leue lyf, my lyues loue' also binds and fuses together. The emotive force of the opening interjection is carried forward via these rhythmical means into a moment of personal reflection. The narrative presents Jesus' saving work in the most intimate of terms: He leads the soul away from woe and into a private and holy 'boure' and birdcage. Such imagery stands in sharp contrast to the horrors of the Passion. Yet it is nevertheless conveyed with the same degree of intensity. Those interjectional cries of woe and sorrow at the sufferings of Christ now become cries of joy and rapture. Due to their similar linguistic nature, such cries echo and connect to each other: they do not cancel each other out, but instead build up a thick and complex emotive charge. Later lines intensify it:

> A swete Ihesu swete leof, my lyues loue my swetyng, þou hast maad me of nouht, fro þe deþ þou hast me bouȝt. From þe world in to þi chaumbre, leue lord þou hast me brouȝt. And more blisse þou hast me hiȝt, þen wiþ herte may be þouȝt. A swete Ihesu my deore lemmon, þat þus muchel hast done for me, what may I þenke, what may I speke, what may I worþly don, for þe loue of þe, what may I ȝelde þe, what may I þole for þe aȝeyn þat þou has þoled for me. (p. 58, ll. 23–30)

This whole passage is predicated upon reiteration. It opens with exactly the same words as the prior passage, but then differs by offering new details and new forms of self-reflection. The opening of the following sentence 'A swete Ihesu my deore lemmon' is almost an inversion of 'my lemmon my deore' in the prior passage. The effect is subtle but powerful. Instead of simply repeating prior lines, this passage uses similarity and near repetition to add depth and texture to the affective states it describes. The reader is caught within a mirrored space that reflects and augments what is described – this is seen especially with the play between 'nouht/bouȝt/brouȝt/þouȝt'. The narrative voice is both rapturous and reflexive, crying out to Jesus in joy then reflecting upon the manifold deeds He has performed. Each interjection expresses this raw affect, with the following lines carefully building upon it. The second 'A swete Ihesu' does not fade out over a series of clauses, but instead contributes to a sense of mounting urgency. The repeated question 'what may I' after this emotive cry functions like a lyrical refrain. Each repetition of this utterance increases the pace of the line, generating a forward momentum and tension that augments the opening interjectional cry. The emotive force of that opening becomes concentrated and reiterated in those repeated questions: like lyrics, they centre the reader's attention upon a point, bringing them back again and again to that sense of urgency. The reader, with the text, is moving beyond compassion into the more complex and layered state of longyng.

When references to the Passion occur at this stage in the text, they do so with an added layer of emotive sophistication. Though Christ is noted to be hung on the Cross with His 'body al on blode, þi limes al to rey3te, þi Ioyntes al to pli3te, þi woundes and þi leoue leor þat was so briht and so cleer ben now mad so grisli', such details are not focused upon for long (p. 60, l. 9–11). Immediately after this observation, the narrative voice notes that by seeing Christ suffer meekly 'þenne fele I redeli a tast wonder ferli of þi derworþe loue, þat precious druri þat fulleþ myn herte so þat al worldliche wo hit makeþ me þinken hony swet' (p. 60, ll. 12–15). Blood and love are mixed here: the horror of the Passion morphs and changes into an occasion for joy and transformation. From this point everything changes. The ghastly sight of Christ crucified becomes the stimulus for a passionate encounter that is sensual and beyond eroticism:

Þenne ginneþ þe loue, to springen at myn herte and glouweþ up in myn brest wonderliche hote, þe loue teres of myn neb runnen ful smerte, my song is likynge of loue al wiþ oute note. I lepe on him raply as grehound on herte, al out of my self wiþ loueliche leete. And cluppe in myn armes þe cros bi þe sterte, þe blood I souke of his feet, þat sok is ful swete I cusse and I cluppe and stunte oþerwhile as mon þat is loue mad, and seek of loue sore. (p. 60, ll. 19–26)

Longyng is a state of antitheses, of strong contrasts and their combinations. The entire passage is dominated by the language of paradox: tears yet joy, pain yet passion, madness yet intensely clear perception. Emotions fold over and into each other, generating new depths of feeling. This is the desire for God, the painful love for Him that occupies and consumes the whole soul: such desire is a complexion of a range of states, not simple erotic enthusiasm. The narrative voice suffers, oscillating between extremes, propelling the reader towards a new level of engagement. Sensory effects of heat and sound slip in and out of reference here, as the narrative jumps between various points of focus. The result is a description of great range and energy that moves beyond evoking simple compassion for Christ. The last line, with its alliteration and imagery of 'loue mad, and seek of loue sore' makes a clear point: longyng is a state so intense that it pushes the soul to its utmost, is a medicine that nearly kills. Lyrical moments like this continue, augmenting and concentrating not simply the narrative's focus on Christ, but also the reader's emotional state. Lines such as 'A swete Ihesu my leoue lyf, my lemmon my gode lord, Mi swetyng my derlyng, swettest over alle þing' use alliteration and repetition to create a meditative focus, a distillation of what essentially one ought to feel about Christ (p. 64, ll. 24–5).

A swete Ihesu swete lef, my deore herte, my lyues loue, Mi lyf, Mi deþ, Mi blisse. For þou ordeyndest me to þi deore lemmon. Bi twene þin armes ley I me. Bi twene myn Armes cluppe I þe. Nou 3if me felyng in þe wiþ outen ending, and hold me in þi kepyng swete Ihesu heuene kyng. Amen. (p. 68, ll. 13–18)

Blurring the lines between prose, lyric and prayer, the close of the text offers an impassioned cry to Christ for continued 'felyng'. Physical proximity to Christ is thus equated with emotional intensity: touch and passion become one and the same. Christ, still hanging on the Cross, can now be embraced. The narrative voice, and thus the reader, can now lie 'Bi twene þin armes'. The crucifixion has become an opportunity for a tender moment, an expression of love. An emotional complex is being carefully generated, as from the pain and suffering of the Cross now comes delight and joy. Yet it is not a replacement of one passion for another. Christ is still suffering, but that pain and the reader's compassion are now made 'hony swet'. It begins with that familiar interjection, and quickly moves into a highly charged paean. The very line begins to break apart in a rush of monosyllabic utterances strung together through the repetition of 'mi'. An urgent pace and forward momentum are generated, compelling the reader into this passionate embrace, into the humble supplication for continued 'felyng' – into longyng for Christ. Such an ending amplifies the reader's engagement with, and emotional response to, the narrative, confining them to a concentrated moment that intensifies feeling by narrowing semantic range and expression. It ends as a charged lyrical prayer, the closing interjection of 'Amen' echoing its opening 'A swete Ihesu' – to the raw cry to God for love, for sowle-hele. The use of lyrical prayer is thus tactical, enabling these strongly contrasting emotions evoked over the course of the text to shade into deeper states, more forceful modes of emotional yearning. It is only prayer, then, that can help the soul reach even greater levels of emotional potency. As the *Cloud* author notes, prayer at its utmost ought to be a raw cry of passion, a 'deuoute entent directe vnto God, for getyng of goodes & remowyng of yuelles'.[33] Such prayer is made not with extensive formulas and texts, but with the mantra-like repetition of a single monosyllabic word full of emotive force and potency. Those who pray at this level must 'crye soche a lityl silable in þe heiȝt & þe depnes, þe lengþe & þe breed of his spirit' as the 'hidous noise of þis crye be alweis herde & holpen of God'.[34]

These prayer words are essentially interjections – words that signify only *per modum affectus*, that can convey and evoke the strongest emotional states within the soul. Lyrical language is best equipped to move the reader into that state. Through it language becomes smaller, more rhythmical, more forceful, better able to push the reader into that complex state of 'loue-longyng'. Such an emotional complex is the soul's final medicine, beyond it lies only prayer and the chance of increasing intimacy with God. The texts explored here are intensely focused on evoking that complex state within the soul, with facilitating the emergence of an intersubjectivity and meekness. Such therapeutic aims are ambitious but, as with all medicines, there exists the potential for health and for harm. When speaking of the prayer of the perfect contemplatives, the text notes that they speak few words but that they are nevertheless 'ful of frute & of fiir'.[35] So too these texts – full of potency and force – have a potential that may be far from therapeutic if not correctly controlled. It is to the idea of dangerous reading, to problematic emotions and the means of controlling them, that the next chapter turns.

5

Dangerous Reading

> Ioie hastow for to muse
> Vpon thy book, and therin stare and poure,
> Til þat it thy wit consume and deuoure.[1]

The act of reading can, sometimes, come at a considerable cost: sanity. Implicit within the exchange between the *Dialogue*'s characters is an acknowledgement of the dangerous and potentially harmful power words can exert over the mind. Made explicit here is the fact that reading is not a passive act but rather a powerful, and to some extent treacherous, activity. The imagery Hoccleve uses to describe it is an inversion of the commonplace medieval understanding of the process of reading – an act comprised of reading, meditation and rumination (*lectio*, *meditatio* and *ruminatio*). Instead of the reader slowly and carefully savouring the book he figuratively eats, it is the book which eats the mind of the reader. Images shift from those of thought and vision ('muse' and 'stare'), to those of fluidity and ingestion ('poure', 'consume', 'deuoure'). The precise meaning of the verb 'poure' is playfully ambiguous, meaning 'to stare intensely/meditate' or 'to pour out a liquid'.[2] It is a deliberate movement aided by the end rhyme between 'poure/deuoure' that conveys the visceral potency and inexorable nature of the act itself – how quickly the book can turn and swallow the reader. What it specifically consumes is the 'wit', a medieval word with a vast range of subtly different meanings from 'the mind', to 'reason' itself, to the 'mental powers comprising intellect', and even 'mature discretion'.[3] Hoccleve's point is that reading can override reason, can manipulate the mind in a way that overwhelms its rational abilities by overly stimulating the soul's emotional powers. He is not the only author to make such observations. His mentor Chaucer also notes the dangers of such emotional manipulation in the *Canturbury Tales*. After listening to the Physician's dour and depressing narrative, Harry Baily exclaims 'but wel I woot thou doost myn herte to erme,/ That I almoost have caught a cardynacle'.[4] He specifies that his 'herte is lost for pitee': the tale's ability to evoke pity has powerfully negative physical consequences.[5]

Similar cautions about the impacts of reading can also be found elsewhere. From the early twelfth century Aelred of Rievaulx notes that reading romances can corrupt the emotional capacities of the soul, misdirecting them and fostering a false and prideful sentimentality.[6] Reading certain texts can bring the emotions into a state of imbalance in physically and spiritually dangerous ways. Yet, such concerns are not strictly confined to medieval romances. Even religious texts, especially those designed to evoke passionate states within the soul, are also subject to warnings:

> And he also erriþ greetli, þat bi vnmesurable and vndiscreet seyinge or synginge of salmes or ympnys, falliþ in-to fransye or in-to woodnes, or in-to bittir heuynes. Þerfore it is good þanne for to stynte fro multitude of wordis, and þinke oonli in þin herte as esily as þou maist.[7]

This text, a translation by Walter Hilton of the work of Dom Lluis de Fontibus (*c.*1383), is clear in its warning on over-abundant reading. A 'multitude of wordis' can cause dangerous psychological problems such as madness, frenzy or depression. Too many words can generate a 'bittir heuynes', a state of emotional intensity that is ultimately poisonous. Far from helping the soul through treating the emotions, immoderate reading and recitation of the Psalter can cause an emotional instability that damages the soul. One of the key words here is the adjective 'vnmesurable', meaning not simply 'limitless', but also 'inordinate', 'immoderate', and 'intemperate'.[8] Any religious reading must, therefore, be carefully calibrated to ensure its salutary effects. As texts such as the Psalter have strong emotive impacts, excessive and uncontrolled reading of them will cause only harm to the soul. As this text asserts, any reading regimen must avoid being 'vndiscreet'. This adjective, which means 'without prudence' and 'extreme' lies at the very centre of comments on the dangers of religious reading.[9] It covers more than simply the frequency of such reading and incorporates the manner, mode and results of its deliberate emotional manipulation.[10] Without discretion, the texts of sowle-hele become dangerous, resulting in physical and spiritual harm rather than health. Ever careful and cautious, Hilton makes clear here that the treatment of the soul through reading must be underpinned at all times with a key virtue: discretion.

It is this virtue that is the central concern of this final chapter. It begins by exploring how reading for sowle-hele can become pathological through the role of the imagination. It then considers texts which note the precise dangers that can result from intense reading: madness, a sorrow that becomes corrupt and seeks to harm both self and others, and a pernicious spiritual pride. Finally, after discussing the pathology of therapeutic reading, this chapter will explore the solution and treatment for it: the virtue of discretion, and the modified penitential subjectivity it seeks to evoke. The chapter explores a range of texts that lie outside the Vernon manuscript, focusing on the most influential texts of spiritual discernment such as the *Chastising of God's Children*, and the texts of the *Cloud* author. Such texts are of great diagnostic value, as they were originally used as sophisticated guides for solitaries. As Gillespie notes, monastic orders (such as the Carthusians) which are 'avowedly contemplative', sought to 'calibrate their machinery for spiritual *probatio* and *discretio*', and used the texts of the *Cloud* corpus and others 'in their own processes of self-assessment and spiritual calibration'.[11] They are concerned with the impacts of emotion on 'sowle-hele', and so their cautions and caveats are invaluable when it comes to understanding how reading can become less than salutary.

A Passionate Pathology

> A good medicyne vn-wyseli taken may be cause of a mannys deth.[12]

Even the best medicine can be dangerous, its effects veering from healthful to harmful through the mode of its usage. Without care, without control, medicine will cause only damage. Such an observation is equally applicable to therapeutic reading and the medicines of the soul it evokes. Dread, penance, compassion and longing – all the emotional medicines that promote sowle-hele – are themselves dangerous and damaging if not correctly used. Their potency is, in part, their problem: any powerful medicine must be used in accordance to set parameters – and emotional medicines generated through reading all the more so. Many texts of spiritual guidance note that while such treatment of the soul is good, it can all too easily become deeply harmful, generating states of mind and even body that are morally and spiritually dangerous. The soul's medicines can quickly 'roten & turnen to corrupcioun' causing the soul not to progress in virtue but rather behave as 'wex whenne hit melteþ'.[13]

Frequent meditation on Christ's suffering, yearning for Him, and contemplation of divinity are fraught with danger, as the cognitive and emotive impacts of these activities can cause individuals to 'trauayle þeire ymaginacion so vndiscreetly, þat at þe laste þei turne here brayne in here hedes'.[14] The mention here of the imagination is crucial, as any act of reading requires the operation of the imaginative faculty to generate memory phantasms. These phantasms are part image and part emotional reaction to that image. Thus, cautions regarding the 'vndiscreet' imagination are, at their core, cautions about the dangers of immoderate emotional states. Such immoderation is the main cause of damage and dissolution to the soul. An overly stimulated imagination will not only run amok, generating bizarre physiological sensations and disturbances such as 'a fals hete', but also act as the main vector by which demonic temptations occur – 'after soche a fals felyng comeþ a fals knowyng in þe feendes scole'.[15] So wary is the *Cloud* that it even refrains from offering any examples of false visions or temptations, for fear they may in fact corrupt those who read of them.[16] The rationale is clear: a mind beset with disordered images will produce similarly disordered emotions. The text clarifies, noting that those 'newe set to þe scole of deuocion' do not grasp how precisely calibrated the emotions of 'sorow' and 'desire' are, and instead 'þei streyne here veynes & here bodily miȝtes so beestly & so rudely, þat with-inne schort tyme þei fallen ouþer into werynes & a maner of vnlisty febilnes in body & in soule'.[17] Immoderate striving in generating these states of sorrow and longing through the imagination is animalistic, and immediately exerts a savage force upon body and soul that is far from salutary. It is advice given repeatedly and with greater detail:

> Streyne not þin hert in þi brest over-rudely, ne oute of mesure; bot wirche more wiþ a list þen wiþ any liþer strengþe. For ever þe more listly, þe more meekly & goostly; & euer þe more rudely, þe more bodely & beestly. & þerfore bewar . . . sekirly soche rude streynynges ben ful harde fastnid in flescelines of bodely felyng, & ful drie fro any wetyng of grace; & þer hurte ful sore þe sely soule, & make it feestre in fantasie feinid of feendes.[18]

To function correctly, medicine must be meticulous. The problem here is not effort, but rather a lack of moderation and proper understanding in that effort. The key word is 'rudely', an adverb which has a range of meanings all operative here, from the obvious of 'roughly', 'violently' and 'forcefully', to the less obvious of 'carelessly', 'unskilfully', and 'without judgement'.[19] The idea of immoderation is inherent in this word choice, and describes here the excess and imprecision of those 'streynynges' of the 'hert'. The passions of the soul – its emotional medicines – are out of order. It is a state contrasted with the better course of treatment – to 'wirche more wiþ a list þen wiþ and liþer strengþe'.

Once again, delimitations are key. This word 'list' has a range of meanings, covering 'desire' and 'love', but also 'cunning' and 'stratagem'.[20] Its usage here conveys the sense of ordered love, of strategically planned and enacted emotion.[21] This is also reflected in the careful structure of the passage, as the use of prose rhythm and rhyme in 'listly/meekly/goostly' enacts the very order it describes. It alone leads to God and treats the soul, whereas the immoderate and rude love causes sickness, making the soul 'feestre in fantasie feinid of feendes'. While the whole passage uses elements of alliteration and prose rhythm, it becomes denser here, falling most strongly on those fricatives which generate a sense of urgency through their sinister sound. The rapid dissent into chaos and sickness is enacted both through the end rhyme of 'rudely/bodely/beestly' and in this cascade of alliteration. Rich in medical meaning is the word 'feestre', which primarily means 'ulceration', but also 'fistula' and 'poisonous decay'.[22] The result of immoderate emotion is made clear: it will cause the imaginative faculty to ulcerate, to become a cognitive and emotional fistula where the emotions become poisons and demonic temptation occurs. Far from helping the soul, the therapeutic emotions of dread, penance, compassion and longing can in fact destroy it. When used 'vndiscreetly', they corrupt the soul in specific ways. As the *Cloud* makes clear, the attempt to treat the soul is beset with dangers. Immoderate and excessive emotions can cause madness, a profoundly self-destructive sorrow, and spiritual pride as demonic as it is subtle. As the text notes, 'it is þe rediest wey to deþ of body & of soule, for it is woodnes & no wisdom, & lediþ a man euen to woodnes'.[23] The soul's emotions exert a force that can compromise cognition, and so harm the mind and ultimately the body. The negative effects are given colourful articulation:

> Some sette þeire iȝen in þeire hedes as þei were sturdy scheep betyn in þe heed, & as þei schulde diȝe anon. Som hangen here hedes on syde, as a worme were in þeire eres. Som pipyn when þei schuld speke, as þer were no spirit in þeire bodies . . . I sey þat þei ben tokenes of pride & coryouste of witte, & of vnordeynde schewyng & couetise of knowyng. & specyaly þei ben verri tokenes of vnstabelnes of herte & vnrestfulnes of mynde, & namely of þe lackyng of þe werk of þis book.[24]

This example of spiritual physiognomy makes it clear that strange countenances and bodily disturbances are the result of corrupt emotions. The imagery used is startling and potent – rolling eyes, brutalised animals, parasites in the ear, and an inability to speak. Such imagery endows the overall diagnosis with a degree of force and gravitas: these overt physical symptoms point to an equally unsettling spiritual problem. It is the emotions that have been corrupted – 'vnstabelnes of herte & vnrestfulnes of mynde' – generating not virtue but the vices of 'pride & coryouste . . . & couetise'. Instability and the reference to beastly behaviour echo prior advice that focuses on immoderate emotion. Yet they go further, noting that the proper operation of the mind and even body have been compromised. Without precision, without order, these emotions corrupt and destroy. Instead of sowlehele there is only further damage to the state of the soul. Madness is the result, a complete breakdown of the inner wits. Hilton's *Of Angels Song*, offers further clarification, and echoes advice found in the *Cloud*. He notes that he who 'ouertravillis be ymagynacion hys wyttes, and be vndiscrete travelynge turnes þe braynes in hys heued & forbrekes þe my3tes & þe wittes of þe saule & of þe body . . . in a fransy'.[25] Once again, a lack of moderation will cause systemic cognitive problems that result in demonic temptation and a kind of spiritual infection. Frenzy or 'fransy' – *phrenesis* or *frenesis* – was understood by medieval medicine as a quasi-chronic brain infection, and is used here to make similar warnings regarding the purification of the emotions.[26] Such advice on the importance of moderation and order is consistent throughout Hilton's writings. In his *Scale of Perfection* he stresses that the reformation of the soul is incremental, subject to precise gradations mediated through equally precise emotions:

> For a man schal not come to goostli delite in contemplacioun of His Godhede, but yif he come first in ymaginacion bi bitirnesse and compassioun and bi stable trouthe and stidefaste mynde of His manhede.[27]

This is an ideal state, difficult to achieve even for the practised. The issue here is not simply the presence of specific emotions, but also the manner of their manifestation. While the soul must experience a 'bitir' penitential sorrow and be tortured through 'compassioun', it must experience these states 'bi stable trouthe and stidefaste mynde': the emotions do not run unchecked, but are here subject to an ordered and calibrated emergence. Emphasis is placed upon this sense of order, as it acts as a barrier to further progress in the treatment of the soul. If there is no order and control in the use of the imagination to generate emotion, then the higher states of spiritual reformation enabled by contemplation cannot be achieved. The implication here is that without stability and steadfastness, the emotional treatment of the soul will be anything but beneficial.

Hilton elaborates upon this elsewhere, noting that 'thei bi undiscrecion, ofte sithes overtravailen hire wittes and breken here bodili myght, and so thei fallen into fantasies and singulere conceites, or into open errours'.[28] A lack of order in the emotional treatment of the soul will in fact damage it, causing sickness, madness, and eventually 'errour' or heterodox opinions. For Hilton, the experience of fear, penance or compassion does not automatically generate positive effects for the soul. Although they can operate as emotional medicines they can just as easily function to generate sin, creating a 'prevei pride and presumpcion of hemself'.[29] In the broadest sense, misused and misapplied emotions can cause both sickness and sin. The texts of the *Cloud*-corpus can provide some clarification. This is a grouping of four letters of spiritual guidance, and three translations and adaptations of other works of spiritual discernment and contemplative guidance.[30] The translation of the *Benjamin Minor* notes:

> Ouer moche drede bryngiþ in dispeyre. And ouer moche sorow castiþ a man into bitternes & heuines of kynde, for þe whiche he is vnable to receyue gostly coumforte. And ouer moche hope is presumpcioun. And outrageous loue is falteryng & glosyng. And outrageous gladnes is dissolucioun and wantonnes. And vntemprid hateredyn of synne is woodnes. And on þis manner þei ben vnordeynd & vnmesured, & þus ben þei tornyd vnto vices.[31]

Excess within the emotions is fatal to the health of the soul. Without order and control even the most salutary emotions turn into poisons that damage and destroy. The whole passage is comprised of a lexis of excess and immoderation, with the constant repetition of 'Ouer moche', 'outrageous', and the echoing sounds of 'vntemprid/vnordeynd/vnmesured'. Here the dangers of a loss of control and moderation are made clear: an emotion evoked too strongly and without sufficient care will become corrupt, corrupting the soul itself. In this manner it moves not closer to the goal of sowle-hele but further from it and from God. Other texts go into more detail regarding these potential dangers, and often focus on a particular emotion.

In the *A Pistle of Preier*, the effects of dread are given sustained attention. This short text of spiritual guidance is beguilingly complex, and while it states that its function is to offer advice on prayer, it immediately specifies that this advice will deal with 'how þou schalt reule þin hert in tyme of þi preier'.[32] From its outset this text is concerned with affective control and moderation during prayer; an activity that would, at first glance, be thought of as only beneficial to the soul. Spiritual practices are not always what they seem, and the text makes it clear that constant vigilance and restraint must be exercised. Its initial counsel is one of imaginative sophistication: to begin prayer by truly believing that 'þou schalt diȝe in þe ende of þi preier'.[33] Such a grim forethought will, the text asserts, 'bring into þin hert a verrey worching of drede'.[34] This drede will stabilise 'þi fals, fleschly, blinde herte', and is 'þe biginnyng of wisdom'.[35] However, while this drede has a useful purpose, it must also be precisely controlled. There is danger with drede even in the practice of prayer:

> Bot for-þi þat þer is no sekir stonding upon drede onliche for drede of sinking into ouer moche heuines, þerefore schalt þou knit to þi first þouȝt . . . a sekir staf of hope to holde þee bi in alle þi good doinges.[36]

Fear can become fathomless. It is figured here as an emotional mire that will soon envelop the soul within its bleak totality. Its limitless nature can cause an 'ouer moche heuines' – a state of spiritual depression and dejection that is all-consuming. The advice here is to seek balance, a form of emotional moderation and control through the evocation of another emotion – hope. Without such a combination, drede will become too strongly felt, and begin to damage the soul and mind. The word used here – heuines – has a range of meanings that show how complex the effects of drede can be. While it is used here primarily to mean a sort of psychological lassitude and oppressive anxiety, it has additional meanings that cover the sin of sloth or spiritual torpor, as well as the emotions of sorrow and despair.[37] Too much drede has, therefore, the potential to generate a corrupted penitential subjectivity – a sorrow that twists into despair. When the text stresses the importance of hope, it is responding to this particular danger: the only hope that can counterbalance drede is 'a certein hope of forȝeuenes'.[38] Problems with the emotions are rarely self-contained, and the dangers of drede can easily overlap with the dangers of other emotions evoked in the treatment of the soul. Thus, although sorrow for sin is of course important, it too must be moderated and kept in check. It is an issue that the *Cloud* author returns to in greater detail over the course of his other works. When dealing with sorrow, he notes how carefully calibrated this state must be:

> Bot in þis sorow nedeþ þee to haue a discrecion on þis maner: þou schalt be ware in þe tyme of þis sorow þat þou neiþer to rudely streyne þi body ne þi spirit, bot sit ful stylle, as it were in a slepynge sleiȝt, all forsobbid & for-sonken in sorow.[39]

While these comments emerge from the *Cloud*'s discussion of advanced contemplation, specifically how the contemplative comes to realise that their own being is the greatest obstacle to full unity with God, they nevertheless are of much wider relevance. Sorrow, as one of the key emotions in the treatment of the soul, must be evoked and experienced with precise care. Here the problem is not with sorrow per se, but rather the level of its intensity: it must not be 'rudely' – or immoderately – evoked. The words used to describe it emphasise moderation, stillness and calm. While the overall goal is to be 'all forsobbid & for-sonken in sorow', it is a sorrow that is 'ful stylle', experienced in a manner akin to 'slepynge'. There is a gentleness and silence to sorrow, a sense of tranquility and repose. There are no roaring tears, no frantic energy, only utter immersion in sorrow.

The use of the intensifier 'for' in 'forsobbid & for-sonken' is significant, as it conveys a potency that has to some extent spent itself: the loose alliteration here suggests a state that is beyond tears – that deep and total sorrow which comes after all tears have been shed. Such language conveys depth not exuberance, a totality of feeling rather than its initial outburst. It is an emotion of utmost delicacy, balanced within itself by the presence of another: like the hope within drede, this sorrow 'is ful of holy desire'.[40] Its composite nature will safeguard against the dangers of excess. As ever 'discrecion' is key. Without it, this sorrow will become disruptive and uncontrollable, overwhelming the soul and leading to sin and demonic temptation. It is a danger the text briefly mentions – 'in al þis sorow he desireþ not to vnbe, for þat were deuelles woodnes & despite vnto God'.[41] If left uncontrolled, sorrow will become corrupted and turn inward, generating a demonic madness that seeks to harm both body and soul. The key word is 'vnbe' – a rejection of existence and life itself. It is easily more harmful than the spiritual depression and lassitude caused by immoderate fear, as this corrupted sorrow generates despair so total that it sees the rejection of sin and the rejection of life as one and the same.[42] It is the utmost corruption of the penitential impulse that other texts explore in more detail:

> Þou shalte hate þi synne, þou shalt not hate þi-selfh as a man, but as a synful man. For-whi, what shul we hate but þat þat is euel & contrarie & noyous to vs. Soþeli not ellis. What is þenne worsh þenne for to reise vp þi-seelf aȝeynst god & what is more contrarie þen for to kast ouȝte þe medicine of cristes blood. And what is to þe more noyous þenne sleynge of þyn owne soule, þus hast þou don to þyn owne seelf & mykel wers þen I can telle þe, þere-fore þourȝe consideracioun of þi vilite, lerne for to hate þi-self as þou hast made þe, and loue þat god hath made.[43]

Initially contrition works to purge sin, and more broadly helps erode pride and self-love. Yet the consideration of one's sins that sorrow entails can soon become problematic. Without careful control, sorrow soon oversteps its boundaries, generating a mental perspective that views sin and life as equivalent. This misapprehension is the root cause of additional problems. Hating the self is, indirectly, a twofold form of rebellion against God. In the first instance, such hatred of the self seeks to harm God's own creation, to the 'sleynge of þyn owne soule', and thus is not really contrition but rather the nihilistic attitude shared by 'þe fende and dampnyd soules'.[44] In the second instance this self-hatred dismisses Christ's sacrifice as, seemingly, neither necessary nor sufficient. Instead of healing the soul, such sorrow rejects the 'medicine of cristes blood' and replaces it with a sinful self-absorption and presumption: it is sacrilegious in the worst possible way, twisting the penitential subjectivity that sorrow ought to generate into a rebuke of Christ's sacrifice. In this way, an immoderate emotion can soon become not simply spiritually damaging, but also pathological – generating sin itself. As Hilton notes, sin is nothing other than a 'fals mysruled love unto thisilf'.[45] Immoderate and uncontrolled emotions will fester, producing sicknesses within the soul both subtle and gross. Pride is first among them, both in terms of danger and frequency.

In *Of Angels Song*, Hilton stresses that even those who experience inner spiritual states by reciting the Holy Name 'may be desceyved be vayn-glorye', as it is their activity that generates these inner states, not a special grace of God.[46] The danger here is presumption of election, an inflation of the self at the expense of others. Those who read moving narratives of Christ's Passion and Nativity are in the same category, open to immoderate passions and the subsequent presence of pride. This is given vivid expression in the *Prickynge of Love*, when the text notes that those who pursue the contemplative life can fall to 'suggestiouns of pride & of presumpcioun'.[47] This pride is seen in medical terms:

> A þis is pryue pestylence bitterer þan deeth, but ȝif a man be war of hit. For-whi, hit dryueth oute criste fro þe soule þat may not suffre presumpcioun ne pride reste wiþ hym . . . þis pride makiþ a soule tome & voide of goostli gladnesse & of grace of deuocioun & of quyknesse of spirite, and kestiþ hym in-to accidie into ydelnesse þat a man leseth affeccioun of charite þat haue to god & to man, and makith hym hard & vnkynde wiþ-outen affeccious, and hit makiþ al þynge þat shulde be referrid to goddis worship, for to be al turned to his owne worshepe & to his owen ese and to þe feendis disseyte.[48]

Like a plague, pride acts as a corrosive and relentless force that consumes everything of spiritual value. Its presence not only halts any progress made in the restoration of the soul, but negates it. Instead of moving closer to that state of health, the soul in fact becomes more diseased. The phrase 'tome & voide' conveys the extent of this damage. For a soul to be 'tome' means that it is not only empty, hollow and uninhabited, but also spiritually deprived.[49] The use of 'voide' enhances this sense of spiritual bareness, and extends it to show additional problems within the soul. The vast semantic range of this word allows various interpretations, such as 'spiritually worthless', 'arrogant', 'devoid of reason' and 'spiritually apostate'.[50] Pride destroys all virtue in the soul, harming rather than healing it. From here, the sin of *accidia* – or spiritual sloth – emerges, and the soul soon is overwhelmed with a lethargy that prohibits any chance of its recovery. Pride and sloth generate a profound indifference within the soul to the needs of others: the emotional powers are unmoved by God or His creation, as the soul in effect becomes completely isolated – locked within a smug and perpetual self-regard. This is potentially the most dangerous state for the soul to be in, as such self-fixation means that it cannot be easily treated again with more moderately applied emotional medicines.

As the treatment of the soul progresses through ever more intensive emotions, the dangers become all the more pressing. Even the most potent medicine of the soul, 'longyng', is subject to warnings:

> A man þat was holde an hiȝ lyuer, ofte was axid for to speke of goostli loue. And þane he bigan for to seye þe falseheed, þe perels and þe disseytis, þat oftsiþis fallen in goostly loue. And he seyde: 'Þer is no þing in al þe world, neiþer man ne feend, ne noon oþer þing, þat I haue so myche suspect as I haue þe affeccioun of loue; ne þat I am so soore a-feerd of, but if it be wel sett. For-whi loue is so passynge a þing and so cleuynge, þat it synkiþ deppir in a soule, þan ony oþir þing may do. And þere is no þing þat so fully occupieþ and byndiþ and ouer-maistriþ a mannys herte, as dooþ loue. Wherfore, it is ful hard, wheþer it be good loue or badde.'[51]

The burning desire for God can all too easily rage out of control. Longyng, that complex blend of love and pain, of fear and hope, is the most powerful – and thus most dangerous – medicine to take. Hilton's words here report only the dangers and hazards of such a state of emotional intensity. The problem lies with its force and nature. This love is 'passynge' – something so extreme and exceedingly intense that it dominates the soul. The words used to describe the effects of such longing – 'occupieþ/byndiþ/ouer-maistriþ' – convey this sense of domination: longyng operates by taking the soul prisoner, completely overpowering and controlling it by virtue of its sheer force. It can do so because of its unique nature. As discussed in the prior chapter, longyng is comprised of multiple emotions that engage multiple parts of the soul – it can 'synkiþ deppir' than any other emotional medicine. Because of this ability to completely pervade the soul, longing can damage its very substance. For Hilton, emotions can corrupt; but emotions that exert a comprehensive and absolute force upon the soul can corrupt it absolutely. The key is moderation, that such longyng 'be wel sett' – ordered, governed and contained with great deliberation and care.

What is needed is a certain form of protection: each person who evokes this powerful emotional complex must 'haue armour of discrecioun bi which he may kepe and gouerne his loue'.[52] Love is dangerous, and requires an almost martial force to keep it in check. The vital virtue of 'discrecioun' is presented here through the concrete and visually striking image of a suit of armour: 'discrecioun' is the life-saving defence required in spiritual combat.[53] Without such protection, longyng will 'liȝtly caste doun þe soule, and make it haue a foule fal'.[54] While the passions can treat the soul, they can all too easily become the source of a greater pathology. There is a fine line between health and harm, and accordingly a number of texts emerge over the course of the period that counsel spiritual discretion. These texts aim to help their readers understand the urgent need of this spiritual armour, its highly specific nature, and how best to acquire it. The soul's treatment continues, taking on a new form and a fresh urgency.

A Discrete Self

> Right as a man that is brought neigh to the deeth thorugh bodili sikenesse, though he resseyve a medicyn bi the whiche he is restorid and sikir of his liyf, he mai not for it as tite risen up and goon to werke as an hool man mai for the feblenesse of his bodi holdeth hym doun, that hym bihoveth to abiden a good while, and kepen hym with medicynes, and dioten hym with mesure aftir the techynge of a leche til he mai fulli recovere bodili heele. Right so goostli . . . yif that he take medicynes of a good leche and use hem in tyme with mesure and descrecion, he schal mykil the sunnere be restorid and reformyd to his goostly strengthe.[55]

The process of obtaining sowle-hele is a delicate one, and cannot be rushed or hastened in any way. Incremental progress, characterised by order and control, is for Hilton the only way the soul can be properly healed. Once again the importance of 'descrecion' is highlighted – without it, no lasting healing can be effected. Hilton's use of medical imagery is apposite, but it also carries additional layers of meaning. Discretion is not itself a medicine, but rather a mode of organising treatment: the soul's medicines must be taken 'in tyme with mesure and descrecion' – in accordance with a specific plan. Its presentation here figures an ordered treatment and specific modes of self-awareness, as the patient must know not to do too much too soon. Crucially, the assistance of another person is also made clear: discretion is not a solitary activity, but rather a communal process requiring the presence and advice of a spiritual doctor. This places an intersubjective dynamic at the very heart of the soul's treatment, one as important as the medicines to be administered. Within this medicinal presentation of discretion, therefore, lies a complete summary of the role it plays in the soul's treatment: it orders and moderates these emotional medicines. It is an understanding of 'descrecion' that builds upon much earlier medieval thought.

The essential concept Hilton is referring to – *discretio spirituum* – has a long history. Initially it is seen as a way to discern angelic spirits from demonic, but is later expanded to incorporate discernment of emotional and interior motivations and thoughts. It overlaps with the concept of *probatio* – or testing – used extensively in the literature of female visionaries. Over the course of the Middle Ages, the ambit of *discretio spiritum* widens to incorporate more pastoral usages for laymen and women.[56] Yet, at its core, this concept engages with the emotional aspects of the religious life. For St Benedict it is the *mater virtutum*, integral to the regulation of both community and self.[57] St Bernard refines this idea, noting that 'discretion is not so much a virtue, as much as it is a certain moderator and charioteer of the virtues, the director of the affections, and the teacher of right living'.[58] Discretion is key in controlling the emotions as it is 'the very principle of order and wisdom within love'.[59] Without it 'virtue becomes vice, and natural affection itself a force that disturbs and destroys nature'.[60] Even when used as medicines, emotions must be subject to a moderating and organising principle. As the *Tretyse of þe Stodye of Wysdome* notes, 'þe vertewe of discrecioun nediþ to be had, wiþ þe whiche alle oþer mowen be gouernyd. For wiþouten it, alle vertewes ben tornid to vices'.[61] As the emotions are the shared fundament between vice and virtue, control of them becomes all the more important. Hilton's understanding of discretion is thus an extension of this idea of judgement married with emotional self-governance. As he states in his *Epistle on the Mixed Life*, 'gode desyre neodeþ to be ruled be discrecion, and medeful werkes to be wrouȝt in ordre of charite'.[62] Without such order, problems soon arise:

> ffor charite vnruled turneþ sumtyme to vice. And þerfore hit is seid in holi writ: Ordinauit in me caritatem, þat is to say: Vre lord ȝaf to me charite set in ordre & in rule, þat hit schulde not be lost þorw myn vndiscrecion.[63]

Even the best and noblest of intentions can quickly fester into vices. While this advice is targeted at a worldly lord embarking on a life that mixes contemplation with active works, the essential message is nevertheless relevant to the practice of therapeutic reading. Unless it is implemented with careful control and calibration, the emotions evoked by texts can become inordinately strong and soon act as an impetus for sin rather than *salus*. The use of the possessive pronoun in 'myn vndiscrecion' highlights how any inordinate or immoderate emotion belongs to the person: inherent within the psychology of mankind is a tendency towards excess. There is implicit here a critique of unchecked enthusiasm – of a state of emotional intensity that goes beyond a divinely appointed order. Discretion is, therefore, essentially a practice that brings order and control to the self and its emotional states. Such an understanding of discretion as a medically framed practice that observes the emotions, and is centred upon humility and an intersubjectivity, is given greater attention by other texts. The most notable is the *Chastising of God's Children*, a discretion text that seeks to ensure the health of the soul, and extols the importance of maintaining a constant inner vigilance over its emotions. Written in the late fourteenth century, this text has much to say about the problems of emotional stimulation.

> Sum, whan þei heere any myschief falle vnto ony womman or man, or heere hem speke ony harde wordis or dredeful bifore her dethe, anon bi temptacion þei fallen into a drede, þat longe tyme aftir þei mowe nat put it fro her herte, for nyȝt and daie, in praier and al oþer þouȝtis and tymes, þei bein so troublid þerwiþ þat verile almost þei wasten awei for drede of þe soule, and makeþ hem desire þe deþ of þe bodi, for to be delyuerd of þat temptacioun, but þat desire wiþout plesynge of god is synne. (p. 119, ll. 16–24)

Such cautions regarding the 'imagynacions of dredeful þinges' recall similar advice in the *Cloud* on the overactive imagination, but there is far greater detail here (p. 118, l.1).[64] While drede is one of the medicines of the soul, its impact here is far from salutary, and goes far beyond a state of 'ouer moche heuines'.[65] Passion becomes pathology, with drede becoming a sinful desire that is utterly self-destructive. Instead of generating a sense of humility, it arrests the mind and generates a desire to neglect the body and wish for death. The danger is pressing, as even prayer cannot shift this emotional fixation: far from beginning the treatment of the soul, such a drede could in fact result in its destruction. The cause of such a state is given precise articulation – 'wordis'. As the text makes clear, any descriptive words – written or spoken – have a direct impact upon the souls of their hearers. Thus, texts of spiritual guidance which contain vividly realised scenes of punishment, trials, or temptations are potentially dangerous. Their imagery may be too much, may evoke emotional states within the soul that are beyond any means of control. However, the text also makes a crucial point: while these verbally mediated images and narratives impact upon the emotions, they do not do so uniformly. Only 'sum' people suffer from inordinate drede and become fixated with a fear that dominates their lives; others do not. What the text articulates here is a model of spiritual physiognomy, an understanding that not everyone will behave in the same way in response to the same stimuli – that different persons will have different emotional dispositions. It is this understanding that underpins the text's dominant preoccupation: the diagnosis of emotional states that have become pathological. From its very outset there is a direct engagement with this connection between the emotional and the medical:

> Hou slouþe and ydelnesse gendren sijkenesse; and hou wirchinge wiþ grace is nedeful; and hou þre kyndes of men fallen bi vnstablenesse; and that vnstablenesse is cause of þe foure goostli feueris, and cause of al oþer errours shewed bifore; and what remedie may be to hem. (p. 94, ll. 3–7)

A diagnostic impulse lies at the very centre of the text that goes beyond simply stating a connection between sin and sickness. Immoderate emotions, or states of 'vnstablenesse', generate a whole host of spiritual pathologies – or 'foure goostli feueris'. The use of medical language here is significant, as medieval medicine understood fever as an affliction (*passio*) of the heart: precise medical language is being used to discern the nature and extent of emotional maladies.[66] The result is that the text conceives of spiritual fevers as highly specific disorders of the emotions – disorders that beset 'þre kyndes of men'. Within this specification is that sense of spiritual physiognomy: immoderate emotions will affect different people in different ways. Variety of persons means a variety of spiritual complexions, and so the need for precision in both emotional stimulation and treatment is all the greater. If the text seeks to function as a 'remedie' for such problems, it must invest considerable energy in understanding the subtle shifts and changes between different spiritual complexions. The language the text uses makes this clear. When it asserts that 'Oure kynde þan of bodili disposicioun be wele ruled aftir discrecioun', and that virtues are 'goostli humours', it deliberately expands the diagnostic ambit of discretion: it is not a form of passive judgement, but a process of constant medical appraisal and action (p. 102, ll. 12–13). To practise spiritual discretion is to be aware of one's own spiritual humours, or emotional complexion – in essence to practise a form of spiritual physiognomy. The text expands upon this greatly in later sections, making a direct comparison between physical and spiritual illnesses. In chapter seven, it notes that when 'wicked humoures bien stired', the body falls 'into dyuers sikenesse', has its 'kyndeli complexion' thrown out of balance, and succumbs to 'perlous feueres' (p. 124, ll. 7–15). Such a medical process is used as an analogy for 'gostli sikenesse' – a state of interior corruption (p. 124, l. 22):

> Þese wicked humours maken þe stomak replete, þat is to sai, fulfillen þe herte wiþ yuel wil, and letten þe sauour of alle goode uertues. Also whan suche men wexen sike for coold, þanne þei fallen into dropesie, and anon þei bien ouercharged wiþ watir, þat is to seie, þei desiren worldli goodis, and the more þei haue þe more þei coueiten, bicause þei bien sike of þe dropesie. Þe bodi, þat is to seie the lust and couetise, wexith and swelliþ grete, but þe þurst is neuer þe les. Þe face, þat is þe consciens, wexeþ leene, for he haþ lost þe sauour of goode metis, þat is to seie lackeþ þe fruyt of grace, for þei wol nat worche wiþ grace, and þis is cause of al þese sickenessis. (p. 125, ll. 14–24)

As with the body, so with the soul. Medical language has a dual function here, elucidating not only pathological problems within the body's physical systems, but also clarifying the nature of a spiritual malaise. The key phrase, 'þat is to seie', structures the entire passage, and is used to forge a conceptual equivalency between physiological and religious pathologies. Through this repeated structure, the medical register deployed in the passage is turned into a diagnostic framework that encompasses sin, desires and interiority within its physiognomic scope. While the specific emotions are not directly mentioned, their corrupted pathological states are. It begins with the problems of 'wicked humours' and 'dropesie' – the equivalents of an 'yuel wil' and an insatiable covetousness. Both are manifestations of corrupt emotions, of desires unchecked and uncontrolled. Yet the diagnosis does not stop here but moves further to cover the body and the face, which figure lust and a weak conscience respectively. Taken collectively, these corrupt emotions and the weak conscience are the 'cause of al þese sickenessis'. Such an assertion makes the point that the causes of spiritual illnesses are complex, manifold, but ultimately emotional. It is a point the text will return to time and again, but with increasingly sophisticated medical terminology. The most precise and detailed way in which the text can diagnose spiritual pathologies – corrupted emotion – is through the language of fever:

> Suche men as I spak of, whiche bien so replete of wiked humours, þat is to seie to vnskilfulli and vnresonabli bien enclyned to lustes and eesis of þe bodi, fallen oft siþes into foure maner of feueres, dyuers men into dyuers feuers as þei bien disposid. (p. 126, ll. 6–10)

Correct diagnosis depends upon adequate models of categorisation and classification. This entire passage is a brilliant synthesis of medical and religious terminology. It begins, as medieval medicine itself does, with the humours. Those 'wiked humours' mentioned earlier in the text are rendered here as initial states that soon develop into more complex and dangerous pathologies. As with prior paragraphs, this one presents these 'wiked humours' as emotional disorders – as inclinations to 'lustes and eesis of þe bodi'. Such states are, at their core, corrupted emotions, sinful desires. Building upon this medical model, the passage soon moves to more complex diagnostic terminology. From the humours we move to complexion theory, as these corrupted states lead to four types of fever that are themselves keyed to 'dyuers' types of persons. The key words here are 'enclyned' and 'disposid' which emphasise this sense of precise diagnosis: they convey the point that while wicked humours – corrupted emotions – are everywhere, they will manifest differently in different types of people. This is the most sophisticated aspect of the passage, as it uses medical terminology to understand, conceptualise and diagnose the emotional disorders besetting religious life. As the text goes on to note, fever is 'propirly in goostli remeuyng a uariaunce of þe herte': such language not only mirrors the medical definition of fever, but also directly applies it to deal with the instabilities and variances within emotional states themselves (p. 126, ll. 11–12). The specification 'propirly' makes it clear that the use of fever is not just a metaphor, but instead a functional equivalent for understanding systemic corruption within the emotions and how they manifest in each person.

The text goes on from here to list each type of fever, specifying 'cotidian', 'tercian' in its two distinct forms, 'quartan', and the doubly dangerous 'double quarteyn' (p. 126, l. 11; p. 127, l. 3; p. 129, l. 11; p. 129, l. 19). Each of these falls roughly into the medieval medical category of interpolated fevers. These are fevers that are not constant, but which wax and wane during a specified time period, and are classified according to their patterns of recurrence within a set number of hours. These terms are used here to make reference to passions that are unstable and inconsistent in their manifestation. Each type of fever is understood in terms of behavioural and psychological factors that depend upon the problems with the emotions. The first, 'cotidian', is essentially a state of emotional instability coupled with a lack of self-knowledge. Those who have it,

> liʒtli þei bien stired and som tyme troubled; her þouʒtes bien ful chaungeable, now heere, now þere, now so, now þus, liche to þe wynde. Þis is a cotidian feuere, for wiþ suche uariaunce þei bien turned and occupied from morwe into euen, and sum tyme in nyʒt, boþ sleepynge and wakyng. Al be it þat þis infirmyte may sum tyme stonde wiþout deedli synne, it lettiþ neþeles gosstli excercises and sauour of god. (p. 126, l. 18 to p. 127, l. 1)

This is a state of discord and dissension brought about through a lack of fixity and focus. The behavioural problems associated with this type of fever are essentially forms of inconsistent religious practice, but they are born out of a psychological problem. As the text notes, those who have this fever are too easily 'stired' – they suffer from an emotional hypersensitivity to both external and internal stimuli. When they are evoked, the emotions lack depth, and so change into others. As a result their 'þouȝtes bien ful chaungeable' and are 'liche to þe wynde': variability in emotions leads to variability in cognition, and eventually to inconstancy in behaviour. Such variability also leads to more damaging spiritual problems, as those who suffer from this fever 'oft siþes þei forȝetten hemsilf': self-knowledge, that key aspect in the treatment of the soul, is utterly corroded through instability in the emotions (p. 126, ll. 15–16).

The next fever 'is clepid a tercian, whiche may be seid inconstaunce or vnstablenesse', and is subdivided into hot and cold forms (p. 127, ll. 3–4). The hot form is a more pernicious version of cotidian fever. Those who have it display no fixity in their actions and behaviours at all: they are the 'fallen of vnstabilnesse' as 'þis dai þei cheesen oo lyueng or oo deuocion, tomorwe þei cheese anoþer' (p. 127, l. 21; p. 127, ll. 12–13). The second form, however, is more explicitly related to the emotions:

> Þe secunde feuer of vnstabilnesse is causid of coold, whiche sum men haue þat gladli wil loue god wiþ sum oþer þing, to þe whiche thynge þei putten her herte vnwiseli, and louen it more þanne nede is. Suche men bien diuided in hemsilf, bicause þei knowen nat wele hemsilf... Faire wordis þei shewen wiþout, but the contrarie is in þe herte. Þei desiren her uertues to be knowe, and for a fewe uertues ȝit þei wolden haue worshyp. (p. 128, l. 12 to p. 129, l. 6)

Method and measure are the problems here. Those afflicted with this form of spiritual fever are overly fixated upon the methods and practices of religious life, and ignore the overall goal: God. The initial impulse of love towards God becomes misdirected among myriad religious practices. Yet, such emotional misdirection does not equate with a lack of intensity. Immoderation in love is also present, as those with this fever love the trappings of religious life 'more þanne nede is': the emotion grows unchecked, with no measure or discretion. As this emotional fever runs its course, the results become increasingly dangerous. The lack of emotional focus and measure generates not only a division within the self, but also a form of spiritual ignorance – 'þei knowen nat wele hemsilf'. This lack of awareness is a key element in the fever's spiritual pathology, and underpins its central danger: pride. Misdirected and immoderate love soon turns inwards, causing a lack of self-knowledge and a pernicious desire to 'haue worshyp' from others. Far from generating a salutary meekness, immoderate emotion becomes the source of a damning spiritual pride.

The presence of pride – the fist and greatest manifestation of self-love – becomes the defining characteristic of the next two spiritual fevers.

> Of an vnresonable inclynenge of þe fleshli kynde, and a derk pride priueli hid, bicause of suche vnstabilnesse in sum men the quartan feuere is causid. Of þis vnstabilnesse, þat is to seie, whan a man is aliened, or wilfulli gooþ out fro god, fro hymsilf, fro al sooþfastnesse and fro al uertues ... Þis sikenesse is more perlous þan ony of þe oþer whiche I haue reherced, for out of þis quarteyn þat is clepid alienacioun sum men fallen into anoþer feuere, þat is clepid double quarteyn,

þat is to seie necligence or sleuth . . . bicasue he is slow and necligent in al maner þinges þat longen to everlastyng hele. (p. 129, ll. 9–23)

The central image in this passage of a dark pride is both compelling and sinister. It conveys with vivid force the insidious nature of these spiritual malaises and their corrupting influence. As with all the other spiritual pathologies, the root cause is 'vnstabilnesse' – a lack of order and control. As it manifests and progresses, such a condition causes further degeneration and problems for the person's spiritual health. Instead of pursuing the health of the soul, such persons pursue their own variable desires and particular vices – they suffer from 'alienacioun'. This word has a range of meanings that cover medical, judicial and theological contexts, two of which are operative here. Medically, the word means 'derangement' or 'insanity', usually due to the presence of fever.[67] Theologically, it means estrangement or desertion from God. This 'quartan feuere' thus combines these senses to figure a form of insanity that results in estrangement from God: a complete – and completely insane – removal 'fro god, fro hymsilf, fro al sooþfastnesse and fro al uertues'. Such a fever results in the negation of all progress in sowle-hele, and begets yet more sins and vices. From it stems the 'double quarteyn', a fever that is not simply pure sin but also the direct opposite of spiritual health itself: from this madness comes the sins of spiritual sloth and lassitude. Each of these fevers are dangerous and to be avoided, but they all share the common cause of 'vnstabilnesse', or lack of control and moderation in the emotions (p. 188, l. 28).

The text, however, does not rest with providing just a diagnosis of spiritual pathologies. Its medicinal frame goes much further than that, and offers remedies as well. As the text makes clear, it 'is goode to see what is þe cause of þese goostli feueris and errouris whiche I haue shewid, and so bi voidaunce of þe cause cast remedie for þe sikenesse' (p. 187, ll. 17–20). To counter the dangers of 'vnstabilnesse' within the emotions requires a specific course of treatment:

Þerfor a souereyn remedie to alle þese goostli feueris, in what degree a man stonde, it is goode to wirche bi counsaile, þat he falle nat fro goode lyueng ne fro his deuocion, ne chaunge nat to worse bi his vnstablenesse. (p. 190, ll. 7–10)

Advice, not emotion, is the best medicine for these dangerous fevers. To 'wirche bi counsaile' is an inherently communal process, one that consists of seeking out and submitting to the advice and wisdom of someone else. Instead of proceeding alone, self-medicating with the emotions without caution or control, such 'counsaile' means that all treatment exists with an endless process of consultation. As Hilton notes, health does not come all at once, but is a gradual process that involves the constant participation and care 'of a good leche'.[68] As the text goes on to clarify, to make real and lasting progress one must seek out a 'confessour . . . and aske oft counseil, and to meke hym to oþer mens preiers' (p. 155, ll. 17–19). This confessor stabilises, makes the treatment of the soul operate within the frameworks of order and moderation.

The treatment offered consists of two levels. The first is this element of intersubjectivity: the self is kept away from solipsistic tendencies and the self-loving dangers of immoderate emotions, by engaging in a consultation with another that extends a penitential subjectivity into a continuous process of self-analysis and monitoring. Related to this is the second element – meekness: to submit to the advice and counsel of this spiritual doctor, to subject all emotions and thoughts to an endless process of scrutiny, is a potent antidote for pride and presumption (p. 174, ll. 1–10). These elements are consistent with the practical application of the virtue of discretion, as they help ensure the salutary presence of humility and work to check any extreme or immoderate emotions. Other texts offer identical advice. For the *Cloud*, the soul's continued development towards God depends upon the 'counsel of sum discrete fader' as this will ensure that the soul's various stirrings are properly understood and controlled.[69] Here confession becomes an activity that extends beyond the sacrament of penance and the evocation of a penitential subjectivity, and moves towards a heightened form of spiritual diagnosis and treatment. The *Treatise of Discrescyon of Spirites* is more explicit:

> Loke þan besily by þe witnes of þi counsel and þi concience, ȝif þou haue be schreuyn and lawfuly amendid, after þe dome of þi confessour, of alle þe consentes þat euer þou consentid to þat kynde of synne þat þi þouȝt is aworde of. And ȝif þou haue not be schreuen, schriue þee þan as trewly as þou maist by grace and by counsel. And þan wite þou riȝt wel þat alle þe þouȝtes þat comen to þee aftir þi schrift, stering þee eft to þe same sinnes, þei ben þe wordes of oþer spirites þan þin owne.[70]

Guided introspection is the key to controlling the soul's various and powerful passions. Here confession is not just about the remission of sin, but rather the creation of specific modalities of self-awareness. It is not sufficient to be aware of the presence of sin in the soul; what is also needed is a deep awareness of the very motivations and impulses of spiritual ascent. The emphasis here lies more on 'þouȝt' than on 'synne'. The psychology of sin is merely an initial stage in obtaining the health of the soul, and must progress into a deeper and more fundamental engagement with the soul's preoccupations and motivations. A distinction between temporal periods undergirds this passage, and brings its subtlety and nuance into sharper relief. Initially, it begins with the self alone, with the unaided and unadvised progress of reformation within the soul. This state is akin to 'vnstabilnesse', as it is full of uncertainty regarding the soul and its motivation: despite any prior progress in the soul's treatment, it is a stage full of 'doute', of 'iuel þouȝtes', of 'vnknouing'.[71] Such internal confusion can only be remedied by the work of 'counsel' and 'concience', which are associated with an 'aftir' time within the soul. This is a temporal period characterised by calm certainty and knowing 'riȝt well' and also communal assistance: the self is not alone here, but guided and assisted by another person. This moment of 'counsel' is one of intense intersubjective engagement, as the thoughts and emotions of the old self become tested, modulated and controlled through the presence of this confessor. While such confessional self-awareness still exists within the sacrament of confession and makes the soul 'as it were, a clene paper leef', it does exert other, more salutary, effects:[72]

> Þe sely soule, at þe licnes of a schip, atteineþ at þe last to þe londe of stabelnes and þe hauen of helþe, þe whiche is þe clere and þe soþfast knowing of himself and of alle his inward disposiciouns; þorow þe whiche knowing he sitteþ quietly in hymself, as a king crouned in his rewme, miȝtly, wisely, and goodly gouernyng himself and alle his þouȝtes & steringes, boþe in body & in soule.[73]

The 'counsel' of confession leads to the health of the soul in ways beyond simply cleansing it from sin. In keeping with the nautical metaphor, the 'hauen of helþe' is reached through what confession promotes within the soul: self-knowledge. This self-knowledge is the essence of discretion, figured here as active knowledge that enables total command over the passions and powers of the soul. Mastery of the waves and waters soon turns into mastery of the self. The metaphors deployed here shift from maritime navigation to those of sovereignty and governance, and function to merge the key concept of 'helþe' with that of 'goodly gouernyng'. Knowledge of the 'inward disposiciouns', a form of spiritual physiognomy, enables all 'þou3tes & steringes' to become subject to precise control and regulation. This is the goal of discretion: a complete harmony within the self, an order and moderation of the emotions that ultimately extends to both body and soul.

Above and beyond order, such introspection generates other important states and virtues within the soul. Confession's intersubjective aspects are vital to the emergence of meekness: the open and honest submission to another person in confession is an act that by its very form encourages humility. As *The Mirror of St Edmund* notes, meekness comes 'þorw knowynge of þi-self: ffor þow mai3t not seon þi-self soþliche w3uch þow art, þat þou ne schald be Meked'.[74] Meekness, therefore, is a key part of discretion's overall impact upon the soul, and is understood as similarly therapeutic. In the *Chastising* true 'lownesse' is seen as 'anoþer remedie' for spiritual ills and fevers.[75] Other texts go into more precise detail, and explore the various constituent parts of discretion and their interrelation. The early fifteenth-century translation of St Catherine's *Dialogue*, the *Orchard of Syon*, offers a whole chapter on this very topic:

> For discrecioun is not ellis but a sooþfast knowyng which a soule schulde haue of hymsilf and of [God]. In þis knowynge discrecioun haldiþ and kepeþ hise rootis . . . This virtue of discrecioun whanne a man haþ knowynge of hymsilf worcehþ ful sikirly, if it be groundid wiþ verry meekness; for if þis mekenes were not in þe soule, as it is seid tofore, þanne were it vttirly vndiscreet. Which indiscrecioun is sett in pryde, as discrecioun is sett in mekenes.[76]

Order depends upon knowledge. Proper control of the self and its emotions requires a profound self-knowledge based upon an equally profound humility. More than simply ordered emotion, discretion is the result of a specific manifestation of a confessional self-awareness that is itself based upon the virtue of meekness. Such a connection is emphasised by the dominant contrast the passage creates between 'discrecioun' and 'indiscrecioun'. Any lack of control, order and self-knowledge in the soul is the result of the sin of pride; any discretion is the result only of meekness. In this way it is a virtuous absolute, not subject to gradation: without meekness the soul is 'vttirly vndiscreet' – there is no intermediate stage when it comes to discretion. Yet, as the texts stresses, discretion is more than simply penitential introspection. This knowledge comes from 'an holy hatrede of hymsilf, by verry mekenes'.[77] The presence of that adjective 'holy' is significant. It qualifies the 'hatrede' mentioned here, and emphasises the key work of discretion. Unlike the corruption of the penitential impulse mentioned by the *Cloud*, this 'holy hatrede' of the self is not self-destructive but rather salutary: only meek self-knowledge will ensure the 'heelþe of soulis'.[78] The text then extends the arboreal metaphor to emphasis their interconnection. It likens discretion to a 'tre þat haþ manye bowes or braunchis', that has its roots 'plauntid in þe erþe of mekenes'.[79] And it is this meekness that 'comeþ of þe knowyng þat a man haþ of hymsilf'.[80] There is a reciprocity and interconnection among discretion, meekness, and self-knowledge that is crucial to the achievement of sowle-hele. Order and moderation of the emotions is the overall goal – to ensure that the soul is not overcome by emotions, but rather uses them to achieve health. While such a concern for moderation and order does not appear so strongly in the texts explored in prior chapters, later materials advocate a reading strategy based upon temperance and knowledge of one's spiritual disposition. The *Myroure of Our Lady*, an early fifteenth-century commentary on the distinctive office of Brigittine Nuns, offers an excellent example:

> Yt is expediente that eche persone vse to rede, and to study in this maner of bokes, suche matters as be moste conuenyeute to hym for the tyme. For yf eny were drawen downe in bytternes of temptacyon or of trybulacyon yt were not spedefull to hym for that tyme to study in bokes of heuynes & drede, though he felte hymselfe wyllyng therto, but rather in suche bokes as mighte sturre vp hys affeccyons to comforte and to hope. And so is yt to be sayde dyuersely after the diuersyte of dysposycions that persones ar sturred wyth for the tyme.[81]

Reading requires not simply a text, but also a self-awareness of one's emotional disposition. Advice is given here, as well as a warning: all reading must be carried out in a manner that ensures moderation and balance of the emotions, otherwise imbalance and harm will result. In practice, the emotional complexion of the person must not only be taken into account but must also frame and guide all reading activity. The key words here are 'tyme' and 'conuenyeute' as they foreground a sense of precision, order and control. The semantic range of 'conuenyeute' is particularly significant, as the word conveys the senses of 'suitable', 'appropriate', 'effective' or 'well suited to function', and 'morally fitting'.[82] To read in this way is to read in the most functionally optimal and morally appropriate manner. Much like the *Cloud*'s emphasis on the importance of 'list' – an ordered stratagem of love – this text extolls the benefits of reading in accordance with a plan, with the level of precision and focus that comes from true self-knowledge. Reading is precisely modulated, tailored to the given emotional disposition of the person as it exists at a given moment.

Emphasis falls upon this idea of precise control: the alliteration in 'dyuersely after the diuersyte of dysposycions' draws attention to the complexity not of a given text but of the person who reads it. This awareness of variability, of constant fluctuation in emotional temperament, is the guiding principle of all reading here. Emotions still exist, and are still evoked by reading, but they all exist within a precisely controlled framework. Instead of amplifying the baseline emotional state of the soul, the reading material ought to contrast with it. The text offers advice that is much like Galenic medicine's concept of *eucrasia*, or balance: the emotions are subject to allopathic treatment, as those with a currently depressive emotional state ought to read material that promotes comfort and hope. To be medicinal, the method of reading must overcome any preferences for it: while the individual may be 'wyllyng' to read all manner of material, all reading must be tailored to the individual's inner state at a given moment. Balance is key, a state given more detailed articulation:

> For yt is written in Vitas patrum that when fendes had longe tempted an holy man; at last they cryed and sayd vnto hym 'Thow hast ouercome vs, for when we wolde lyfte the vp by to moche

hope, thou berest downe thy selfe in drede and sorow of thy synnes, & when we wolde brynge the in ouer moche drede and heuynes, then thou rerest vp thyselfe to hope, & comforte of mercy'.[83]

The lives of the Desert Fathers were ones of exemplary control, judgement and discretion in all areas – especially in regards to their emotions. The advice here shows the potential benefit of precisely moderating and balancing the emotions. Such emotional *eucrasia* moves the soul into a state of harmony and accord, endowing it with an emotional robustness that is conducive to sowle-hele: through control and discretion the soul establishes an immunity to demonic temptation. Yet, it is an immunity brought about through carefully calibrated reading. Discretion is key, and here forms a reading practice that is thoroughly integrated into the person's psychological and emotional condition. Therapeutic reading in this mode is reading enabled and constrained by the emotions themselves. To read in this way is to be attuned to one's inner state, and to seek out reading material that stimulates the emotions into harmony, not excess. Such complexional reading offers treatment that is more bespoke and directed than explored heretofore. To read in this manner is to heal, but not through extremes. Fear, penance, compassion and longing all have their place, but to ensure they do not corrupt and harm the soul they must be finely attuned to the state of the soul, evoked and experienced only as and when necessary. When used discretely, the texts of sowle-hele will treat the soul and its emotions, but they will do so through ordering those emotions, bringing a harmony to the soul that moves it towards a deep humility and calm – towards complete health: salvation.

Conclusion: Sowle-hele

The Crucifix of San Marcello, in all its black and gold splendour, is an object of religious art and devotion that sheds light on the sheer complexity of premodern ideas of healing. As its social history makes clear, religion and medicine are deeply linked in premodern cultures. Moreover, it makes the case that religious artefacts from this era and earlier have a functional sophistication to them that is lost to modern eyes. So too the texts of sowle-hele. The Vernon manuscript is an exquisite example of the medieval relationship between religion, medicine and reading. Its vast pharmacy of texts, of *verbi medicina*, are there for a specific reason – they aim to treat the soul, to enable *salus animae* through their arresting images and emotional potency. To understand this requires a careful analysis of those texts that incorporates a range of medieval perspectives on theology, literature and emotion.

This book has attempted to explore these connections and interconnections over its course, and has focused on a number of key areas. One of the most significant is that of emotion as a form of treatment. While medieval studies has explored the therapeutic potential of reading, it has only done so in regard to secular works – not vernacular devotional texts. As a result, our understanding of the connection between reading and healing is dominated by the medical account of the non-naturals and the importance it attributes to positive emotions. While joy and laughter are important, this book has shown that other emotions can perform therapeutic work as well. This becomes apparent when medieval theology's engagement with the emotions and their connection to vice and virtue is made clear. Habituated emotions – the very essence of virtue and vice – play a key role in the overall health of the soul. As a result, emotions understood by medieval medicine as dangerous are now directly useful in furthering *salus animae*: fear, penance, pity, compassion, remorse, shame and longing can all play a role in treating the soul. This book has shown how vernacular devotional texts which evoke such emotions operate within a contemporary therapeutic model. The Vernon manuscript, with its claim to provide 'sowle-hele', is situated directly within this contextual model. Its array of texts evoke only the most difficult and intense of emotional states – all for the purposes of treating the soul. Thus, when religious texts mention their medicinal function, it is not an arch conceit but rather a signal of the emotional and, by extension, therapeutic impacts they seek to enable. As a form of treatment, reading is an integral part of the religious and devotional life of the medieval period, as fascinating and as beguiling as any of its others. This book has explored the extent to which emotion, reading, medicine and religion go hand-in-hand, and in so doing it has shed light on this important aspect of medieval religious culture. And yet, as with the Cross of San Marcello, every light casts a shadow: religious emotions can become dangerously intense.

The texts in Vernon come from earlier points in medieval England's literary history, and show different languages and degrees of emotional intensity. As the last chapter of this book has shown, while there are no bad emotions when it comes to treating the soul, there are dangerously immoderate ones. Every medicine has its measure, and to exceed it can damage the health of the soul just as much as vice. The rise of texts of *discretio spiritum*, especially outside monastic circles, is a key signal that the emotional impacts of religious writing became subject to some important caveats and conditions. Reading for sowle-hele becomes more moderated and moderate in the decades after Vernon's production. A series of shifts in attitude and approach are detectable within the vernacular religious texts of the early fifteenth century. The scope of this book does not permit a full study here, but there is room for an illustrative example. Another manuscript full of devotional writings and similarly concerned with the health of the soul is the Audelay manuscript (Oxford, Bodleian Library, MS Douce 302). It was written, according to the scribe, in 1426 (fol. 22vb) by a blind chaplain. Its contents cannot match Vernon in terms of length or diversity, but it nevertheless has an identical interest in a state it calls 'soule-hele'. A therapeutic agenda underpins its overall composition and purpose, with the health of the soul being one of its fundamental preoccupations. It contains a number of texts that signal such a purpose. A text in the edition titled 'Carol number 17: Jesus flower of Jesse's Tree' presents its core subject matter – Jesus – as 'most of hele'.[1] Its exposition of the *Pater Noster* contains seven points, the sixth of which 'is moste salve to the soule' (p. 217, l. 57). So too in a section of *The Counsel of Conscience* called 'Gabriel's Salutations to the Virgin' Jesus is 'hele of al monkyn', and is the 'blessid burthe of hele'; a similar phrase occurs earlier, in the 'Virtues of the Mass' when the mass is noted to provide 'helth to al monkynd' (p. 155, l. 10, l. 28; p. 80, l. 3).

To achieve this goal of soule-hele, this collection of texts also seeks to stir the emotions. However, in so doing it shows that it is far more moderate and less intense, and is concerned not with pushing the soul to its emotional limits, but with evoking an elaborate penitential subjectivity. Key differences in approach and content are given, such as its instructions for reading: the manuscript encourages its readers to 'rede thys offt, butt rede hit sofft, / And whatt thou redust, forgeete hit noght' (p. 211, ll. 1–2). Softness and delicacy characterise these texts, and form a framework for understanding them and their therapeutic ambitions. The emotional range of the texts in the manuscript, while incorporating compassion and other emotions, is far less extreme – subject not to rapid peaks and troughs, but rather to a steady and avowedly penitential rhythm. This is evident upon close inspection of *The Counsel of Conscience*, a large combination of a range of devotional, penitential and liturgical texts. In a section called 'Prayer for Pardon After the Levation', the Passion is mentioned but not focused upon. After noting that Jesus took flesh and blood from Mary, it brings the imagery of the Passion into the verse, but only for a moment:

CONCLUSION 155

> And that same blod be grace
> Thou chidist out of thi presious syde,
> Hongyng on cross with wondis wyde.
> Fore our hele hit was. (p. 79, ll. 3–6)

Suffering is static, suspended in a moment that is strictly confined and managed. Blood flows only by implication, and not direct pictorial representation. The image of Christ on the Cross is silent and semi-glorified – 'presious' and full of grace. Unlike other, earlier, depictions of the Passion, this one is measured and managed, filled not with an abundance of images, colours or sounds, but instead the mute postures of the dead. It is powerful in its own way, but any and all emotive charge is channelled into the penitential response of that final line – all that suffering, literally unspeakable, was and is for our soule-hele. That this text is prefaced by a short verse instruction on how to pray which encourages the reader to reflect on his or her sins, only adds to the sense of emotional control and measure: penance is the focus, not the agony of Christ ('Instructions for Prayer 5', p. 79, ll. 5–6).

Similar shifts in focus are evident elsewhere. In section 'XXIII Visiting the Sick and Consoling the Needy', the Passion and ideas of soule-hele combine:

> And thenk apon his Passion –
> That fore thi love here wold he dey
> With cros, spere, nayle, and croune –
> Fore in him is al consolacion,
> And may thee hele of thi sekenes,
> And grawnt thee here now remission,
> And of thi syns foregifnes. (p. 99, ll. 249–55)

The Passion is confined to its implements, to 'cros, spare, nayle, and croune'. Any mention of the person at its centre, with His torn and broken body, does not occur. Pain and suffering are, in a sense, an absent presence here when compared with earlier treatments on the same theme. Instead, the Passion here is fragmentary, with only a procession of loosely connected images: the implements of the Passion are out of sequence, and so do not build the same emotive charge. Any mention of Jesus and emotion is confined to 'consolacion'. In this way the Passion and the emotions it evokes are not foregrounded; rather, they form a backdrop for the real focus of the stanza: penance. The last four lines form an interconnected unit, one that stresses that the sickness of the soul will be remedied through an act not of compassion but of penitential sorrow: 'remission' is connected with 'consolacion', just as 'sekenes' will eventually lead to 'foregifnes'. Such a rendering of the Passion is essentially milder, more exhortative than emotive. It has a softer tone and tenor, and is consistent with other texts.

The section called 'XVI The Seven Bleedings of Christ' would seem to provide ample sources of vivid emotional imagery. However, while this is clearly a text predicated upon the suffering of Christ, it is nevertheless focused and directed towards penitential subjectivity. Its Latin opening 'De effusione sanguinis Christi in remissione peccatorum' frames the rest of the text and provides what will be its main emotional arc. After listing each occasion on which Christ bled, the text devotes a stanza to each occasion. Yet, the overall focus is not His pain or misery, but the reader's appropriately penitential response:

> O Jhesu, fore thi scharp croune,
> That mad the blod to ren adoune
> About thi fayre face,
> Ther Proud in Her I have be,
> Lord, unbuxum to thee,
> Grawnt mercé and grace. (p. 68, ll. 37–42)

The pain and suffering of Christ generate a moment of self-reflection. While there is imagery here, it is diffuse and opaque: the crown of thorns is simply mentioned as 'scharp', and sharp enough to make blood run down the face. No further details are provided, no reactions or reflections on it or its effects – Jesus simply has it on His head. The result is powerful in its own way, but it is not overstated. Any emotional significance this image has is not permitted to develop and grow. Instead, it is subject to careful control through narrative pacing and progression. A certain brisk speed prevents the key emotional effect of earlier accounts of the Passion – intensity: the image cannot linger and deepen in its emotive charge, but instead acts only as a foil to the subsequent penitential section of the stanza. Time, like emotion, is controlled. The narrative pivots with precision between the time-past of the Passion and the time-present of penance. It is a pattern repeated in the remaining stanzas: objects of the Passion, or tokens of His suffering, are excerpted from their original narrative moment and brought into a new one where a concern for penance modulates and controls their overall emotional impact. Here, as elsewhere in the manuscript, there is no focus on the anguish of Christ or Mary, no use of what Rolle terms techniques of 'wexenge manyfold with hepynge sorewys'.[2] What there is, however, is a focus on behaviour, on correct religious observance, and the importance of correct feeling creating correct action.

The brief mentions of 'soule-hele' in the Marcolf and Solomon section of *The Counsel of Conscience* focus on behaviour – 'ye schul schew good ensampyl to the soule-hele' and 'thai schowe youe good ensampil to the soulehele' – of both persons and curates (p. 48, l. 526; p. 57, l. 798). Similarly, in Audelay's *Epilogue to the Counsel of Conscience*, the reference that 'few ther bene that sechen soulehele' is set within the wider concern for proper behaviour and the need to stay true to the fundamental readings of the faith – the 'pistill and gospel, the Sauter, treuly' (p. 136, l. 105; p. 140, l. 258). Here, soule-hele is more akin to 'þe ground of helþe, þat is cristen mannes bileeue': not intensive emotional treatment, but correct belief, correct practice, and with constant penitential self-scrutiny.[3]

In the decades after Vernon, sowle-hele changes and becomes something more moderate and less intensive. Treating the soul through the emotional manipulation reading provides still occurs, but the overall character and methods of enabling this state change. The medieval 'medicyne of words' is not always the same. But for this book, and for the interactions between medieval medicine, theology and reading it sought to explore, one point is clear: treating the soul in medieval England was a goal to be achieved by reading vernacular devotional texts; texts full of beautiful imagery and sound, of force and potency. As the Vernon manuscript shows, sowle-hele will not be achieved through texts that evoke just joy, but rather through reading material of painful intensity, through texts that evoke fear, penance, compassion and a desperate longing to be healed: *salus animae* requires the best medicines, and the best medicines are always the bitterest.

Notes

Introduction

1. For a fuller discussion of the 1522 plague see Sheryl E. Reiss, 'Adrian VI, Clement VII, and Art', in Kenneth Gouwens and Sheryl E. Reiss (eds), *The Pontificate of Clement VII: History, Politics, Culture* (Aldershot: Ashgate, 2005), pp. 341–63 (p. 344); Julia Haig Gaisser, *Pierio Valeriano on the Ill Fortune of Learned Men* (Ann Arbor: University of Michigan Press, 1999), p. 107 n. 31. For the history of the crucifix, see the Rome City Council's public website *http://www.comune.roma.it/pcr/it/newsview.page?contentId=NEW107963* accessed on 14 Dec. 2016.
2. Naoë Kukita Yoshikawa (ed.), *Medicine, Religion and Gender in Medieval Culture* (Cambridge: D. S. Brewer 2015), pp. 1–27 (p. 7).
3. Yoshikawa, *Medicine, Religion and Gender in Medieval Culture*, p. 17.
4. Leonard Boyle, 'The Fourth Lateran Council and Manuals of Popular Theology', in Thomas J. Heffernan (ed.), *The Popular Literature of Medieval England* (Knoxville: University of Tennessee Press, 1985), pp. 30–43 (pp. 40–3).
5. Jeremy Catto, 'Theology after Wycliffism,' in Jeremy Catto and Ralph Evans (eds), *The History of the University of Oxford*, vol. 2. (Oxford: Oxford University Press, 1992), pp. 263–80 (p. 265).
6. Richard Rolle, *English Psalter*, ed. Hope Emily Allen, *English Writings of Richard Rolle, Hermit of Hampole* (Oxford: Clarendon Press, 1931), p. 5.
7. This is by no means an exhaustive list, but for a selection of some of the most influential recent publications in medieval studies, see Peregrine Horden, 'Religion as Medicine: Music in Medieval Hospitals', in Peter Biller and Joseph Ziegler (eds), *Religion and Medicine in the Middle Ages* (York: York Medieval Press, 2001), pp. 135–54, his 'A Non-natural Environment: Medicine without Doctors and the Medieval European Hospital', in Barbara S. Bowers (ed.), *The Medieval Hospital and Medical Practice* (Aldershot: Ashgate, 2007), pp. 133–45; Naoë Kukita Yoshikawa, *Medicine, Religion and Gender in Medieval Culture*; her 'Holy Medicine and Diseases of the Soul: Henry of Lancaster and Le Livre de Seyntz Medicines', *Medical History*, 53 (2009), 397–414; Virginia Langum, *Medieval and the Seven Deadly Sins in Late Medieval Literature and Culture* (New York: Palgrave Macmillian, 2016); Catherine Batt, 'Henry, Duke of Lancaster's Book of Holy Medicines: The Rhetoric of Knowledge and Devotion', *Leeds Studies in English*, ns, 37 (2006), 407–14; Elena Carrera (ed.), *Emotions and Health 1200–1700* (Leiden: Brill, 2013); Carole Rawcliffe, *Communal Health in Late Medieval English Towns and Cities* (Cambridge: Boydell and Brewer, 2013); Marion Turner (ed.), 'Medical Discourse in Premodern Europe', *Journal of Medieval and Early Modern Studies*, 46/1 (2016); Naama Cohen-Hanegbi, *Caring for the Living Soul: Emotions, Medicine and Penance in the Late Medieval Mediterranean*

(Leiden: Brill, 2017); and Jeremy J. Citrome, *The Surgeon in Medieval English Literature* (New York: Palgrave Macmillan, 2006).
8   Glending Olson, *Literature as Recreation in the Later Middle Ages* (Ithaca: Cornell University Press, 1985). He revisits some of these themes in a later publication: 'The Profits of Pleasure', in Alistair Minnis and Ian Johnson (eds), *The Cambridge History of Literary Criticism Volume Two: The Middle Ages* (Cambridge: Cambridge University Press, 2005), pp. 275–90.
9   Brian Stock, 'Healing Meditation, and the History of Reading', *New Literary History*, 37 (2006), 503–13, and Brian Stock, 'Minds, Bodies, Readers', *New Literary History*, 37 (2006), 489–501.
10 This is not an exhaustive list, only a selection of the most pertinent and influential contributions that have informed scholarship in medieval studies. For a useful overview of these terms, see Melissa Gregg and Gregory Seigworth (eds), *The Affect Theory Reader* (Durham, NC: Duke University Press, 2010); William M. Reddy, 'Against Constructionism: The Historical Ethnography of Emotions', *Current Anthropology*, 38 (1997), 327–51; Reddy, *The Navigation of Feeling: A Framework for the History of Emotions* (New York: Cambridge University Press, 2001); Reddy, 'Historical Research on the Self and Emotions', *Emotion Review*, 1 (2009), 302–15; Reddy, 'Neuroscience and the Fallacies of Functionalism', *History and Theory*, 49 (2010), 412–25; Sara Ahmed, *Cultural Politics of Emotion* (New York: Routledge, 2004); Luc Ciompi, *Die emotionalen Grundlagen des Denkens: Entwurf einer fraktalen Affektlogik* (Göttingen: Vandenhoeck und Ruprecht, 1997); Barbara H. Rosenwein, *Emotional Communities in the Early Middle Ages* (Ithaca, NY: Cornell University Press, 2006); Peter King, 'Emotions in Medieval Thought', in Peter Goldie (ed.), *The Oxford Handbook of the Emotions* (Oxford: Oxford University Press, 2010), pp. 167–88; Simo Knuuttila, *Emotions in Ancient and Medieval Philosophy* (Oxford: Oxford University Press, 2004), his 'Emotion', in Robert Pasnau (ed.), *The Cambridge History of Medieval Philosophy: Volume One* (Cambridge: Cambridge University Press, 2010), pp. 428–40, his 'Medieval Theories of the Passions of the Soul', in Henrik Lagerlund and Mikko Yrönsuuri (eds), *Emotions and Choice from Boethius to Descartes* (Dordrecht: Kluwer Academic Publishers, 2002), pp. 49–84, and his exceptionally useful 'Emotions from Plato to the Renaissance', in Simo Knuuttila and Juha Sihvola (eds), *Sourcebook for the History of the Philosophy of Mind: Philosophical Psychology from Plato to Kant* (London: Springer, 2014), pp. 463–98; Martin Pickavé and Lisa Shapiro (eds), *Emotion and Cognitive Life in Medieval and Early Modern Philosophy* (Oxford: Oxford University Press, 2012); Naama Cohen-Hanegbi, 'A Moving Soul: Emotions in Late Medieval Medicine', *Osiris*, 31/1 (2016), 46–66; and Damien Boquet and Piroska Nagy, 'Medieval Sciences of Emotions during the Eleventh to Thirteenth Centuries: An Intellectual History', *Osiris*, 31/1 (2016), 21–45.
11 Brian Massumi, 'The Autonomy of Affect', *Cultural Critique*, 31 (1995), 83–109; Ruth Leys, 'The Turn to Affect: A Critique', *Critical Inquiry*, 37 (2011), 434–72; Joseph LeDoux, 'Rethinking the Emotional Brain', *Neuron*, 72 (2012), 653–76.
12 Mirko D. Grmek, *Diseases in the Ancient Greek World*, tr. Mireille Muellner and Leonard Muellner (Baltimore: John Hopkins University Press, 1989), p. 1.
13 See Naama Cohen-Hanegbi, Damien Boquet and Piroska Nagy in *Osiris*, 31/1.
14 Knuuttila, *Emotions*, p. 3.
15 Knuuttila, *Emotions*, p. 3.
16 Boquet and Nagy, 'Medieval Sciences of Emotions', p. 24.
17 Vincent Gillespie: 'Lukynge in haly bukes: Lectio in some Late Medieval Spiritual Miscellanies', *Analecta Cartusiana*, 106/2 (1984), 1–27; 'Strange Images of Death: The Passion in Later Medieval English Devotional and Mystical Writing', *Analecta Cartusiana*, 117 (1987), 111–59; 'Mystic's Foot: Rolle and Affectivity', in Marion Glasscoe (ed.), *The Medieval Mystical Tradition in England: Volume Two* (Exeter: Exeter University Press, 1982), pp. 199–230; 'The Senses in Literature: The Textures of Perception', in Richard G. Newhauser (ed.), *A Cultural History of the Senses in the Middle Ages* (London: Bloomsbury, 2016), pp. 153–73; 'The Songs of the Threshold: Enargeia and the Psalter', in Francis Leneghan and Tamara Atkin (eds), *The Psalms and Medieval English Literature: From the Conversion to the Reformation* (London: Boydell & Brewer, 2017), pp. 271–97.

Alistair Minnis, 'Affection and Imagination in *The Cloud of Unknowing* and Walter Hilton's *Scale of Perfection*', *Traditio*, 39 (1983), 323–66. William F. Pollard and Robert Boeing (eds), *Mysticism and Spirituality in Medieval England* (Cambridge: Boydell & Brewer, 1997).

[18] Nicholas Watson, *Richard Rolle and the Invention of Authority* (Cambridge: Cambridge University Press, 1991); Denis Renevey, *Language, Self, and Love: Hermeneutics in the Writings of Richard Rolle and the Commentaries on the Song of Songs* (Cardiff: University of Wales Press, 2001).

[19] Jennifer Bryan, *Looking Inward: Devotional Reading and the Private Self in Late Medieval England* (Philadelphia: University of Pennsylvania Press, 2008). Michelle Karnes, *Imagination, Meditation and Cognition in the Middle Ages* (Chicago: University of Chicago Press, 2011).

[20] Mark Amsler, *Affective Literacies: Writing and Multilingualism in the Late Middle Ages* (Turnhout: Brepols, 2011), p. 11.

[21] Ayoush Lazikani, *Cultivating the Heart: Feeling and Emotion in Twelfth and Thirteenth Century Religious Texts* (Cardiff: University of Wales Press, 2015), p. 4. Her idea of 'co-feeling' is interesting, though it is limited to discussion of the emotions. I pursued a similar, though broader idea, which I termed 'co-experience' in my Ph.D. thesis: Daniel B. McCann, 'Possible Selves: Imagined Experience, Narrative Transformation, and Late Medieval Religious Literature' (unpublished Ph.D. thesis, Queen's University Belfast, 2010).

[22] Sarah McNamer, *Affective Meditation and the Invention of Medieval Compassion* (Philadelphia: University of Pennsylvania Press, 2010), p. 12; pp. 50–70.

[23] McNamer, 'The Literariness of Literature and the History of Emotion', *PMLA*, 130/5 (2015), 1433–42. Her work draws from the work of Keith Oatley, 'A Taxonomy of the Emotions of Literary Response and a Theory of Identification in Fictional Narrative', *Poetics*, 23 (1994), 53–74; Jenefer Robinson, *Deeper than Reason: Emotion and Its Role in Literature, Music, and Art* (Oxford: Oxford University Press, 2005); Suzanne Keen, 'Introduction: Narrative and the Emotions', *Poetics Today*, 32 (2011), 1–53; and Patrick C. Hogan, *Affective Narratology: The Emotional Structure of Stories* (Lincoln: University of Nebraska Press, 2011).

[24] McNamer, 'The Literariness of Literature', 1436.

[25] Brian Boyd, *On the Origin of Stories: Evolution, Cognition, and Fiction* (Cambridge: Harvard University Press, 2009).

[26] A useful analogy is Chaucer's *Canterbury Tales* – a work which is concerned with the inter-relationship between tales, between tellers, and between tellers and tales: such inter-relations and inter-textual reactions can be seen as a parallel for the dynamic emergence of intersubjectivity through reading highly emotive medieval texts.

[27] McNamer, 'The Literariness of Literature', 1436.

[28] Mary Carruthers, *The Experience of Beauty in the Middle Ages* (Oxford: Oxford University Press, 2013), p. 168.

[29] Jeremy Catto, '1349–1412: Culture and History,' in Vincent Gillespie and Samuel Fanous (eds), *The Cambridge Companion to Medieval English Mysticism* (Cambridge: Cambridge University Press, 2011), pp. 113–31 (p. 126).

[30] Oxford, Bodleian Library, MS Eng. poet. a. 1, fol. 1.

[31] Rolle, *English Psalter*, p. 5.

[32] See Rawcliffe, 'On the Threshold of Eternity: Care for the Sick in East Anglian Monasteries', in Christopher Harper-Bill, Carole Rawcliffe and Richard G. Wilson (eds), *East Anglia's History: Studies in Honour of Norman Scarfe* (Woodbridge: The Boydell Press, 2002), pp. 41–72.

[33] Vivian Nutton, 'God, Galen, and the Depaganization of Ancient Religion', in Peter Biller and Joseph Ziegler (eds), *Religion and Medicine in the Middle Ages* (York: York Medieval Press, 2001), pp. 15–32 (25).

[34] Elisabeth Hsu and Stephen Harris (eds), *Plants, Health, and Healing: On the Interface of Ethnobotany and Medical Anthropology* (New York: Berghahn, 2010).

[35] See *Timaeus* 86b–90d, and also *Phaedo* 107c.

[36] Celsus, *De Medicina*, ed. and tr. W. G. Spencer (Cambridge, MA: Harvard University Press, 1956), p. 16.

37 Faith Wallis (ed.), *Medieval Medicine: A Reader* (Toronto: Toronto University Press, 2010), p. 544.
38 Celsus, *De Medicina*, p. 25.
39 Celsus, *De Medicina*, p. 25.
40 The precise origin of this schema in Galen is subject to revision and debate, as Galen revised many of his ideas over his lifetime. For an analysis of this theory in Galen see L. J. Rather, 'The "six things non-natural": A Note on the Origins and Fate of a Doctrine and a Phrase', *Clio Medica*, 3 (1968), 337–47; P. Niebyl, 'The Non-Naturals', *Bulletin of the History of Medicine*, 45/5 (1971), 486–92; and Luis Garcia-Ballester, 'On the Origin of the "Six Non-natural Things" in Galen', in Jutta Kollesch and Diethard Nickel (eds), *Galen und das hellenistische Erbe. Verhandlungen des IV. Internationalen Galen-Symposiums* (Stuttgart: Franz Steiner Verlag, 1993), pp. 105–15.
41 This list is far from static, and over the course of the medieval period there were variations in translation, some of which expand the therapeutic potential of the non-naturals greatly. See Pedro Gil Sotres, 'The Regimens of Health', in Mirko Grmek (ed.), *Western Medical Thought from Antiquity to the Middle Ages* (Cambridge, MA: Harvard University Press, 1998), pp. 291–319. A more extensive analysis of the non-naturals is in Arnald of Vilanova's *Regimen sanitatis ad regem Aragonum*, in *Arnaldi de Villanova Opera medica omnia*, ed. Luis Garcia-Ballester, vol. 10/1 (Barcelona: Pagès Editors, 1996), pp. 321–27. I am grateful to Dr William MacLehose for bringing this to my attention.
42 Jean Leclercq, *The Love of Learning and the Desire for God: A Study of Monastic Culture*, tr. Catherine Misrahi (New York: Fordham University Press, 1982), pp. 16–20.
43 *Secretum Secretorum: Nine English Versions*, ed. M.A. Manzalaoui, EETS O. S. 276 (Oxford: Oxford University Press, 1977), p. 8, ll. 32–5.
44 Olson, *Literature as Recreation*, p. 57.
45 Johannitius, *Isagoge*, in Faith Wallis (ed.), *Medieval Medicine: A Reader* (Toronto: University of Toronto Press, 2010), p. 146.
46 This division has a long history in philosophy, but Avicenna was writing with a more medical focus and agenda here. See Knuuttila, *Sourcebook*, pp. 478–9.
47 *Avicenna Latinus: Liber de Anima seu Sextus de Naturalibus, IV–V*, ed. Gerard Verbeke (Leiden: Brill,1968), 4, p. 58. The translation is from Knuuttila, *Sourcebook*, p. 479.
48 Olson, *Literature as Recreation*, p. 112.
49 Carruthers, *Beauty*, p. 30.
50 Two of the non-naturals – sleep and waking, and the air and environment – are not really included but more alluded to. For instance, Jerome notes in a letter to Eustochium 'let sleep steal upon you with a book in your hand, and let the sacred page catch your drooping head' (Jerome, *Selected Letters*, tr. F. A. Wright (Cambridge, MA: Harvard University Press, 1933), p. 22, l. 17). Similarly, Cassian likens such reading to being at rest 'as it were immersed in the stupor of sleep' – see *John Cassian: The Conferences*, tr. Boniface Ramsey (New York: Paulist Press, 1997), p. 515; for Hugh of St Victor, meditation can be like 'a strong gust of air' (*flatu vehementioris*), see his *Homiliae in Ecclesiasten* 1, PL 175, cols 117C–118A.
51 For more detailed information on their interrelationship, see Jay M. Hammond, 'Contemplation and the Formation of the *Vir Spiritualis* in Bonaventure's *Collationes in Hexaemeron*', in Timothy J. Johnson (ed.), *Franciscans at Prayer* (Leiden: Brill, 2007), pp. 123–65 (124–28); Brian Stock, *After Augustine: The Meditative Reader and the Text* (Philadelphia: University of Pennsylvania Press, 2001), pp. 105–14.
52 This was not always a fourfold schema. For Hugh of St Victor there is a fifth stage between *oratio* and *contemplatio*: *operatio*, a state characterised by performance. See Hugh's *Didascalicon* in *The Didascalicon of Hugh of St Victor*, tr. Jerome Taylor (New York: University of Colombia Press, 1991), 5, 9, p. 132. This is given some attention in Duncan Robertson, *Lectio Divina: The Medieval Experience of Reading* (Minnesota: Liturgical Press, 2011), pp. 205–13.
53 Mary Carruthers, *The Book of Memory: A Study of Memory in Medieval Culture* (Cambridge: Cambridge University Press), p. 165.

54 Leclercq, *The Love of Learning*, p. 73. This is given powerful expression by Anselm, who notes that true mediation consists of a ruminative process: 'mande cogitando, suge intelligendo, gluti amando et gaudendo' (*Meditationes* 3.10–11). See his *Orationes sive meditationes* in *St Anselmi Cantuariensis archiepiscopi opera omnia, tomus 2:2–91*, ed. Franciscus Salesius Schmitt (Stuttgart: Frommann, 1968).

55 Carruthers, *The Book of Memory*, p. 166.

56 Augustine, *Sermo 32: Psalmum CXLII: De Golia et David ac de contemptu mundi*, PL 38, col. 197. In this quotation from Augustine, I use the Latin translation from Shelley Annette Reid, 'The First Dispensation of Christ Is Medicinal: Augustine and Roman Medical Culture' (unpublished Ph.D. thesis, University of British Columbia, 2008), 206.

57 See references in Chapter Three of this book.

58 Augustine, *Enarratio in Psalmos*, 66.7, PL 36, col. 809. For the translation see *St Augustine: Expositions on the Psalms*, Nicene and Post-Nicene Fathers, First Series, 8, ed. Philip Schaff and tr. J. E. Tweed (repr. New York: Cosimo, 2007), p. 284.

59 Augustine, *Enarratio in Psalmos*, 76.14, PL 36, col. 978. For the translation see *Augustine: Expositions on the Psalms*, p. 364.

60 Carruthers, *The Book of Memory*, p. 329, n. 50.

61 Jacques Rousse, Hermann Sieben and André Boland (eds), 'Lectio divina et lecture spirituelle', *Dictionnaire de Spiritualité*, 9 (Paris: Beauchesne, 1976), cols 470–510.

62 Hammond, 'Contemplation', p. 124.

63 Stock, 'Minds, Bodies, Readers', 510.

64 Stock, *Augustine the Reader: Meditation, Self-Knowledge, and the Ethics of Interpretation* (Cambridge, MA: Harvard University Press, 1996), pp. 68–9; Hammond, 'Contemplation', p. 128.

65 Stock, 'Minds, Bodies, Readers', 510.

66 Augustine, *Confessions*, I.15, ed. and tr. R. S. Pine-Coffin (Harmondsworth: Penguin Books, 1961), pp. 35–6.

67 Cited in Leclercq, *The Love of Learning*, p. 135. For the original see 'Les divertissements poétiques d'Itier de Vassy', *Anal. S. Ord. Cist* (1956), 296–304.

68 Phyllis Hodgson and Gabriel M. Liegey (eds), *The Orchard of Syon*, EETS O.S. 258 (Oxford: Oxford University Press, 1966), p. 1.

69 John Henry Blunt (ed.), *The Myroure of Our Lady*, EETS E. S. 19 (London: N. Trübner and Co., 1873), pp. 68–9.

70 See *MED* entries for 'stirre' (v.) and 'quicken' (v.).

71 M. C. Seymour and Malcolm Andrew (eds), *On the Properties of Things: John Trevisa's translation of Bartholomeus Anglicus's* De Proprietatibus Rerum (Oxford: Clarendon Press, 1975), 7, 6, p. 350.

72 Luke Demaitre, *Medieval Medicine: The Art of Healing, From Head to Toe* (Santa Barbara: Praeger, 2013), p. 1, p. 11.

73 Knuuttila, *Emotions*, p. 173; and his 'Emotions from Plato to the Renaissance', pp. 476–7.

74 Origin, *Commentary on Matthew*, XV.16, in *Commentarius in Matthaeum, Die griechischen christlichen Schriftsteller der ersten drei Jahrhunderte 40*, ed. E. Klostermann and E. Benz (Leipzig: J Hinrichssche Buchhandlung, 1935–37), pp. 396.25–398.1. The translation is from Knuuttila in 'Emotions from Plato to the Renaissance', p. 476.

75 William, *De natura corporis et animae*, PL 180, cols 695–726. For the English translation, see *Three Treatises on Man: A Cistercian Anthropology*, ed. and tr. Bernard McGinn (Kalamazoo: Cistercian Publications, 1977), pp. 103–52. Isaac of Stella, *Epistola de anima*, PL 194, col. 1878D.

76 'Medieval Sciences of Emotions', 39.

77 *The Twelve Patriarchs*, in *Richard of St Victor*, tr. Grover A. Zinn (New York, Paulist Press, 1979), p. 60. For the Latin see, Richard of St Victor, *Benjamin Minor*, PL 196, col. 5C.

78 Richard of St Victor, *De quatuor gradibus violentae caritatis*, PL 196, cols 1207C–24D (cols 1209C–12D).

79 Boquet and Nagy, 'Medieval Sciences of Emotions', 40.

80 Dag Hasse, *De Anima in the Latin West: The Formation of a Peripatetic Philosophy of the Soul 1160–1300* (London: Warburg Institute, 2000), pp. 47–8.
81 Knuuttila, *Emotions*, p. 232.
82 J. G. Bougerol (ed.), *Summa De Anima: Textes philosophiques du moyen âge 19* (Paris: Vrin, 1995), 107, p. 262: 'Sicut enim uirtutis apprehensiue sensibilis organum est cerebrum principale, ita uirtutis motiue organum est cor, sicut dicunt physici.' Translation is my own.
83 P. Michaud-Quantin (ed.), *Tractatus de divisione multiplici potentiarum animae: Textes philosophiques du moyen âge 11* (Paris, Vrin, 1964), 50, pp. 126–7.
84 *Summa*, 107, p. 256. Latin text reads: 'concupiscere, desiderare, gaudere, letari, amare, diligere'.
85 *Summa*, 107, p. 256. Latin text reads: 'fastidire quod est contrarium concupiscere, abhominari quod est contrarium desiderare, dolere quod contrariatur gaudere, tristari quod est contrarium letari, odire quod est contrarium amare et diligere'.
86 *Summa*, 107, p. 257. Latin text reads: 'Sed quia misereri est contristari in alienis malis, inuidere tristari in alienis bonis, ideo continentur sub tristicia'.
87 *Summa*, 107, pp. 259–60. Latin text reads: 'Secundum hoc ergo sunt actus ambicio et spes, superbia, dominacio, contemptus . . . irascibilis, audere scilicet, et irasci et insurgere'.
88 *Summa*, 107, pp. 260–1.
89 See Eileen C. Sweeney, 'Aquinas on the Seven Deadly Sins: Tradition and Innovation', in Richard G. Newhauser and Susan J. Ridyard (eds), *Sin in Medieval and Early Modern Culture: The Tradition of the Seven Deadly Sins* (York: York Medieval Press, 2012), pp. 85–106 (87); Silvana Vecchio, 'The Seven Deadly Sins Between Pastoral Care and Scholastic Theology: The *Summa de vitiis* by John of Rupella', tr. Helen Took, in Richard G. Newhauser (ed.), *In the Garden of Evil: The Vices and Culture in the Middle Ages* (Toronto: Pontifical Institute of Medieval Studies, 2005), pp. 104–27 (104).
90 Vecchio, 'The Seven Deadly Sins', pp. 110–11.
91 Vecchio, 'The Seven Deadly Sins', p. 118. See John of la Rochelle, *Summa de Vitiis*, in Paris, Bibliotheque Nationale MS. lat.16417 fols 113rb–44va.
92 *Conciliorum oecumenicorum decreta*, ed. Giuseppe Alberigo, J. A. Dossetti, P. Joannou, C. Leonardi and P. Prodi, 3rd edn (Bologna: Istituto per le Scienze Religiose, 1973), p. 248. For a fuller exploration of the history of this quotation, see Joseph W. Goering, *William de Montibus (c.1140–1213): The Schools and the Literature of Pastoral Care* (Toronto: Pontifical Institute of Medieval Studies, 1992), p. 58, nn. 1–3; p. 95.
93 Christopher Mierow (tr.), *The Letters of Saint Jerome, Vol. 1* (New York: Newman Press, 1963), p. 118.
94 'The Constitution "Cum ex eo" of Boniface VIII: Education of Parochial Clergy', *Mediaeval Studies*, 24 (1962), 263–302.
95 Boyle, 'The Fourth Lateran Council and Manuals of Popular Theology', pp. 30–43.
96 Robert Grosseteste, *Templum Dei*, ed. Joseph W. Goering and F. A. C. Mantello (Toronto: Pontifical Institute of Medieval Studies, 1984), p. 41; p. 38.
97 *Templum Dei*, p. 38.
98 Richard C. Trexler (ed.), *The Christian at Prayer: An Illustrated Prayer Manual Attributed to Peter the Chanter* (New York: Medieval and Renaissance Texts and Studies, 1987), ll. 2005–10.
99 *Peter the Chanter*, ll. 2000–10.
100 Avicenna, *Liber de Anima*, IV.4, p. 58, l. 26. The translation is from Knuuttila, *Sourcebook*, p. 479.
101 Carruthers, *The Book of Memory*, pp. 59–60.
102 Gillespie, 'The Songs of the Threshold', p. 279.
103 Carruthers, *The Book of Memory*, pp. 57–60.
104 The concept of *enargeia* enjoys a wider dissemination in the *Rhetorica ad Herrenium* as the term 'demonstration'. See Gillespie, 'The Songs of the Threshold', p. 280.
105 For this text see Lynn Mooney, 'A Middle English Text on the Seven Liberal Arts', *Speculum*, 68 (1993), 1027–52; ll. 139–45.

106 See Deborah L. Black's 'The "Imaginative Syllogism" in Arabic Philosophy: A Medieval Contribution to the Philosophical Study of Metaphor', *Mediaeval Studies*, 51 (1989), 242–67; 107 Minnis, 'Medieval imagination and memory', in A. Minnis and I. Johnson (eds), *The Cambridge History of Literary Criticism*, pp. 237–74; Gillespie, 'The Senses in Literature: The Textures of Perception', p. 165.

107 Mary Theresa Brady, '*The Pore Caitif*: Edited from Ms Harley 2336 With Introduction and Notes' (unpublished Ph.D. thesis, Fordham University, 1954), 1, l. 9. Hereafter *Pore Caitif*.

108 *Pore Caitif*, 2, ll. 27–8.

109 *Pore Caitif*, 162, ll. 7–1.

110 *Pore Caitif*, 9, ll. 2–11.

111 *Pore Caitif*, 46, ll. 26–47, l. 3.

112 Martin Irvine with David Thomson, '*Grammatica* and Literary theory', in Minnis and Ian Johnson (eds), *The Cambridge History of Literary Criticism*, pp. 13–41. See also James J. Murphy, 'Literary implications of instruction in the verbal arts in fourteenth century England', *Leeds Studies in English*, n.s. 1 (1967), 119–35.

113 Donatus, *Ars grammatica*, in *Grammatici latini, 4*, ed. Heinrich Keil (Leipzig, 1857), pp. 391, ll. 25–392, l. 3. Translated in Rita Copeland and Ineke Sluiter (eds), *Medieval Grammar and Rhetoric: Language Arts and Literary Theory, AD 300–1475*, (Oxford: Oxford University Press, 2009), p. 93.

114 Priscian, *Institutiones grammaticae*, in *Grammatici latini, 2*, ed. Heinrich Keil (Leipzig, 1857), p. 53, l. 27. Translated in *Medieval Grammar and Rhetoric*: 'two parts of speech, noun and verb, because these by themselves, when combined with each other, may form a complete sentence. The other parts they called *syncategoremata*, i.e. Co-signifiers', p. 176.

115 St Augustine, *De sermone domini in monte libri duo*, ed. Almut Mutzenbecher, Corpus Christianorum Series Latina, 35 (Turnhout: Brepols, 1967), p. 24.

116 See Jean Leclercq, 'Le De grammatica de Hugues de Saint Victor', in *Archives d'histoire doctrinale et littéraire du moyen âge*, 20 (1945), 288, ll. 23–6. Thomas Aquinas, *Sententia libri politicorum tabula libri ethicorum*, in *Sancti Thomae de Aquino Opera omnia*, 48 ed. P. Minge (Rome: Commissio Leonina, 1971), pp. 128–37. Albertus Magnus, *Super Mattheum*, in *Alberti Magni Opera omnia, cura et studio Instituti Alberti Magni*, vol. 21/1, ed. Bernardus Schmidt (Münster: Aschendorff, 1987), p. 134.

117 See Ria Van Der Lecq, 'Modistae', in Henrik Lagerlund (ed.), *Encyclopedia of Medieval Philosophy* (Dordrecht: Springer, 2011), pp. 806–8 (p. 807).

118 K. M. Fredborg, Lauge Nielsen and Jan Pinborg (eds), 'An unedited part of Roger Bacon's *Opus maius: De signis*', *Traditio*, 34 (1978), 75–136 (para. 10). Translation: Thomas S. Maloney (ed.), *On Signs: Opus maius, Part 3, Chapter 2*, Medieval Sources in Translation, 54 (Toronto: Pontifical Institute of Medieval Studies, 2013), p. 41.

119 Roger Bacon, *Communia naturalium*, in *Opera hactenus inedita II*, ed. Robert Steele (Oxford: Clarendon Press, 1905), p. 110, ll. 25–32. Translation from *On Signs*, p. 121.

120 Pseudo-Kilwardby, *Commentum super Priscianum maiorem*, in Irene Rosier-Catach, *La Parole comme acte* (Paris: Vrin, 1994), p. 75. Latin: Dicendum quod vox interiectionalis potest considerari dupliciter. Uno modo prout refertur ad significatum et modum significandi quem habet ex institutione, et sic significat ratione dominante et sensualitate succumbente ... Vel potest considerari in comparatione ad utentes voce interiectionali. Illi autem utuntur ea quandoque ex vehementi motu prosperi vel adversi apprehensi subito sensualitate dominante et ratione subcumbente. Aliquando enim ex vehementi motu prosperi vel adversi ratio que est coniuncta sensualitate quasi prosternitur vel saltem non cohibet sensualitatem nec moderatur eam in suo motu, sicut patet in apprehensione valde tristi ut in morte patris ve aciluius excellentis boni prosperi, et sic prorumpit homo in voce que re vera illud significat ex institutione ad quod significandum homo utitur quasi naturaliter, quia ratione subcumbente et sensualitate dominante.

121 K. Reichl (ed.), *Tractatus de grammatica eine falschlich Robert Grosseteste zugeschriebene spekulative Grammatik: Edition und Kommentar*, Veröffentlichungen 122 des Grabmann-Institutes, 28 (Munich: Schoningh, 1976), p. 59.

122 *Tractatus de grammatica*, p. 60.
123 Knuuttila, *Emotions*, p. 211.
124 Similar comments on prayer are in Augustine's *De doctrina christiana*, Corpus Christianorum Series Latina, 32 (Turnhout, 1962), p. 42.
125 Bacon, *Opus tertium*, in *Opera quaedam hactenus inedita: Opus tertium, Opus minus, Compendium studii philosophiae, Epistola de secretis operibus Artis et Naturae, et de nullitate Magiae*, ed. J. S. Brewer (London: Longman, 1965), p. 96. The translation is from Nancy Van Deusen, 'Roger Bacon on Music', in Jeremiah Hackett (ed.), *Roger Bacon and the Sciences: Commemorative Essays*, Studien und Texte zur Geistesgeschichte des Mittelalters 57 (Leiden: Brill, 1997), pp. 223–42 (240).
126 Traugott Lawler (ed.), *The Parisiana poetria of John of Garland* (New Haven: Yale University Press, 1974), p. 112 (translation p. 113).
127 IMEV 4087 and IMEV 3242. See S. H. Thomson, 'The Date of the Early English Translation of the "Candet Nudatum Pectus"', *Medium Aevum*, 4/2 (1935), 104; and Rosemary Woolf, *The English Religious Lyric in the Middle Ages* (Oxford: Clarendon Press, 1968), nos 29, 36; Thomas G. Duncan (ed.), *Medieval English Lyrics and Carols*, rev. edn (Cambridge: D.S. Brewer, 2013), I, no. 86; Ralph Hanna, 'Editing Middle English Lyrics: The Case of *Candet Nudatum Pectus*', *Medium Aevum*, 80/2 (2011), 189–200.
128 *Pore Caitif*, 70, ll. 18–20.
129 *Pore Caitif*, 136, ll. 1–10.
130 *MED*, 'drenchen' (v.).
131 *Cloud*, p. 166, l. 25.
132 *Revelation*, p. 54.
133 Bryan, *Looking Inward*, p. 14; more broadly Derek Pearsall (ed.), *Studies in the Vernon Manuscript* (Cambridge: D. S. Brewer, 1990); more recently Wendy Scase (ed.), *The Making of the Vernon Manuscript: The Production and Contexts of Oxford, Bodleian Library, MS Eng. poet. a. 1* (Turnhout: Brepols, 2013).
134 Vincent Gillespie, 'Morality Touched by Emotion: the Lyrics of the Vernon Manuscript' (unpublished B.Litt. thesis, University of Oxford, 1976), 5.

1: Apprehensive Medicine

1 G. R. Morgan (ed.), 'A Critical Edition of Caxton's *The Art and Craft to Know Well to Die*, and *Ars Moriendi* Together with the Antecedent Manuscript Material' (unpublished Ph.D. thesis, University of Oxford, 1972), 33, ll. 8–13. Hereafter *The Craft of Dying*.
2 For recent explorations of this text and the diffuse nature of its impact, see Amy Appleford, *Learning to Die in London, 1380–1540* (Philadelphia: University of Pennsylvania Press, 2015), and Vincent Gillespie, 'Seek, Suffer and Trust: Ese and Disese in Julian of Norwich', *Studies in the Age of Chaucer*, 39 (2017), 129–58.
3 *The Craft of Dying*, 44, ll. 10–1.
4 *The Craft of Dying*, 44, ll. 13–44; 45, ll. 1–2.
5 *The Craft of Dying*, 45, ll. 2–3.
6 *MED*, 'drede' (n.)
7 Carl Horstmann (ed.), *The Mirror of St Edmund*, in *Yorkshire Writers: Richard Rolle of Hampole, an English Father of the Church, and His Followers*, 1/2 (London: Swan Sonnenschein, 1895–96), pp. 240–61 (247).
8 *Mirror*, p. 247.
9 See Jeremiah 5:22; Isaiah 8:12–13, 11:2–3; Psalms 111:10; Proverbs 9:10, 28:14, 14:27; Job 28:28; 2 Corinthians 7:1.

10 See Clement of Alexandria's *Stromata* in *The Stromata or Miscellanies*, ed. A. Robert and J. Donaldson, The Ante-Nicene Fathers 2 (Grand Rapids, MI: Eerdmans, 1967), 2–12.

11 Basil *Regulae Fusius Tractatae* in PG 3, cols 889–1052; Gregory of Nazianzus, *Adversus Iram*, PG 37, col. 813–51; *Gregory of Nyssa: Life of Moses*, ed. A. Malherbe, tr. E. Ferguson (New York: Paulist Press, 1978), 2.320.

12 Peter Lombard, *Sententiae in IV Libris Distinctae*, 2 vols, Spicilegium Bonaventurianum, 3rd edn, ed. Ian Brady (Grottaferrata: Editiones Collegii S. Bonaventurae ad Claras Aquas, 1971–1981), 3.34.4; 3.34.9.

13 It is repeated by William Peraldus in his *Summae virtutum ac vitiorum*, 2 vols, (Antwerp: Philippus Nutius, 1571), 4. 1. 3. For an excellent engagement with the theology of fear in medieval culture, see Eric J. Johnson, 'In dry3 dred and daunger: The Tradition and Rhetoric of Fear in *Cleanness* and *Patience*' (unpublished Ph.D. thesis, University of York, 2000), 24.

14 St John Damascene, *De fide orthodoxa*, PG 94, cols 781–1228, (2, 15); Bonaventure, *Commentaria in Quatuor Libros Sententiarum Magistri Petri Lombardi*, Opera Omnia vol. 3, ed. R. P. Aloysii A Parma (Collegium S. Bonaventurae: Quaracchi, 1882–1902), pp. 769–70.

15 Johnson, 'In dry3 dred and daunger', 32.

16 As Bonaventure notes, 'Timor enim aut est ex natura, aut ex libidine sive concupiscentia, aut ex gratia', in *Commentaria*, p. 768.

17 Bonaventure, *Commentaria*, pp. 769–70.

18 *Glossa ordinaria: Biblia sacra cum glossis et postillis Nicoli Lyrani*, vol. 1 (Lyon, 1545), fol. 154va. Translation is from Johnson, 'In dry3 dred and daunger', 43.

19 'De erubescentia, dicit Ioannes Damascenus, quod est optima passio ... Sine verecundia nihil rectum esse potest, nihil honestum.' *Summae virtutum ac vitiorum*, 6, 3, 3. See Johnson, 'In dry3 dred and daunger', 34.

20 Johnson, 'In dry3 dred and daunger', 35; 47.

21 Bonaventure, *Collationes de septem donis Spiritus sancti*, in Opera Omnia vol. 5, Collatio 2, 7, p. 464: Oritur autem timor Dei in nobis primo ex consideratione sublimitatis divinae potentiae, secundo, ex consideratione perspicacitatis divinae sapientiae, tertio, ex consideratione severitatis divinae vindictae; see Johnson, 'In dry3 dred and daunger', 48 for a translation.

22 Bonaventure, *Commentaria*, 3. 34. 2 (p. 765): 'Et propterea potest adhuc aliter dici, quod duplex est usus ipsius timoris gratuiti: unus, inquam, quo cor hominis sollicitatur ex consideratione suae fragilitatis; alius, quo humiliatur ex consideratione suae parvitatis et divinae magnitudinis'.

23 Bonaventure, *Commentaria*, 3. 34. 2 (p. 766).

24 *Glossa ordinaria*, Romans 8:15, 6, fol. 18va; the translation is from Johnson, 'In dry3 dred and daunger', 53.

25 Bonaventure, *Commentaria*, 3. 34. 2 (p. 758): 'sic timor servilis, cum quis timet incurrere aeterna tormenta, est ex amore aeternae salutis et beatitudinis'. The translation is from Johnson, 'In dry3 dred and daunger', 55.

26 Peter Lombard, *Sententiae*, 3. 34. 5.

27 Johnson, 'In dry3 dred and daunger', 59–61.

28 Bonaventure, *Commentaria*, 3. 34. 2 (p. 769): 'obiectum magis principale'.

29 Bonaventure, *Commentaria*, 3. 34. 2 (pp.762–6).

30 St Bernard, *Sermones in Cantica Canticorum*, in PL 183, 38.3, col. 976.

31 W. Nelson Francis (ed.), *The Book of Vices and Virtues: A Fourteenth Century English Translation Of The Somme le roi of Lorens d'Orléans*, EETS O. S. 217 (London: Oxford University Press, 1945), p. 126, ll. 3–6.

32 *MED*, 'proprelie' (adv.).

33 For further comments on this, see my 'Medicine of Words: Purgative Reading in Richard Rolle's Meditations on the Passion', *The Mediaeval Journal*, 5/2 (2015), 53–83 (60f).

34 *Vices and Virtues*, p. 12, ll. 3–5.

35 *Vices and Virtues*, p. 127, ll. 14–19.

36 *MED*, 'turblen' (v.).

[37] *Scale*, 1, ll. 2557–60.
[38] Hugh of St Victor, *De arca Noe morali*, PL 176, 3. 2. col. 648c. The translation is from *Hugh of Saint Victor: Selected Spiritual Writings*, ed. and tr. Aelred Squire (London: Harper and Row, 1962), p. 96.
[39] Margaret Connolly (ed.), *The Contemplations of the Drede and Love of God*, EETS O. S. 303 (Oxford: Oxford University Press, 1993), p. 9, ll. 50–6.
[40] *MED*, 'waxen' (v.).
[41] *Contemplations of the Drede and Love of God*, p. 8, ll. 4–5.
[42] *Prickynge*, p. 90, ll. 6–13.
[43] *Stodye*, p. 17, ll. 4–13–p. 18, ll. 1–3.
[44] *Stodye*, p. 18, l. 16.
[45] *Scale*, 1, ll. 619–23.
[46] *MED*, 'knitten' (v.).
[47] *MED*, 'stāblen' (v.(1)).
[48] Rosemond Tuve, *Allegorical Imagery: Some Mediaeval Books and their Posterity* (Princeton: Princeton University Press, 1966), pp. 94–5.
[49] *PoC*, xxxvii.
[50] *MED*, 'unsted-fast' (adj.).
[51] *MED*, 'priken' (v.)
[52] As noted by Howell Chickering, 'Rhetorical *Stimulus* in the *Prick of Conscience*', in Stephanie Hayes-Healy (ed.), *Medieval Paradigms: Essays in Honour of Jeremy du Quesnay Adams*, The New Middle Ages Series 1 (New York: Palgrave Macmillan, 2005), pp. 191–230 (203–8). Her article offers an interesting engagement with medieval rhetorical concepts in this text.
[53] Mary Carruthers, *The Experience of Beauty in the Middle Ages* (Oxford: Oxford University Press, 2013) pp. 134–64.
[54] *MED*, 'driven' (.v).
[55] *MED*, 'stiren' (v.).
[56] Vincent Gillespie, 'Anonymous Devotional Writings', in A. S. G. Edwards (ed.), *A Companion to Middle English Prose* (Cambridge: D. S. Brewer, 2004), pp. 127–49.

2: Lyrical Treatment

[1] Chaucer, *Troilus and Criseyde*, in *The Riverside Chaucer*, 3rd edn, gen. ed. Larry D. Benson (Oxford: Oxford University Press, 1988).
[2] The contextual penitential significance of this scene has been explored by Henry Ansgar Kelly, 'Penitential Theology and Law at the Turn of the Fifteenth Century', in Abigail Firey (ed.), *A New History of Penance* (Leiden: Brill, 2008), pp. 239–318 (244).
[3] Gillespie, 'Moral and Penitential Lyrics', in Thomas G. Duncan (ed.), *A Companion to the Middle English Lyric* (Cambridge: D. S. Brewer, 2005), pp. 68–95 (70).
[4] Carl Horstmann (ed.), *Twelve Profits of Tribulation*, in *Yorkshire Writers: Richard Rolle of Hampole, an English Father of the Church, and His Followers*, 2/2 (London: Swan Sonnenschein, 1895–96), pp. 391–406 (394).
[5] *Twelve Profits of Tribulation*, p. 394.
[6] *Twelve Profits of Tribulation*, p. 394.
[7] Canon 21–2, in Alberigo Giuseppe (ed.), *Conciliorum Oecumenicorum Decreta* (Basel: Herder, 1962), pp. 215–16.
[8] Jessalynn Bird, 'Medicine for Body and Soul: Jacques de Vitry's Sermons to Hospitallers and their Charges', in Peter Biller and Joseph Ziegler (eds), *Religion and Medicine in the Middle Ages* (York: York Medieval Press, 2001), pp. 91–108.

NOTES

9   See Peter Biller, 'Confession in the Middle Ages: An Introduction', in Peter Biller and A. J. Minnis (eds), *Handling Sin: Confession in the Middle Ages* (York: York Medieval Press, 1998), pp. 1–34 (8); and Leonard E. Boyle, 'Robert Grosseteste and the Pastoral Care', in Boyle (ed.), *Pastoral Care, Clerical Education and Canon Law, 1200–1400* (London: Variorum, 1981), pp. 3–51.

10 Hugo de Folieto, *De medicina anime*, in PL 176, col. 1198. The translation is from Dr Cohen-Hanegbi, 'Accidents of the Soul: Physicians and Confessors on the Conception and Treatment of Emotions in Italy and Spain, Late Twelfth–Fifteenth Centuries' (unpublished Ph.D. thesis, The Hebrew University, 2011), 30–1.

11 Faith Wallis (ed.), *Medieval Medicine: A Reader* (Toronto: University of Toronto Press, 2010), p. 14.

12 William de Montibus, *Peniteas Cito*, in *William de Montibus (c.1140–1213)*, ed. Joseph Goering (Toronto: Pontifical Institute of Medieval Studies, 1992), pp. 107–38 (107–11).

13 William of Auvergne, *Guilelmi Alverni Episcopi Parisiensis*, in Opera omnia vol. 1 and Supplementum, ed. F. Hotot and B. Le Feron (Orléans and Paris, 1674; reprint Frankfurt, 1963), I, 487aB. I am grateful to Dr Cohen-Hanegbi for bringing this quotation to my attention; I use her translation.

14 *Robertus Grosseteste: Dicta*, ed. Joseph Goering, www.grosseteste.com (accessed June 2013). Translation is from 'On true compassion and Alms', *Robert Grosseteste: The Complete Dicta in English vol. 1*, ed. and tr. Gordon Jackson (Lincoln: Asgill Press, 2003), p. 11.

15 Grosseteste, *Templum Dei*, ed. Joseph W. Goering and F. A. C. Mantello (Toronto: Pontifical Institute of Medieval Studies, 1984), p. 64.

16 I. M. Resnick, 'Ps.-Albert the Great on the Physiognomy of Jesus and Mary', *Mediaeval Studies*, 64 (2002), 227–40 (227).

17 *Templum Dei*, p. 38.

18 *The Twelve Patriarchs*, in *Richard of St Victor*, tr. Grover A. Zinn (New York: Paulist Press, 1979), p. 123.

19 *Regulae de Sacra Theologia*, PL 210, cols 665B–65C. Translation is from Howell Chickering, 'Rhetorical *Stimulus* in the *Prick of Conscience*', in Stephanie Hayes-Healy (ed.), *Medieval Paradigms: Essays in Honour of Jeremy du Quesnay Adams*, The New Middle Ages Series 1 (New York: Palgrave Macmillan, 2005), pp. 191–230 (228–9).

20 'Dico ergo quod attritio ad contritionem sic est, sicut vulneratio non laetalis ad occisionem' in William of Auvergne, *De sacramento poenitentiae*, in *Opera Omnia* vol. 1, 6. 466H–67A. The translation is from Chickering, p. 229.

21 William notes an additional stage to this process – compunction – a word with heavy medical connotations. It is based on the feelings of fear and sorrow, and ought to include some form of tears. The choice of this word is significant, and includes the idea of puncturing the heart. See Jean Leclercq, *The Love of Learning and the Desire for God: A Study of Monastic Culture*, tr. Catherine Misrahi (New York: Fordham University Press, 1982), pp. 29–30.

22 Richard Rolle, *Ego Dormio*, in *English Writings of Richard Rolle, Hermit of Hampole*, ed. Hope Emily Allen (Oxford: Clarendon Press, 1931), p. 64, ll. 92–102.

23 Richard Rolle, *Oleum Effusum*, in *Uncollected Prose and Verse with Related Northern Texts*, ed. Ralph Hanna, EETS O. S. 329 (Oxford: Oxford University Press, 2007), p. 5, ll. 59–63.

24 Richard Rolle, *Incendium Amoris*, in *The Fire of Love and the Mending of Life, or the Rule of Living*, ed. Ralph Harvey, EETS O. S. 106 (London: Oxford University Press, reprint 1973), p. 66, l. 40; p. 5, l. 7.

25 Richard Rolle, *Form of Living*, in *Richard Rolle: Prose and Verse*, ed. S. J. Ogilvie-Thomson, EETS O. S. 293 (Oxford: Oxford University Press, 1988), p. 13, ll. 399–400.

26 *The Commandment*, in *Richard Rolle: Prose and Verse*, p. 38, ll. 183–7.

27 See *The Prayers and Meditations of Saint Anselm with the Proslogion*, tr. Benedicta Ward (London: Penguin Books, 1973), p. 53.

28 *Scale*, 2, ll. 862–4.
29 *Scale*, 1, ll. 2499–502.
30 *Scale*, 1, ll. 1556–8.
31 *Revelation*, p. 40.
32 *Revelation*, p. 126.
33 Rolle, *English Psalter*, p. 5.
34 Gillespie, 'Moral and Penitential Lyrics', p. 80.
35 Cassiodorus notes that 'at one time some psalms endowed with health-giving instruction lead louring and stormy spirits into a bright and most peaceful way of life' in *Cassiodorus: Explanation of the Psalms: Volume 1*, tr. P. G. Walsh (New York: Paulist, 1991), p. 24. Peter Lombard emphasises their penitential function (see *Petri Lombardi in psalmos Davidicos commentarii praefatio*, PL 191, cols 55–62). He divides the Psalter 'into three groups of fifty, by which are signified the three conditions of the Christian religions. The first is the condition of penitence; the second of justice; the third, that of praise of eternal life' in A. J. Minnis and A. B. Scott (eds), *Medieval Literary Theory and Criticism c.1100–1375: The Commentary Tradition* (Oxford: Clarendon Press, 1988), p. 107. Rolle makes an identical point in his *English Psalter*, stating that 'þis boke es distynged in thris fyfty psalmes in þe whilke iij states of Cristens mans religioun ere signyfyed; þe first in penaunce, þe toþer in rightwisenes, þe thrid in lovynge of endeles lyf' (p. 6).
36 Cassiodorus: *Explanation of the Psalms*, p. 24. For the Latin see *In Psalterium Praefatio*, PL 70, col. 9: 'Tanta enim illie est pulchritudo sensuum et stillantium medicina verborum'.
37 *In Psalterium Praefatio*, cols 10–11.
38 *In Psalterium Praefatio*, col. 11B.
39 Augustine notes that there are two senses to the word 'pricked' – as either penitential or based on fervent desire. Augustine, *Enarratio in Psalmos*, PL 36, Psalm 4.6, cols 80–1: 'Compungimini autem, aut ad poenitentiæ dolorem refertur, ut se ipsam anima puniens compungat, ne in Dei judicio damnata torqueatur; aut ad excitationem, ut evigilemus ad videndam lucem Christi, tanquam stimulis adhibitis.'
40 Richard Rolle, *The Psalter or Psalms of David and Certain Canticles with a Translation and Exposition in English by Richard Rolle of Hampole*, ed. H. R. Bramley (Oxford: Clarendon Press, 1884), Psalm 37.5, p. 138.
41 Annie Sutherland, *English Psalms in the Middle Ages*, 1300–1450 (Oxford: Oxford University Press, 2015), pp. 39–40.
42 *MPP*, l. 8.
43 Carl Horstmann (ed.), *Maidstone's Paraphrase of Psalm L*, in *The Minor Poems of the Vernon MS Part 1*, EETS O. S. 98 (London: Kegan Paul, Trench Trübner and Co., 1892), pp. 12–16.
44 *MPP*, ll. 105–12.
45 John A. Alford, 'Rolle's *English Psalter* and Lectio Divina', *Bulletin of the John Rylands Library*, 77/3 (1995), 47–60 (52–9).
46 *Revelation*, pp. 39–40.
47 Gillespie, 'Moral and Penitential Lyrics', p. 86.
48 Oxford, Bodleian Library Rawlinson G.22.
49 Thomas G. Duncan (ed.), *Medieval English Lyrics and Carols* (Cambridge: D. S. Brewer, 2013), I. 36, p. 87.
50 Oxford, Bodleian Library, MS Digby 2.
51 Carleton Brown (ed.), *English Lyrics of the Thirteenth Century* (Oxford: Clarendon Press, 1932), no. 65.
52 *English Lyrics of the Thirteenth Century*, p. 217.
53 Gillespie, 'Moral and Penitential Lyrics', p. 87.
54 *Medieval English Lyrics and Carols*, p. 332.
55 F. J. Furnivall (ed.), 'Sayings of Saint Bernard: Man's Three Foes', in *The Minor Poems of the Vernon MS Part II*, EETS O. S. 117 (London: Kegan Paul, Trench Trübner and Co., 1901), pp. 511–22.

56   *MED*, 'warant' (n.).
57   'Merci God and Graunt Merci', in *The Minor Poems of the Vernon MS Part II*, pp. 696–9.
58   Gillespie, 'Moral and Penitential Lyrics', p. 86.

3: Compassionate Healing

1   This lyric is from Oxford, Bodleian Library, MS Bodley 42. See Carleton F. Brown (ed.), *Religious Lyrics of the XIV Century*, 2nd edn (Oxford: Clarendon Press, 1924), no. 1, pp. 1–2. Gillespie notes the imagistic power and force of this small lyric and its Latin original, stressing that the 'reader almost drowns in a welter of blood and suffering', that such writing 'produces a kind of affective overload of the imagination which is designed to generate extremities of compassion', in 'Strange Images of Death', in *Looking in Holy Books: Essays on Late Medieval Religious Writing in England* (Turnhout: Brepols, 2012), pp. 209–42 (225). Another version of this lyric in Cambridge, St John's College, MS A 15, f. 72r, sits beside the composite medical/theological table in Grosseteste's *Templum Dei* (p. 41). The combination is far from accidental, and shows the close connection between *salus animae* and the very texts which seek to evoke it. I am grateful to Ms Samira Lindstedt for the reference.
2   *Revelation*, p. 54.
3   Michael G. Sargent (ed.), *The Mirror of the Blessed Life of Jesus Christ: A Reading Text* (Exeter: University of Exeter Press, 2004), p. 9, ll. 21–8.
4   *Prickynge*, p. 11, ll. 8–17.
5   Faith Wallis (ed.), *Medieval Medicine: A Reader* (Toronto: University of Toronto Press, 2010), pp. 177–8.
6   *MED*, 'compassioun' (n.); also, Sarah McNamer, *Affective Meditation and the Invention of Medieval Compassion* (Philadelphia: University of Pennsylvania Press, 2010), pp. 11–12.
7   M. C. Seymour and Ralph Hanna (eds), *On the Properties of Things: John Trevisa's translation of Bartholomeus Anglicus's* De Proprietatibus Rerum (Oxford: Clarendon Press, 1975), 5, 1, p. 166, ll. 12–16.
8   For a full list of references see my 'Purgative Reading in Richard Rolle's Meditations on the Passion A', *The Mediaeval Journal*, 5/2 (2015), 53–83 (57); also Shelley Annette Reid, 'The First Dispensation of Christ Is Medicinal: Augustine and Roman Medical Culture' (unpublished Ph.D. thesis, University of British Columbia, 2008), 206; Rudolph Arbesmann, 'The Concept of "Christus Medicus" in St Augustine', *Traditio*, 10 (1954), 1–28; and Thomas F. Martin, 'Paul the Patient: Christus Medicus and the "Stimulus Carnis" (2 Cor. 12:7): A Consideration of Augustine's Medical Christology', *Augustinian Studies*, 32/2 (2001), 219–56.
9   One of the key aspects of the *Christus Medicus* concept is the related idea of Christ as a surgeon. For further information, see Virginia Langum, 'The Wounded Surgeon: Devotion, Compassion, and Metaphor in Medieval England', in Larissa Tracy and Kelly DeVries (eds), *Wounds and Wound Repair in Medieval Culture* (Leiden: Brill, 2015), pp. 269–90, and Karl Whittington, 'Picturing Christ as Surgeon and Patient in British Library MS Sloane 1977', *Mediaevalia*, 35 (2014), 83–115.
10 Augustine, *In Epistolam Joannis ad Parthos*, Tract. 9. 4, PL 35, col. 2048. The Translation is from Arbesmann, p. 22 (n. 102).
11 Calix passionis amarus est, sed omnes morbos poenitus curat; calix passionis amarus est, sed prior eum bibit medicus, ne bibere dubitaret aegrotus': *Serm Mai* 19.2, in *Miscellanea Agostiniana: Testi e Studi* 1, ed. Germain Morin (Rome: Tipografia poliglotta vaticana, 1930), p. 310. The translation is from Arbesmann, p. 15.
12 Arbesmann, 'The Concept of *Christus Medicus*', pp. 15–20.
13 Gregory the Great, *Homiliarum in Evangelia Liber II, Homilia 37*, PL 76, col. 1277: 'Crux quippe a cruciatu dictur. Et duobus modis crucem Domini bajulamus, cum aut per abstinentiam carnem

afficimus, aut per compasionem proximi necessitatem illius nostrum putamus.' For a fascinating engagement with this concept and the specific translation of the word as torture, see C. Matthew Phillips, 'Crux a cruciatu dictur: Preaching Self-Torture as Pastoral Care in Twelfth-Century Religious Houses', in Ronald J. Stanbury (ed.), *A Companion to Pastoral Care in the Late Middle Ages 1200–1500* (Leiden: Brill, 2010), pp. 285–310 (286).

14 Bernard of Clairvaux, *Sententiae*, 3.74 in *Sancti Bernardi Opera* 6/2, ed. Jean Leclercq, Henri Rochais, Charles H. Talbot (Rome: Editiones Cistercienses, 1957–77), p. 115.

15 In his *Meditation Five*, he notes that when 'I look at the cross of your passion, the nails of fear of you pierce me' – see his *On Contemplating God, Prayer, Meditations*, tr. Sister Penelope Lawson (Shannon: Irish University Press, 1971), p. 119.

16 Richard Rolle, 'A Salutation to Jesus', in *English Writings of Richard Rolle, Hermit of Hampole*, ed. Hope Emily Allen (Oxford: Clarendon Press, 1931), p. 48, l. 1.

17 *Meditations on the Passion*, in *English Writings*, p. 22, l. 110.

18 *Revelation*, p. 3.

19 *Revelation*, pp. 30–31.

20 Augustine, *Sermo* 175. 8. 9, PL 38, col. 949. The translation is from Martin, 'Paul the Patient', p. 221.

21 Augustine, *Sermo* 87. 12. 15, PL 38, col. 538: 'Habemus exempla. Persequebatur membra ejus jam sedentis in coelo Saulus: persequebatur graviter in phrenesi, mente perdita, morbo nimio. At ille una voce de coelo clamans ei, *Saule, Saule, quid me persequeris?* percussit phreneticum, erexit sanum; occidit persecutorem, vivificavit prædicatorem.' The translation is from Arbesmann, p. 18.

22 Augustine, *Enarratio in Psalmos*, PL 36, 58.2, col. 709. The translation is from Martin, 'Paul the Patient', p. 229.

23 Augustine, *Enarratio in Psalmos*, PL 37, 98.13, col. 1269: 'Ecce quomodo propitius erat Deus, vindicans in omnes affectiones ejus.' The translation is from Martin, 'Paul the Patient', p. 234.

24 Odilo of Cluny, *De sancta cruce*, Sermo 15, PL 142, col.133; Peter Damian, *Sermo 18*, in Corpus Christianorum Continuatio Medievalis 57, ed. Giovanni Luchessi (Turnholt: Brepols, 1983), pp. 119–20; Bruno, *Commentaria in Matthaeum, Pars Tres*, PL 165, cols 215D–16. See Phillips, 'Crux a cruciatu dictur', pp. 289–91 for more information.

25 *Revelation*, p. 16.

26 This has been explored by Gillespie in 'Seek, Suffer and Trust: Ese and Disese in Julian of Norwich', *Studies in the Age of Chaucer*, 39 (2017), 129–58.

27 *MED*, 'sufferen' (v.); 'travailen' (v.).

28 *Revelation*, p. 54.

29 Carl Horstmann (ed.), *Twelve Profits of Tribulation*, in *Yorkshire Writers: Richard Rolle of Hampole, an English Father of the Church, and His Followers*, vol. 2 (London: Swan Sonnenschein, 1895–96), pp. 391–406 (405).

30 *Prickynge*, p. 27, ll. 16–20.

31 *Twelve Profits of Tribulation*, p. 405.

32 *Twelve Profits of Tribulation*, p. 403.

33 *Pore Caitif*, 122, ll. 6–15.

34 *Pore Caitif*, 122, l. 18.

35 *Chastising*, p. 199, ll. 3–4.

36 *Chastising*, p. 199, l. 5.

37 *MED*, 'serchen' (v.) – specifically sense 6.

38 W. Nelson Francis (ed.), *The Book of Vices and Virtues: A Fourteenth Century English Translation of The Somme le roi of Lorens d'Orléans*, EETS O. S. 217 (London: Oxford University Press, 1945), p. 143, ll. 5–13.

39 See Nancy Siraisi, *Medieval and Early Renaissance Medicine* (Chicago: University of Chicago Press, 2009), pp. 118–19; Joseph Ziegler, 'Medicine and Immortality in Terrestrial Paradise', in Peter Biller and Joseph Ziegler (eds), *Religion and Medicine in the Middle Ages* (York: York

Medieval Press, 2001), p. 216; Naöe Kukita Yoshikawa (ed.), *Medicine, Religion, and Gender in Medieval Culture* (Cambridge: D. S. Brewer, 2015), p. 3.

40 *MED*, 'proprelīce' (adv.).

41 This is proposed by John of la Rochelle in Chapter 75 of his *Summa De Anima*. See J. G. Bougerol (ed.), *Summa De Anima: Textes philosophiques du moyen âge 19* (Paris: Vrin, 1995). He is, however, drawing from Saint John of Damascus' *De fide et Orthodoxa*. See Denise Ryan, 'An Examination of a Thirteenth-Century Treatise on the Mind/Body Dichotomy: Jean de La Rochelle on the Soul and its Powers' (unpublished Ph.D. thesis, National University of Ireland, Maynooth, 2010), 151.

42 *Prickynge*, p. 50, ll. 14–17.

43 *Prickynge*, p. 49, ll. 14–18.

44 *Prickynge*, p. 49, ll. 11–12.

45 *Prickynge*, p. 49, ll. 18–25.

46 *MED*, 'wonderli' (adv.).

47 *Prickynge*, p. 50, ll. 23–4.

48 Richard Rolle, *The Psalter or Psalms of David and Certain Canticles with a Translation and Exposition in English by Richard Rolle of Hampole*, ed. H. R. Bramley (Oxford: Clarendon Press, 1884), Psalm 115.4, p. 405.

49 *Prickynge*, p. 27, ll. 9–11.

50 *Scale*, 2, ll. 1149–52.

51 *Scale*, 2, l. 1158.

52 *Scale*, 1, ll. 472–4.

53 *Twelve Profits of Tribulation*, pp. 398–9.

54 Augustine, *Enarratio in Psalmos*, 66. 7, PL 36, col. 809. For the translation see *St Augustine: Expositions on the Psalms*, ed. Philip Schaff and tr. J. E. Tweed, Nicene and Post-Nicene Fathers, First Series, 8 (repr. New York: Cosimo, 2007), p. 284.

55 Carl Horstmann (ed.), *A Tretise of Ghostly Battle*, in *Yorkshire Writers: Richard Rolle of Hampole, an English Father of the Church, and His Followers*, vol. 2 (London: Swan Sonnenschein, 1895–96), pp. 420–36 (426).

56 For the definitive analysis of the Latin text, see Falk Eisermann's survey in *Stimulus amoris: Inhalt, lateinische Überlieferung, deutsche Übersetzungen, Rezeption*. Münchener Texte und Untersuchungen 118 (Tübingen: M. Niemeyer, 2001).

57 Jennifer Bryan, *Looking Inward: Devotional Reading and the Private Self in Late Medieval England* (Philadelphia: University of Pennsylvania Press, 2008), pp. 128–9. This is not to say that there is no concern with spiritual health in the *Stimulus Amoris*. On the contrary, there are moments in the text that show a concern with the health of the soul – or the lack thereof – and with Christ as a healer: Christ is the shop full of spices (pp. 634–5) who provides a healing bath in His side-wound (p. 641). See the *Stimulus Amoris*, in *S. Bonaventura Opera Omnia*, ed. A. C. Peltier, vol. 12 (Paris: Ludovicus Vivès, 1868) pp. 631–703. The *Prickynge*, however, enhances these core images and themes.

58 The medical lexis is consistent across many manuscript witnesses; see vol. 2 of Kane's edition: pp. 327–9.

59 These medical terms are consistent with other witnesses; see Kane, vol. 2, p. 335.

60 *MED*, 'shelle' (n.). While consistent across manuscript witnesses, this word is a unique addition of the translator. The Latin *Stimulus Amoris* uses 'flagellum' or 'whip' (p. 636).

61 *MED*, 'paren' (v.(1)).

62 These medical terms are consistent across the majority of manuscripts – see Kane, vol. 2, pp. 293–4.

63 This is probably what Rolle has in mind when he makes reference to the 'letwary' of love. See his *Incendium Amoris*, in *The Fire of Love and the Mending of Life, or the Rule of Living*, ed. Ralph Harvey, EETS O. S. 106 (London: Oxford University Press, reprint 1973), p. 7, l. 12.

64 *MED*, 'licour' (n.) – sense 3.

65   *MED*, 'lumpe' (n.).
66   *Revelation*, p. 54.

4: Longing for Health

1. *The Book of Privy Counselling*, p. 138, l. 28 to p. 139, l. 10. The importance of touching Christ is often mentioned in texts which deal with advanced practices of meditation and contemplation. In Julian's *Revelation*, touch provides not simply context between her and God, but also a form of emotive response: she has 'contrition be the blisfull touching of the Holy Gost' (p. 119), and that 'contrition takyth hym be touchyng of the Holy Gost' (p. 53). Moreover, she notes a connection between touching and longing for God: the 'kinde yernings of the soule' come 'by the touching of the Holy Gost' (p. 7).
2. *MED*, 'plat' (adj.), 'pleyn' (adj.).
3. *MED*, 'longen' (v.(1)).
4. *Cloud*, p. 84, ll. 3–7.
5. Richard Rolle, *The Psalter or Psalms of David and Certain Canticles with a Translation and Exposition in English by Richard Rolle of Hampole*, ed. H. R. Bramley (Oxford: Clarendon Press, 1884), Psalm 12, p. 45.
6. Richard of St Victor, *De quatuor gradibus violentae caritatis*, PL 196: 1207C–24D; *Of the Four Degrees of Passionate Charity*, in *Richard of Saint Victor: Selected Writings on Contemplation*, tr. C. Kirchberger (London: Faber & Faber, 1957), pp. 213–33. I follow Andrew Kraebel's translation of the title as *Four Degrees of Violent Love* rather than *Four Degrees of Violent Charity*. He, rightly to my mind, notes that the Latin is itself meant to seize attention, to offer a 'jarring' moment for the reader. See Kraebel's excellent introduction to *The Four Degrees of Violent Love*, in *On Love: A Selection of Works of Hugh, Adam, Achard, Richard, and Godfrey of St Victor: Victorine Texts in Translation Vol. 2*, ed. H. Feiss (Turnhout: Brepols, 2012), p. 263 n. 2.
7. *Four Degrees*, p. 215, 'Nonne tibi corde percussus videtur, quando igneus ille amoris aculeus mentem hominis medullitus penetrat' (col. 1209C).
8. *Four Degrees*, pp. 215–16, 'Primum enim gradum diximus qui vulnerat, secundum qui ligat' (col. 1209D); and 'sed acutæ febris more continuo ardore animum urit' (col. 1210B).
9. *Four Degrees*, pp. 217–18, 'omnem alium affectum excludit' (col. 1211A) and 'In hoc autem gradu amoris nimietas ad languoris similitudinem manus ac pedes enervat' (col. 1211C).
10. *Four Degrees*, p. 219, 'Hic gradus quia humanae possibilitatis metas semel excessit, crescendi, ut caeteri, terminum nescit, quia semper invenit quod adhuc concupiscere possit' (col. 1212C).
11. *Four Degrees*, p. 219, 'Quid, quaeso, est quod cor hominis profundius penetret, acerbius cruciet, vehementius exagitet?' (col. 1212D).
12. *Four Degrees*, p. 219. Latin: col. 1212D.
13. *Four Degrees*, p. 224, 'quarto animus exit propter Deum, et descendit sub semetipsum. In primo animus ingreditur ad seipsum, in secundo transgreditur semetipsum. In primo pergit in seipsum, in tertio pergit in Deum suum. In primo ingreditur propter seipsum, in quarto egreditur propter proximum. In primo intrat meditatione, in secundo ascendit contemplatione, in tertio retroducitur in jubilatione, in quarto egreditur ex compassione' (col. 1217D).
14. *Pistle*, p. 50, l. 23 to p. 51, l. 5.
15. *MED*, medlen (v.).
16. Similar comments are found in related works of the *Cloud* author. In *A Tretyse of þe Stodye of Wysdome*, the figure of Rachel is used as analogy for the emotional nature of contemplative aspirations: she 'whetteþ hir desires, iche desire on desire, so þat at þe laste, in greet habundaunce of brennyng desires and sorow of þe delaiing of hir desire, Beniamyn is borne, and his moder Rachel diȝeþ', p. 45, ll. 3–6. Longyng for God requires an emotional complex of the utmost power, and will push the soul to a state akin to death.

17	*PoC*, l. 345.
18	*PoC*, ll. 9490–7.
19	*PoC*, ll. 9495–9.
20	*PoC*, ll. 9498–9.
21	Such an understanding can be found in the work of John of la Rochelle. See J. G. Bougerol (ed.), *Summa De Anima: Textes philosophiques du moyen âge 19* (Paris: Vrin, 1995), 108, 7–14: 'Vnde affectiones multiplicantur secundum quattuor differencias, et hoc secundum sanctos et philosophos, scilicet gaudium seu leticia, dolor seu tristicia, cupiditas seu spes, metus seu timor; quarum patet numerus. Nam due sunt ex comprehensione boni, due ex comprehensione mali. Ex comprehensione boni, gaudium seu leticia, cupiditas seu spes. Sed gaudium siue leticia est de bono presenti, cupiditas uel spes de futuro. Due ex comprehensione mali, dolor seu tristicia de presenti malo, timor uel metus de futuro.'
22	*SV*, ll. 1625–8.
23	*SV*, ll. 1663–4.
24	*Revelation*, pp. 118–19.
25	*Revelation*, p. 119.
26	*Revelation*, p. 106.
27	*Revelation*, p. 54.
28	*Pore Caitif*, p. 164, ll. 12–13.
29	*Pore Caitif*, p. 167, l. 13.
30	*Chastising*, p. 164, ll. 1–112.
31	*Chastising*, p. 207, ll. 9–10.
32	*Cloud*, p. 77, ll. 6–16. See also my 'Words of Fire and Fruit: The Psychology of Prayer Words in *The Cloud of Unknowing*', *Medium Aevum*, 84/2 (2015), 213–30.
33	*Cloud*, p. 77, ll. 4–5.
34	*Cloud*, p. 76, ll. 1–3.
35	*The Book of Privy Counselling*, p. 166, l. 25.

5: Dangerous Reading

1	Thomas Hoccleve, 'A Dialogue', in *'My Compleinte' and Other Poems*, ed. Roger Ellis (Exeter: University of Exeter Press, 2001), ll. 404–6.
2	*MED*, 'pouren' (v.(1+2)).
3	*MED*, 'wit' (n.).
4	'The Introduction to the Pardoner's Tale', in *The Riverside Chaucer*, 3rd edn, gen. ed. Larry D. Benson (Oxford: Oxford University Press, 1988), p. 194, ll. 312–13.
5	'The Introduction to the Pardoner's Tale', l. 317.
6	Ad haec verba quodam ille pudore perfusus, demisso capite, fixisque in terram luminibus: 'Verissime, inquit, verissime. Nam et in fabulis, quae vulgo de nescio quo finguntur Arcturo, memini me nonnunquam usque ad effusionem lacrymarum fuisse permotum. Unde non modicum pudet propriae vanitatis, qui si forte ad ea quae de Domino pie leguntur, vel cantantur, vel certe publico sermone dicuntur, aliquam mihi lacrymam valuero extorquere, ita mihi statim de sanctitate applaudo, ut si magnum aliquid ac inusitatum mihi miraculum contigisset. Et revera vanissimae mentis judicium est, pro his affectibus, si forte pro pietate contingant, vana gloria ventilari: quibus in fabulis et mendaciis solebat compungi (in *Speculum caritatis*, in PL 195, col. 565D). For the translation see Tahkokallio's 'Fables of King Arthur', *Mirator*, 9/1 (2008), 25–6: 'At these words the novice blushed and, with his head bowed and his eyes fixed on the ground, he said: 'Truly so, very truly so. For also when (listening to/reading) fables that are popularly made up about that Arthur, whoever he is, I remember I was sometimes moved to the point of shedding tears. Therefore I feel greatly ashamed of my vanity, for when I succeed in squeezing out a tear listening to things that are, with piety, read, chanted or indeed preached about our Lord, I

immediately congratulate myself as if some great and extraordinary miracle had happened to me. And it is, in fact, the mark of a very vain mind to become puffed up with vainglory because of these affections that, even though they accidentally come up in relation to piety, used to move my mind when (reading/listening to) fables and lies.'

7   *Eight Chapters on Perfection*, p. 8, ll. 113–18.
8   *MED*, 'unmesurable' (adj.).
9   *MED*, 'undiscreete' (adj.).
10 This is in part due to the psychological nature of its operation. As Jean Leclercq notes, religious reading causes 'a kind of chain reaction of associations which will bring together words that have no more than a chance connection, purely external, with one another', as such the order of the reading process 'really follows a psychological development, determined by the plan of associations, and one digression may lead to another or even to several others' (*Love of Learning*, p. 74). In essence, such reading is potentially problematic as it is psychologically ungovernable. Such concerns are made during the period as well. As Guigo II notes in the *Scala Claustralium*, anyone who practises *lectio divina* must take care: 'Sed caveat sibi iste ne post contemplationem istam, qua elevatus fuerit usque ad coelos, inordinato casu corruat usque ad abyssos' (PL 184, col. 483B) ('but let such a man beware, after having reached contemplation, in which he was raised to the heavens, lest he fall back in disorder to the depths'). The translation is in *The Ladder of Monks, A Letter on the Contemplative Life, and Twelve Meditations*, ed. and tr. Edmund Colledge and James Walsh (Kalamazoo: Cistercian Publications, 1981), p. 83. Without the modulating influence of habitual order and practice, reading can become dangerous. Moreover, he makes it clear that reading is not inherently beneficial: 'Legere enim et meditari tam bonis quam malis commune est' (PL 184, col. 478A) ('The good and the wicked alike can read and meditate') (p. 72). As reading is, in terms of its psychological operation, morally neutral, great care must be taken.
11 Vincent Gillespie, 'Dial M for Mystic: Mystical Texts in the Library of Syon Abbey and the Spirituality of the Syon Brethren', in Marion Glasscoe (ed.), *The Medieval Mystical Tradition in England VI* (Boydell & Brewer: Cambridge, 1999), pp. 241–68 (244–6).
12 *Prickynge*, p. 138, ll. 9–11.
13 *Prickynge*, p. 148, ll. 6–13.
14 *Cloud*, p. 96, ll. 22–4.
15 *Cloud*, p. 86, l. 10; p. 86, ll. 17–18.
16 *Cloud*, p. 86, ll. 24–7.
17 *Cloud*, p. 85 l. 23 – p. 86 l.2.
18 *Cloud*, p. 87, ll. 5–15.
19 *MED*, 'rudeli' (adv.).
20 *MED*, 'list' (n.(2+3)).
21 René Tixier notes that this phrase is also a proverb used frequently by the author in his works and translated from Richard of Saint Victor, see '"Good gamesumli pley": Games of Love in *The Cloud Of Unknowing*', *The Downside Review*, 108 (1990), 235–53 (251 n.3).
22 *MED*, 'festren' (v.).
23 *Cloud*, p. 96, ll. 10–12.
24 *Cloud*, p. 97, l. 21 to p. 100, l. 2.
25 *Angels Song*, pp. 179–80.
26 Luke Demaitre, *Medieval Medicine: The Art of Healing, From Head to Toe* (Santa Barbara: Praeger, 2013), p. 133.
27 *Scale*, 1, ll. 922–4.
28 *Scale*, 1, ll. 722–4.
29 *Scale*, 1, ll. 722–5.
30 Tixier, '"Þis louely blinde werk": Contemplation in the *Cloud of Unknowing* and Related Treatises', in William F. Pollard and Robert E. Boenig (eds), *Mysticism and Spirituality in Medieval England* (Cambridge: D. S. Brewer, 1997), pp. 107–38 (107 n. 1).

NOTES 177

31 *Stodye*, p. 38, l. 11 to p. 39, l. 1.
32 *Pistle*, p. 48, ll. 1–2.
33 *Pistle*, p. 48, l. 7.
34 *Pistle*, p. 48, l. 16.
35 *Pistle*, p. 48, ll. 18–19; p. 49, l. 9.
36 *Pistle*, p. 49, ll. 11 to p. 50, l. 12.
37 *MED*, 'hevinesse' (n.).
38 *Pistle*, p. 59, ll. 3–4.
39 *Cloud*, p. 83, ll. 14–27.
40 *Cloud*, p. 84, l. 7.
41 *Cloud*, p. 84, ll. 20–2.
42 Such emotional problems beset monastic life. As Alexander Murray notes, there is a wealth of stories of suicidal melancholy that focus on those in religious orders (p. 333), and such stories – as well as texts which explore psychological and emotional problems – 'are part of the monks' professional equipment' (p. 333). Theologically, such a desire to 'vnbe' is akin to a breach of obedience, a refusal to accept God's will (*fiat volutas tua*) and to despair enough to take one's own life – which belongs only to God. For more on the monastic rules against suicide, see Murray's *Suicide in the Middle Ages: Volume II: The Curse on Self-Murder* (Oxford: Oxford University Press, 2008).
43 *Prickynge*, p. 96, ll. 2–12.
44 *Prickynge*, p. 96, ll. 1–2.
45 *Scale*, 1, l. 1556.
46 *Angels Song*, p. 181.
47 *Prickynge*, p. 139, l. 9.
48 *Prickynge*, p. 139, l. 16 to p. 140, l. 8.
49 *MED*, 'tome' (adj.).
50 *MED*, 'voide' (adj.).
51 *Eight Chapters on Perfection*, p. 17, ll. 260–70.
52 *Eight Chapters on Perfection*, p. 18, ll. 273–5.
53 The *Cloud* has a similar image: the 'scharpe double eggid dreedful swerde of discrecion', p. 68, ll. 10–12.
54 *Eight Chapters on Perfection*, p. 18, ll. 275–6.
55 *Scale*, 2, ll. 866–78.
56 Vincent Gillespie and Samuel Fanous (eds), *The Cambridge Companion to Medieval English Mysticism* (Cambridge: Cambridge University Press, 2011), p. 292.
57 *The Rule of St Benedict: Latin and English*, tr. Luke Dysinger, O. S. B. (Santa Ana, CA: Source Books, 1997, rep. 2003), 64, p. 153.
58 *Sermones super Cantica Canticorum*, in *Sancti Bernardi Opera Omnia*, ed. Jean Leclercq, Henri Rochais, Charles H. Talbot, 2 (Rome: Editiones Cistercienses, 1957–1977), *Sermo* 49 2. 5: 'Est ergo discretio non tam virtus, quam quaedam moderatrix et aurigam virtutum, ordinatrixque affectuam, et morum doctrix'. The translation is from Ann W. Astell, 'A Discerning Smell: Olfaction among the Senses in St Bonaventure's *Long Life of St Francis*', 59 *Franciscan Studies*, 67 (2009), 91–131 (108 n. 68).
59 Astell, 'A Discerning Smell', p. 109.
60 Bernard of Clairvaux, *On the Song of Songs III*, Cistercian Fathers Series 31 (Kalamazoo: Cistercian Publications, 1979), p. 25, 'Tolle hanc, et virtus vitium erit; *Sermo* 29, PL 183, col. 1018D.
61 *Stodye*, p. 39, ll. 6–8.
62 *Mixed Life*, p. 267.
63 *Mixed Life*, p. 267.
64 *Cloud*, p. 86, ll. 24–7.
65 *Pistle*, p. 49, ll. 11–13.

66 Demaitre, *Medieval Medicine*, p. 38.
67 *MED*, 'alienacioun' (n.), specifically senses 2 and 3.
68 *Scale*, 2, l. 878.
69 *Cloud*, p. 92, ll. 12–13.
70 *Discrescyon of Spirites*, p. 88, ll. 13–20.
71 *Discrescyon of Spirites*, p. 88, l. 11; p. 88, l. 11; p. 88, l. 8.
72 *Discrescyon of Spirites*, p. 90, l. 22.
73 *Discrecioun of Stirings*, p. 64, ll. 17–23.
74 Carl Horstmann (ed.), *The Mirror of St Edmund*, in *Yorkshire Writers: Richard Rolle of Hampole, an English Father of the Church, and His Followers*, vol. 1 (London: Swan Sonnenschein, 1895–96), p. 261.
75 *Chastising*, p. 112, ll. 4–5.
76 Phyllis Hodgson and Gabriel M. Liegey (eds), *The Orchard of Syon*, EETS O. S. 258, (Oxford: Oxford University Press, 1966), p. 37, l. 17 to p. 38, l. 14.
77 *Orchard*, p. 37, l. 1.
78 *Orchard*, p. 37, l. 3.
79 *Orchard*, p. 37, l. 22; p. 37, l. 24.
80 *Orchard*, p. 38, ll. 34–5.
81 John Henry Blunt (ed.), *The Myroure of Our Lady*, EETS E. S. 19 (London: N. Trübner & Co, 1873), p. 69.
82 *MED*, 'convenient' (adj.).
83 *Myroure*, p. 69.

Conclusion

1 Susanna Fein (ed.), *John the Blind Audelay: Poems and Carols* (Kalamazoo: Medieval Institute Publications, 2009), p. 198, l. 55.
2 Richard Rolle, *Meditations on the Passion*, in *English Writings of Richard Rolle, Hermit of Hampole*, ed. Hope Emily Allen (Oxford: Clarendon Press, 1931), p. 22, l. 110.
3 *Pore Caitif*, 1, l. 10.

Select Bibliography

Primary

Manuscripts

Cambridge, St John's College, MS A 15.
Oxford, Bodleian Library, MS Bodley 42.
Oxford, Bodleian Library, MS Digby 2.
Oxford, Bodleian Library, MS Digby 55.
Oxford, Bodleian Library MS Douce 302.
Oxford, Bodleian Library, MS Eng. poet. a. 1.
Oxford, Bodleian Library Rawlinson G.22.
Paris, Bibliotheque Nationale MS. lat.16417.

Editions

Aelred of Rievaulx, *Speculum caritatis*, in PL 195.
Alanus de Insulis, *Regulae de Sacra Theologia*, in PL 210.
Albertus Magnus, *Super Mattheum*, in *Alberti Magni Opera omnia, cura et studio Instituti Alberti Magni*, ed. Bernardus Schmidt, vol. 21/1 (Münster: Aschendorff, 1987).
Anselm, St, *Orationes sive meditationes*, in *St Anselmi Cantuariensis archiepiscopi opera omnia*, ed. Franciscus Salesius Schmitt (Stuttgart: Frommann, 1968).
— , *The Prayers and Meditations of Saint Anselm with the Proslogion*, tr. Benedicta Ward (London: Penguin Books, 1973).
Aquinas, Thomas, *Sententia libri politicorum tabula libri ethicorum*, in *Sancti Thomae de Aquino Opera omnia*, ed. P. Minge, 48 (Rome: Commissio Leonina, 1971).
Arnald of Vilanova, *Regimen sanitatis ad regem Aragonum, Arnaldi de Villanova Opera medica omnia*, ed. Luis Garcia-Ballester, vol. 10/1 (Barcelona : Pagès Editors, 1996).
Augustine, *De doctrina christiana*, ed. Almut Mützenbecher, Corpus Christianorum Series Latina, 32 (Turnhout: Brepols, 1962).
— , *De sermone domini in monte libri duo*, ed. Almut Mützenbecher, Corpus Christianorum Series Latina, 35 (Turnhout: Brepols, 1967).

—, *Enarratio in Psalmos*, in PL 36.
—, *Ex Sermonibus ab Angelo Mai Editis*, in *Miscellanea Agostiniana: Testi e Studi*, ed. Germain Morin, vol. 1 (Rome: Tipografia poliglotta vaticana, 1930).
—, *Expositions on the Psalms*, ed. Philip Schaff, tr. J. E. Tweed, Nicene and Post-Nicene Fathers, First Series, 8 (repr. New York: Cosimo, 2007).
—, *In Epistolam Joannis ad Parthos*, in PL 35.
—, *Sermones*, in PL 38.
Avicenna, *Avicenna Latinus: Liber de Anima seu Sextus de Naturalibus, IV–V*, ed. Gerard Verbeke and Simone Van Riet (Leiden: Brill, 1968).
Bacon, Roger, *Communia naturalium*, in *Opera hactenus inedita II*, ed. Robert Steele (Oxford: Clarendon Press, 1905).
—, *On Signs: Opus maius, Part 3, Chapter 2*, ed. Thomas S. Maloney, Medieval Sources in Translation, 54 (Toronto: Pontifical Institute of Medieval Studies, 2013).
—, *Opus tertium*, in *Opera quaedam hactenus inedita: Opus tertium, Opus minus, Compendium studii philosophiae, Epistola de secretis operibus Artis et Naturae, et de nullitate Magiae*, ed. J. S. Brewer (London: Longman, 1965).
Basil, St, *Regulae Fusius Tractatae*, PG 31.
Bazire, Joyce, and Colledge, Eric (eds), *The Chastising of God's Children, and The Treatise of Perfection of The Sons of God* (Oxford: Basil Blackwell, 1957).
Benedict, St, *The Rule of St Benedict: Latin and English*, tr. Luke Dysinger, O. S. B. (Santa Ana, CA: Source Books, 1997, rep. 2003).
Bernard of Clairvaux, *On the Song of Songs III*, Cistercian Fathers Series 31 (Kalamazoo, MI: Cistercian Publications, 1979).
—, *Sententiae*, in *Sancti Bernardi Opera Omnia* 6/2, ed. Jean Leclercq, Henri Rochais, Charles H. Talbot (Rome: Editiones Cistercienses, 1957–77).
—, *Sermones in Cantica Canticorum*, in PL 183.
Bestul, Thomas H. (ed.), *The Scale of Perfection* (Kalamazoo, MI: Medieval Institute Publications, 2000).
Blunt, John Henry (ed.), *The Myroure of Our Lady*, EETS E. S. 19 (London: N. Trübner & Co., 1873).
Bonaventure, St, *Collationes de septem donis Spiritus sancti*, in *Opera Omnia*, vol. 5.
—, *Commentaria in Quatuor Libros Sententiarum Magistri Petri Lombardi*, in *Opera Omnia*, vol. 3, ed. R. P. Aloysii A. Parma (Collegium S. Bonaventurae: Quaracchi, 1882–1902).
—, *Stimulis Amoris*, in *St Bonaventura Opera Omnia*, vol. 12, ed. A. C. Peltier (Paris: Ludovicus Vivès, 1868).
Brady, Mary Theresa, '*The Pore Caitif*: Edited from MS Harley 2336 With Introduction and Notes' (unpublished Ph.D. thesis, Fordham University, 1954).
Bramley, H. R. (ed.), *The Psalter or Psalms of David and Certain Canticles with a Translation and Exposition in English by Richard Rolle of Hampole* (Oxford: Clarendon Press, 1884).
Brown, Carleton F. (ed.), *English Lyrics of the Thirteenth Century* (Oxford: Clarendon Press, 1932).
— (ed.), *Religious Lyrics of the Fourteenth Century*, 2nd edn (Oxford: Clarendon Press, 1924).
Bruno of Segni, *Commentaria in* Matthaeum, PL 165.
Cassian, John, *The Conferences*, tr. Boniface Ramsey (New York: Paulist Press, 1997).

Cassiodorus, *Explanation of the Psalms: Volume 1*, tr. P. G. Walsh (New York: Paulist, 1991).
— , *In Psalterium Praefatio*, PL 70.
Celsus, *De Medicina*, tr. W. G. Spencer (Cambridge, MA: Harvard University Press, 1956).
Chaucer, Geoffrey, 'The Introduction to the Pardoner's Tale', in *The Riverside Chaucer*, 3rd edition, gen. ed. Larry D. Benson (Oxford: Oxford University Press, 1988).
— , *Troilus and Criseyde*, in *The Riverside Chaucer*, 3rd edn, gen. ed. Larry D. Benson (Oxford: Oxford University Press, 1988).
Clement of Alexandria, *Stromata*, in *The Stromata or Miscellanies*, ed. A. Robert and J. Donaldson, The Ante-Nicene Fathers 2 (Grand Rapids, MI: Eerdmans, 1967).
Conciliorum oecumenicorum decreta, 3rd edn, ed. Giuseppe Alberigo, J. A. Dossetti, P. Joannou, C. Leonardi and P. Prodi (Bologna: Istituto per le Scienze Religiose, 1973).
Connolly, Margaret (ed.), *The Contemplations of the Drede and Love of God*, EETS O. S. 303 (Oxford: Oxford University Press, 1993).
Copeland, Rita, and Sluiter, Ineke (eds) and tr., *Medieval Grammar and Rhetoric: Language Arts and Literary Theory, AD 300–1475* (Oxford: Oxford University Press, 2009).
Damascene, John St, *De fide orthodoxa*, PG 94.
Damian, Peter, *Sermones*, ed. Giovanni Luchessi, Corpus Christianorum Continuatio Medievalis 57 (Turnholt: Brepols, 1983).
Donatus, *Ars grammatica*, in *Grammatici latini, 4*, ed. Heinrich Keil (Leipzig, 1857).
Duncan, Thomas G. (ed.), *Medieval English Lyrics and Carols*, rev. edn (Cambridge: D. S. Brewer, 2013).
Edden, Valerie (ed.), *Richard Maidstone's Penitential Psalms: Edited from Bodleian MS Rawlinson A.389* (Heidelberg: Carl Winter, 1990).
Fein, Susanna (ed.), *John the Blind Audelay: Poems and Carols* (Kalamazoo, MI: Medieval Institute Publications, 2009).
Francis, W. Nelson (ed.), *The Book of Vices and Virtues: A Fourteenth Century English Translation of The Somme le roi of Lorens d'Orléans*, EETS O. S. 217 (London: Oxford University Press, 1945).
Fredborg, K. M., Nielsen, Lauge, and Pinborg, Jan (eds), 'An unedited part of Roger Bacon's *Opus maius: De signis*' Traditio, 34 (1978), 75–136.
Furnivall, F. J. (ed.), *The Minor Poems of the Vernon MS Part II*, EETS O. S. 117 (London: Kegan Paul, Trench Trübner & Co., 1901).
Glossa ordinaria: Biblia sacra cum glossis et postillis Nicoli Lyrani, vol. 1, (Lyon: 1545).
Gregory the Great, *Homiliarum in Evangelia Liber II*, PL 76.
Gregory of Nazianzus, *Adversus Iram*, PG 37.
Gregory of Nyssa, in *Gregory of Nyssa: Life of Moses*, ed. A. Malherbe and E. Ferguson (New York: Paulist Press, 1978).
Grosseteste, Robert, *Dicta*, in *Robertus Grosseteste: Dicta*, ed. Joseph Goering, www.grosseteste.com.
— , *Templum Dei*, ed. Joseph W. Goering and F. A. C. Mantello (Toronto: Pontifical Institute of Medieval Studies, 1984).
— , *The Complete Dicta in English vol. 1*, ed. and tr. Gordon Jackson (Lincoln: Asgill Press, 2003).
Guigo II, *Scala Claustralium*, PL 184.

—, *The Ladder of Monks, A Letter on the Contemplative Life, and Twelve Meditations*, ed. and tr. Edmund Colledge and James Walsh (Kalamazoo, MI: Cistercian Publications, 1981).

Hanna, Ralph (ed.), *Speculum Vitae: A Reading Edition*, EETS O. S. 331 (Oxford: Oxford University Press, 2008).

—, *Uncollected Prose and Verse with Related Northern Texts*, EETS O. S. 329 (Oxford: Oxford University Press, 2007).

Hanna, Ralph, and Wood, Sarah (eds), *Richard Morris's Prick of Conscience: A Corrected and Amplified Reading Text*, EETS O. S. 342 (Oxford: Oxford University Press, 2013).

Harvey, Ralph (ed.), *The Fire of Love and the Mending of Life, or the Rule of Living* EETS O. S. 106, (London: Oxford University Press, reprint 1973).

Hoccleve, Thomas, 'A Dialogue', in *'My Compleinte' and Other Poems*, ed. Roger Ellis (Exeter: University of Exeter Press, 2001).

Hodgson, Phyllis (ed.), *Deonise hid Divinite and Other Treatises on Contemplative Prayer related to The Cloud of Unknowing*, EETS O. S. 231 (London: Oxford University Press, 1955).

— (ed.), *The Cloud of Unknowing and The Book of Privy Counselling*, EETS, O. S. 218 (London: Oxford University Press, 1944).

Hodgson, Phyllis, and Liegey, Gabriel M. (eds), *The Orchard of Syon*, EETS O.S 258 (Oxford: Oxford University Press, 1966).

Horstmann, Carl (ed.), *Epistle on the Mixed Life*, in *Yorkshire Writers: Richard Rolle of Hampole, an English Father of the Church, and His Followers*, 2 vols (London: Swan Sonnenschein, 1895–96), vol. 1, pp. 264–92.

— (ed.), *Of Angels Song*, in *Yorkshire Writers: Richard Rolle of Hampole, an English Father of the Church, and His Followers*, 2 vols (London: Swan Sonnenschein, 1895–96), vol. 1, pp. 175–82.

Hugo de Folieto, *De medicina anime*, PL 176.

Hugh of St Victor, *De arca Noe morali*, PL 176.

—, *Homiliae in Ecclesiasten* 1, PL 175.

—, *Selected Spiritual Writings*, ed. Alered Squire (London: Harper and Row, 1962).

—, *The Didascalicon of Hugh of St Victor*, tr. Jerome Taylor (New York: Columbia University Press, 1991).

Isac of Stella, *Epistola de anima*, PL 194.

Jerome, St, *Selected Letters*, tr. F. A. Wright (Cambridge, MA: Harvard University Press, 1933).

—, *The Letters of Saint Jerome, Vol. 1*, tr. Christopher Mierow (New York: Newman Press, 1963).

John of La Rochelle, *Summa De Anima: Textes philosophiques du moyen âge 19*, ed. J. G. Bougerol (Paris: Vrin, 1995).

—, *Tractatus de divisione multiplici potentiarum animae: Textes philosophiques du moyen âge 11*, ed. P. Michaud-Quantin (Paris: Vrin, 1964).

Julian of Norwich, *A Revelation of Love*, ed. Marion Glasscoe (Exeter: University of Exeter Press, 1976).

Kane, Harold (ed.), *The Prickynge of Love*, 2 vols (Salzburg: Institut für Anglistik und Amerikanistik der Universität Salzburg, 1983).

Kuriyagawa, Fumio (ed.), *Walter Hilton's Eight Chapters on Perfection* (Tokyo: Keio University, 1967).
Lawler, Traugott (ed.), *The Parisiana poetria of John of Garland* (New Haven: Yale University Press, 1974).
Leclercq, Jean, 'Le De grammatica de Hugues de Saint Victor', in *Archives d'histoire doctrinale et littéraire du moyen âge,* 20 (1945).
Lombard, Peter, *Petri Lombardi in psalmos Davidicos commentarii praefatio*, PL 191.
— , *Sententiae in IV Libris Distinctae*, 2 vols, Spicilegium Bonaventurianum, 3rd edn, ed. Ian Brady (Grottaferrata: Editiones Collegii S. Bonaventurae ad Claras Aquas, 1971–1981)
Manzalaoui, M. A. (ed.), *Secretum Secretorum: Nine English Versions*, EETS O. S. 276 (Oxford: Oxford University Press, 1977).
McGinn, Bernard (ed.), *Three Treatises on Man: A Cistercian Anthropology* (Kalamazoo, MI: Cistercian Publications, 1977).
Minnis, A. J., and Scott, A. B. (eds), *Medieval Literary Theory and Criticism c.1100–1375: The Commentary Tradition* (Oxford: Clarendon Press, 1988).
Mooney, Lynn, 'A Middle English Text on the Seven Liberal Arts', *Speculum*, 68 (1993), 1027–52.
Morgan, G. R., 'A Critical Edition of Caxton's *The Art and Craft to Know Well to Die*, and *Ars Moriendi* Together with the Antecedent Manuscript Material' (unpublished Ph.D. thesis, University of Oxford, 1972).
Odilo of Cluny, *De sancta cruce*, PL 142.
Ogilvie-Thomson, S. J. (ed.), *Richard Rolle: Prose and Verse*, EETS O. S. 293 (Oxford: Oxford University Press, 1988).
Origin, *Commentary on Matthew*, in *Commentarius in Matthaeum, Die griechischen christlichen Schriftsteller der ersten drei Jahrhunderte 40*, ed. E. Klostermann and E. Benz (Leipzig: J. Hinrichssche Buchhandlung, 1935–37).
Patrologia cursus completus series Graeca, ed. J. P. Migne, 161 vols (Paris: Garnier Frères, 1857–1905).
Patrologia cursus completus series Latina, ed. J. P. Migne, 221 vols (Paris: Garnier Frères, 1844–1905).
Peraldus, William, *Summae virtutum ac vitiorum*, 2 vols (Antwerp: Philippus Nutius, 1571).
Plato, *Phaedo*, ed. and tr. David Gallop (Oxford: Clarendon Press, 1975).
— , *Timaeus*, ed. and tr. John Warrington (London: Dent, 1965).
Priscian, *Institutiones grammaticae*, in *Grammatici latini, 2*, ed. Heinrich Keil (Leipzig: Teubner, 1857).
Pseudo-Kilwardby, *Commentum super Priscianum maiorem*, in *La Parole comme acte*, ed. Irene Rosier-Catach (Paris: Vrin, 1994).
Reichl, K. (ed.), *Tractatus de grammatica eine falschlich Robert Grosseteste zugeschriebene spekulative Grammatik: Edition und Kommentar*, Veröffentlichungen des Grabmann-Institutes, 28 (Munich: Schoningh, 1976).
Richard of St Victor, *Benjamin Minor*, PL 196.
— , *De quatuor gradibus violentae caritatis*, PL 196.
— , *Of the Four Degrees of Passionate Charity*, in *Richard of Saint Victor: Selected Writings on Contemplation*, tr. C. Kirchberger (London: Faber & Faber, 1957).
— , *The Twelve Patriarchs*, tr. Grover A. Zinn (New York: Paulist Press, 1979).

Rolle, Richard, *English Writings of Richard Rolle, Hermit of Hampole*, ed. Hope Emily Allen (Oxford: Clarendon Press, 1931).

Sargent, Michael G. (ed.), *The Mirror of the Blessed Life of Jesus Christ: A Reading Text* (Exeter: University of Exeter Press, 2004).

Seymour, M. C., and Andrew, Malcolm (eds), *On the Properties of Things: John Trevisa's translation of Bartholomeus Anglicus's* De Proprietatibus Rerum (Oxford: Clarendon Press, 1975).

Trexler, Richard C. (ed.), *The Christian at Prayer: An Illustrated Prayer Manual Attributed to Peter the Chanter* (New York: Medieval and Renaissance Texts and Studies, 1987).

Wallis, Faith (ed.), *Medieval Medicine: A Reader* (Toronto: Toronto University Press, 2010).

Westra, Salvina (ed.), *A Talking of the Love of God* (The Hague: Martinus Nijhoff, 1950).

William of Auvergne, *De sacramento poenitentiae,* in *Guilelmi Alverni Episcopi Parisiensis, Opera omnia vol. 1 and Supplementum*, ed. F. Hotot and B. Le Feron (Orléans and Paris, 1674; reprint Frankfurt, 1963).

William de Montibus, *Peniteas Cito*, in *William de Montibus (c.1140–1213): The Schools and the Literature of Pastoral Care*, ed. Joseph Goering (Toronto: Pontifical Institute of Medieval Studies, 1992).

William of St Thierry, *De natura corporis et animae*, PL 180.

—, *On Contemplating God, Prayer, Meditations*, tr. Sister Penelope Lawson (Shannon: Irish University Press, 1971).

Secondary

Alford, John A., 'Rolle's *English Psalter* and Lectio Divina', *Bulletin of the John Rylands Library* 77/3 (1995), 47–60.

Amsler, Mark, *Affective Literacies: Writing and Multilingualism in the Late Middle Ages* (Turnhout: Brepols, 2011).

Arbesmann, Rudolph, 'The Concept of "Christus Medicus" in St Augustine', *Traditio*, 10 (1954), 1–28.

Astell, Ann W., 'A Discerning Smell: Olfaction among the Senses in St Bonaventure's *Long Life of St Francis*', *Franciscan Studies*, 67 (2009), 91–131.

Biller, Peter, 'Confession in the Middle Ages: An Introduction', in Peter Biller and A. J. Minnis (eds), *Handling Sin: Confession in the Middle Ages* (York: York Medieval Press, 1998), pp. 1–34.

Boquet, Damien, and Nagy, Piroska, 'Medieval Sciences of Emotions during the Eleventh to Thirteenth Centuries: An Intellectual History', *Osiris*, 31/1 (2016), 21–45.

Boyle, Leonard, 'The Fourth Lateran Council and Manuals of Popular Theology', in Thomas J. Heffernan (ed.), *The Popular Literature of Medieval England* (Knoxville: University of Tennessee Press, 1985), pp. 30–43.

Bryan, Jennifer, *Looking Inward: Devotional Reading and the Private Self in Late Medieval England* (Philadelphia: University of Pennsylvania Press, 2008).

Carruthers, Mary, *The Book of Memory: A Study of Memory in Medieval Culture* (Cambridge: Cambridge University Press, 1990).

—, *The Experience of Beauty in the Middle Ages* (Oxford: Oxford University Press, 2013).

Catto, Jeremy, 'Theology after Wycliffism', in Jeremy Catto and Ralph Evans (eds), *The History of the University of Oxford*, vol. 2 (Oxford: Oxford University Press, 1992), pp. 263–80.

—, '1349–1412: Culture and History', in Vincent Gillespie and Samuel Fanous (eds), *The Cambridge Companion to Medieval English Mysticism* (Cambridge: Cambridge University Press, 2011), pp. 113–31.

Cohen-Hanegbi, Naama, 'Accidents of the Soul: Physicians and Confessors on the Conception and Treatment of Emotions in Italy and Spain, Late Twelfth–Fifteenth Centuries' (unpublished Ph.D. thesis, the Hebrew University, 2011).

—, 'A Moving Soul: Emotions in Late Medieval Medicine', *Osiris*, 31/1 (2016), 46–66.

Chickering, Howell, 'Rhetorical *Stimulus* in the *Prick of Conscience*', in Stephanie Hayes-Healy (ed.), *Medieval Paradigms: Essays in Honour of Jeremy du Quesnay Adams*, The New Middle Ages Series 1 (New York: Palgrave Macmillan, 2005), pp. 191–230.

Demaitre, Luke, *Medieval Medicine: The Art of Healing, From Head to Toe* (Santa Barbara, CA: Praeger, 2013).

Gillespie, Vincent, 'Dial M for Mystic: Mystical Texts in the Library of Syon Abbey and the Spirituality of the Syon Brethren', in Marion Glasscoe (ed.), *The Medieval Mystical Tradition in England VI* (Cambridge: Boydell & Brewer, 1999), pp. 241–68.

—, 'Moral and Penitential Lyrics', in Thomas G. Duncan (ed.), *A Companion to the Middle English Lyric* (Cambridge: D. S. Brewer, 2005), pp. 68–95.

—, 'Morality Touched by Emotion: the Lyrics of the Vernon Manuscript' (unpublished B.Litt. thesis, University of Oxford, 1976).

—, 'Seek, Suffer and Trust: Ese and Disese in Julian of Norwich', *Studies in the Age of Chaucer*, 39 (2017), 129–58.

—— 'Strange Images of Death: The Passion in Later Medieval English Devotional and Mystical Writing', *Analecta Cartusiana*, 117 (1987), 111–59.

—— 'The Senses in Literature: The Textures of Perception', in Richard G. Newhauser (ed.), *A Cultural History of the Senses in the Middle Ages* (London: Bloomsbury, 2016), pp. 153–73.

—— 'The Songs of the Threshold: Enargeia and the Psalter', in Francis Leneghan and Tamara Atkin (eds), *The Psalms and Medieval English Literature: From the Conversion to the Reformation* (London: Boydell & Brewer, 2017), pp. 271–97.

Gillespie, Vincent, and Fanous, Samuel (eds), *The Cambridge Companion to Medieval English Mysticism* (Cambridge: Cambridge University Press, 2011).

Grmek, Mirko D., *Diseases in the Ancient Greek World*, tr. Mireille Muellner and Leonard Muellner (Baltimore: John Hopkins University Press, 1989).

Hammond, Jay M., 'Contemplation and the Formation of the *Vir Spiritualis* in Bonaventure's *Collationes in Hexaemeron*', in Timothy J. Johnson (ed.), *Franciscans at Prayer* (Leiden: Brill, 2007), pp. 123–65.

Hasse, Dag, *De Anima in the Latin West: The Formation of a Peripatetic Philosophy of the Soul 1160–1300* (London: Warburg Institute, 2000).

Johnson, Eric J., 'In dry3 dred and daunger: The Tradition and Rhetoric of Fear in *Cleanness* and *Patience*' (unpublished Ph.D. thesis, University of York, 2000).

Kelly, Henry Ansgar, 'Penitential Theology and Law at the Turn of the Fifteenth Century', in Abigail Firey (ed.), *A New History of Penance* (Leiden: Brill, 2008), pp. 239–318.

Knuuttila, Simo, *Emotions in Ancient and Medieval Philosophy* (Oxford: Oxford University Press, 2004).

—, 'Emotions from Plato to the Renaissance', in Simo Knuuttila and Juha Sihvola (eds), *Sourcebook for the History of the Philosophy of Mind: Philosophical Psychology from Plato to Kant* (London: Springer, 2014), pp. 463–98.

Lazikani, Ayoush, *Cultivating the Heart: Feeling and Emotion in Twelfth and Thirteenth Century Religious Texts* (Cardiff: University of Wales Press, 2015).

Leclercq, Jean, *The Love of Learning and the Desire for God: A Study of Monastic Culture*, tr. Catherine Misrahi (New York: Fordham University Press, 1982).

Martin, Thomas F., 'Paul the Patient: Christus Medicus and the "Stimulus Carnis" (2 Cor. 12:7): A Consideration of Augustine's Medical Christology', *Augustinian Studies*, 32/2 (2001), 219–56.

McCann, Daniel, 'Medicine of Words: Purgative Reading in Richard Rolle's Meditations on the Passion', *The Mediaeval Journal*, 5/2 (2015), 53–83.

McNamer, Sarah, *Affective Meditation and the Invention of Medieval Compassion* (Philadelphia: University of Pennsylvania Press, 2010).

—, 'The Literariness of Literature and the History of Emotion', *PMLA*, 130/5 (2015), 1433–42.

Murray, Alexander, *Suicide in the Middle Ages: Volume II: The Curse on Self-Murder* (Oxford: Oxford University Press, 2008).

Nutton, Vivian, 'God, Galen, and the Depaganization of Ancient Religion', in Peter Biller and Joseph Ziegler (eds), *Religion and Medicine in the Middle Ages* (York: York Medieval Press, 2001), pp. 15–32.

Olson, Glending, *Literature as Recreation in the Later Middle Ages* (Ithaca: Cornell University Press, 1985).

Phillips, C. Matthew, 'Crux a cruciatu dictur: Preaching Self-Torture as Pastoral Care in Twelfth-Century Religious Houses', in Ronald J. Stanbury (ed.), *A Companion to Pastoral Care in the Late Middle Ages 1200–1500* (Leiden: Brill, 2010), pp. 285–310.

Reid, Shelley Annette, 'The First Dispensation of Christ Is Medicinal: Augustine and Roman Medical Culture' (unpublished Ph.D. thesis, University of British Columbia, 2008).

Reiss, Sheryl E., 'Adrian VI, Clement VII, and Art', in Kenneth Gouwens and Sheryl E. Reiss (eds), *The Pontificate of Clement VII: History, Politics, Culture* (Aldershot: Ashgate, 2005), pp. 341–63.

Resnick, I. M., 'PS.-Albert the Great on the Physiognomy of Jesus and Mary', *Mediaeval Studies*, 64 (2002), 227–40.

Robertson, Duncan, *Lectio Divina: The Medieval Experience of Reading* (Minnesota: Liturgical Press, 2011).

Rousse, Jacques, Sieben, Hermann, and Boland, André (eds), 'Lectio divina et lecture spirituelle', *Dictionnaire de Spiritualité*, 9 (Paris: Beauchesne, 1976).

Stock, Brian, *After Augustine: The Meditative Reader and the Text* (Philadelphia: University of Pennsylvania Press, 2001).

—, *Augustine the Reader: Meditation, Self-Knowledge, and the Ethics of Interpretation* (Cambridge, MA: Harvard University Press, 1996).

—, 'Healing Meditation, and the History of Reading', *New Literary History*, 37 (2006), 503–13.

—, 'Minds, Bodies, Readers', *New Literary History*, 37 (2006), 489–501.

Sutherland, Annie, *English Psalms in the Middle Ages*, 1300–1450 (Oxford: Oxford University Press, 2015).

Tahkokallio, Jaakko, 'Fables of King Arthur: Aelred of Rievaulx and Secular Pastimes', *Mirator*, 9/1 (2008), pp. 19–35.

Tixier, René, '"Good gamesumli pley": Games of Love in *The Cloud Of Unknowing*', *The Downside Review*, 108 (1990), 235–53.

— , '"Þis louely blinde werk": Contemplation in the *Cloud of Unknowing* and Related Treatises', in William F. Pollard and Robert E. Boenig (eds), *Mysticism and Spirituality in Medieval England* (Cambridge: D. S. Brewer, 1997), pp. 107–38.

Tuve, Rosemond, *Allegorical Imagery: Some Mediaeval Books and their Posterity* (Princeton: Princeton University Press, 1966).

Van Der Lecq, Ria, 'Modistae', in Henrik Lagerlund (ed.), *Encyclopedia of Medieval Philosophy* (Dordrecht: Springer, 2011), pp. 806–8.

Van Deusen, Nancy, 'Roger Bacon on Music', in Jeremiah Hackett (ed.), *Roger Bacon and the Sciences: Commemorative Essays*, Studien und Texte zur Geistesgeschichte des Mittelalters 57 (Leiden: Brill, 1997), pp. 223–42.

Vecchio, Silvana, 'The Seven Deadly Sins Between Pastoral Care and Scholastic Theology: The *Summa de vitiis* by John of Rupella', tr. Helen Took, in Richard G. Newhauser (ed.), *In the Garden of Evil: The Vices and Culture in the Middle Ages* (Toronto: Pontifical Institute of Medieval Studies, 2005), pp. 104–27.

Yoshikawa, Naōe Kukita (ed.), *Medicine, Religion and Gender in Medieval Culture* (Cambridge: D. S. Brewer, 2015).

Ziegler, Joseph, 'Medicine and Immortality in Terrestrial Paradise', in Peter Biller and Joseph Ziegler (eds), *Religion and Medicine in the Middle Ages* (York: York Medieval Press, 2001), pp. 201–42.

Index

A
Aelred of Rievaulx 133
  Speculum caritatis 175
affect 3, 13, 16, 21–2, 30; *see also* emotion
Albertus Magnus 13, 165, 169
Alcher of Clairvaux 13
Alexander of Hales 15, 16
Allen, Hope Emily 159, 169, 172, 178
allopathic 53, 150
amore 14, 164, 167; *see also* love
ambicio (ambition) 15, 164
anger 7, 15, 41, 53, 119; *see also* emotion
Anselm of Bec 56, 163, 169
antidote 53
apathy 39, 106
apprehension 22, 27, 34, 39, 48, 113–15, 165; *see also* fear
Aquinas, St Thomas 13, 164–5
Arabic 7, 165
Aristotle 18
Arnald of Vilanova 162
ars artium 16; see also *cura animarum*
Ars Moriendi 27
attrition (*attritio*) 51, 55–7, 68; *see also* 'penaunce'
Audelay, John 154–6, 178
  The Counsel of Conscience 154–6
Augustine, St 8–12, 21, 82–6, 91,
  Enarratio in Psalmos 91, 163, 170, 172, 173
  Epistolam Joannis ad Parthos 84, 171
Aurelius Cornelius Celsus 6, 161–2
Averroes 12, 18
Avicenna 7, 12, 18, 162–4
Awe 28–31, 36, 94, 109, 56, 90; *see also* fear

B
Bacon, Roger 21–3, 165–6
  De signis 21
  Communia naturalium 165
  Opus maius 23, 165
  Opus tertium 166
Bartholomeus Anglicus 12, 163, 171
Basil, St 29, 167
beatitudes 15–16, 38, 55, 167
belching 8
belief 41–2, 94, 156
belly 54
Benedict, St 142, 169, 177
Bernard of Clairvaux 20, 27, 31, 46, 84, 142, 163–5, 172, 177
  Sermones super Cantica Canticorum 172, 177
Blood (blode) 43, 52, 64, 81–2, 86, 94–5, 100, 127, 131
Blund, John 13
  Tractatus de anima 13
Boethius 160
Bonaventure, St 13, 29–31, 162, 167, 167, 173
  Collationes de septem donis Spiritus sancti 30, 167
  Commentaria in Quatuor Libros Sententiarum Magistri Petri Lombardi 167, 173
  Stimulus Amoris 92, 173
Boniface, Pope 164
Book of the Craft of Dying 27–8, 166
Book of Vices and Virtues 31, 88, 167, 172
boxynge (medical procedure) 52
brain 14, 135–7
Brigittine Nuns 11, 150
Bruno of Segni 86, 172
Buridan, John 13

C

'cadeance' 122–3
Calcidius 9
Cappadocian Fathers 52
Carthusians 134
Cassian, John 162
Cassiodorus 58–9, 170
catarrh 7
catechetical 15, 28, 39, 74
catharsis 9
Catherine, St 11, 149, 159, 162, 169
  Dialogue 11, 149
Chaucer, Geoffrey 51, 133, 161, 168, 175
Chastising of God's Children 26, 88, 117, 134, 143, 149, 172–8
Christus Medicus 9, 26, 32, 52, 60–1, 82–8, 90–107, 171
  as surgeon 9, 84, 92, 171
clara lectio 6–8
Clement of Alexandria 12, 167
  Stromata 167
Cloud Author, the 26, 113, 132, 138, 174
  A Pistle of Discrecioun of Stirings 148, 178
  A Treatise of Discrescyon of Spirites 148, 178
  A Pistle of Preier 113, 115, 138, 142, 174, 177
  A Tretyse of þe Stodye of Wysdome þat Men Clepen Beniamyn 33, 142, 168, 174, 177
  The Cloud of Unknowing 112, 161, 175, 176
co-experience 87, 161
compassion 25–6, 68, 79, 81–113, 120–37, 151–7, 171; *see also* pain
  etymology 83–4
  as emotional complex 86–92; *see also* emotional complex
complexion 54, 144–5, 150–1
compounds (medical) 83, 97
comprehensio 18
compunction 17, 56, 169; *see also* 'penaunce'
concupiscible 7, 13–15, 22, 114, 164, 167, 174; *see also* powers (of the soul)
conscience 9–10, 43, 48–54, 62, 92–6, 112–13, 144
contemplation (*contemplatio*) 113–20, 135–42, 174, 176
Contemplations of the Drede and Love of God 32, 168
contemptus mundi 46–7, 164
contraries, medicine of 53–5, 82

contrition (*contritio*) 17, 25, 32, 51–9, 62–8, 70–4, 93, 139, 169, 174; *see also* 'penaunce'
conversion, as cure 85–6
cordis 17, 53
  ore 8
  dilatio 89
corruption 9, 14, 44, 66, 139, 144, 145, 149
covetousness 56–7, 77, 82–3, 117–19, 136, 144
cupiditas (greed) 22, 175
  as illness 54
Cura animarum 1, 2, 15–16, 28, 35
cure 9, 16, 28, 53–4, 78, 84–6, 156, 171

D

Damien, Peter 160
despair 15, 85, 138–9, 177
diagnose 31, 49, 70, 134, 144–5
digestion 6–8
discernment (spiritual) 26, 134–7, 142
  discretio spirituum 142, 154
  as *mater virtutum* 142
  'discrecion' 139, 141–2, 148, 177, 178
dolor (sorrow) 21–3, 55, 84, 164, 170, 175; *see also* emotions
dominacio (imperiousness) 15, 164; *see also* emotions
Donatus 23, 165
drede *see* fear
Duns Scotus 13

E

Edmund of Abingdon 28
  Speculum Ecclesiae 28
  The Mirror of St Edmund 149, 166, 176, 178
ekphrasis 18
emotions
  critical history of 3–5
  evocation through language 4, 21–25; *see also* interjections
  as 'feelyng/felyng' 34, 57, 91, 118–19, 121, 126, 131–135
  medical theories of 7
  medieval terms for 3
  moderation of *see* discretion
  and reading 11–12, 150
  and prayer 17–18
  emotional complex 36–7, 40, 43, 85, 97, 107, 112–17, 127, 130–2, 141
  as 'reuerent affeccioun' 114–16
empathy in compassion 83
enargeia 18, 164
eructation 8; *see also* belching

INDEX

eucrasia 7, 150, 151
evacuation 7, 9, 53, 53
exegematic narration 51, 61, 108, 125

F
faculties, of the soul 18, 22, 135, 136
fear
  as *admiratio* 29–30, 167
  as drede 11–12, 27–51, 90–4, 102, 108, 114–16, 138–9, 143, 150–1, 166
  as *erubescentia* 29–30, 167
  as *reuerencia* 15, 35
  as *segnities* 29–30, 167
  as *stupor* 29–30, 167
  as *timor filialis* 29, 31, 37, 114, 116
  as *timor servilis* 29, 30, 31, 114, 167
  theology of 22–5, 28–31, 29, 30, 167
  as *verecundia* 29–30, 167
fever 53, 54, 144–9
  cotidian 145–6
  tercian 145–6
  quartan 145–7
  double quarteyn 145–7
  as emotional disorder 144–6
fomenta verborum 9, 92
food 6, 7, 11, 18, 44
frenesis (phrenesis) 134, 137; *see also* fever
  as spiritual infection 137

G
Galen 7, 150
gaudere (joy) 8, 22, 164, 175; *see also* ioie
Glossa Ordinara 30, 167
gostli sikenesse 144
grammarians *see Modistae*
greed (as spiritual illness) 54; *see also* ydropisi
Gregory the Great 56, 84, 171
Gregory of Nyssa 29, 167
Gregory of Nazianzus 29, 167
grief 13, 22, 105; *see also* emotions
Grosseteste, Robert
  De Artibus Liberalibus 18
  Dicta 54, 169
  Templum Dei 16, 54, 164, 169, 171
  Pseudonymous grammar text 22, 165
Guigo II 176

H
habitus (as habituated emotion) 13, 16
harmony
  physical 7
  spiritual/emotional 149, 151
hate 13–14; *see also* emotion
Henry of Lancaster 159

'heuines' (as spiritual pathology) 137–8, 143, 150–1
hilaritas 8, 11
Hippocrates 7
Hoccleve, Thomas 133
  Dialogue 133, 175
Hugh of Saint Cher 16
Hugh of St Victor
  Didascalicon 162, 165
  Homiliae in Ecclesiasten 162
Hugo of Fouilloy 53, 169
humblenesse 31; *see also* meekness
humilitas (humility) 15–16, 31; *see also* poverty of Spirit
humours 7, 9, 32, 52, 83, 92, 144–5

I
illnesses (spiritual) 17, 27, 54, 82, 144, 145
infirmitas 15, 16, 86, 145
imagination 4, 8, 18, 70, 75, 134, 135, 137, 143, 161, 165, 171; *see also* 'ymaginacion'
imbalance (emotional) 134, 150
immoderation (emotional) 135, 136, 138; *see also* 'vndiscrecion'
indeclinable parts of speech 22
instability (emotional) 134, 145, 146
intention
  through words 17, 23
  as part of memory phantasm 18
interjection (part of speech) 20–3, 165
  interjectional cry 67, 71, 125, 130
intersubjectivity 4, 26, 33–7, 60, 79, 83, 89–98, 104–6, 112–20, 128, 132, 142–9, 161
'ioie' 19, 97, 102, 112
irascible 7, 8, 12–15, 22–3, 38, 94, 115, 164; *see also* powers (of the soul)
irrational soul 21, 24, 89, 90
Isaac of Stella 13, 163
  Epistola de anima 13, 164
Isagoge ad Techne Galieni 7, 162
Itier of Vassy 11, 163

J
Jerome, St 16, 162
'Jhesu' (as healer) 117–19
John of Damascene, St 29, 167
  De fide orthodoxa 29, 167, 173
John of Garland 23, 166
John of La Rochelle (Rupella) 13, 16, 164, 173, 175
  Summa de anima 13, 14, 164, 173
  Summa de vitiis 15, 164

Tractatus de divisione multiplici potentiarum animae 13, 14, 164
John Trevisa 12, 163, 171
Julian of Norwich 25, 57, 71, 85, 86, 87, 109, 111, 116, 117, 174
Revelation of Divine Love 57, 86, 111, 116, 166, 170–5

K
Kenosis 91, 109, 124; *see also* meekness

L
Lateran IV 16, 39, 52
Leclercq, Jean 162, 163, 165, 169, 172, 176, 177
lectio divina 2, 8–10, 70, 162, 163, 170, 176
lectio spiritualis 8–11
'letuarie' (medicinal drink) 83, 173
'longynge' 91, 109, 112, 118, 130
Lombard Peter 29, 58, 167, 170
Sententiae in IV Libris Distinctae 29, 165, 167, 172

M
madness 12, 26, 85, 131, 134, 136, 137, 139, 147; *see also* 'woodnes'
Maidstone, Richard 26, 52, 59, 70, 170
'medelid' 33, 93–4, 97, 114–15
Medicus animarum 52
'medicinable' 9, 91, 117, 118, 141
meditatio (meditation) 2, 8–10, 26, 82–92, 98, 104, 108, 120, 124, 133–5, 160, 162, 163, 174
meekness 34, 40, 57, 91, 109, 116–20, 129, 132, 146–50
melancholia 8, 12, 177
memory phantasm 18, 135
Modistae 21, 23, 165
Myroure of Our Lady 150, 163, 178

N
natura lapsa 12, 29
non-naturals (*res non-naturales*) 7, 8, 11, 153, 162
air and the environment 7, 162
diet 8–11
exercise/rest 6–8, 11
sleeping and waking 7
evacuation and repletion 7, 9
passions/accidents of the soul 8–10; *see also* passions

O
Odilo of Cluny 86, 172
Olson, Glending 2, 160

oratio 8, 17, 20–3, 162; *see also* prayer
Orchard of Syon 11, 149, 163, 178
Origen 12

P
Pantegni 14
Passions *see* emotions, medieval terms for
pastoralia 16, 54
pathology 13, 26, 60, 134, 141, 143, 146–7
'penaunce' 19, 59, 170
Peraldus, William 30, 167
Peter the Chanter 16, 17, 164
pain 7, 10, 21–9, 31, 36, 37, 47, 60–7, 73–6, 82–113, 119, 120–4; *see also* emotions
phantasia 18
pharmaceutical 9, 11, 82
phlebotomy 49, 52, 79
physicians 2, 6
physiognomy 54, 136, 143, 144, 149
pity 14, 16, 20, 62–8, 83; *see also* emotions
as medicine 62, 87, 88, 89
and intersubjectivity 90–100, 107, 112
as 'reuthe' 89, 93
poisons 32, 56, 57, 134, 136, 138
Pope Adrian VI 1
Pope Innocent III 44
Pore Catiff 18–19, 117
poverty of Spirit 15, 31, 38; *see also* beatitudes
powers (of the soul) 22, 114, 149
prayer 10, 17, 23, 35–9, 61– 79, 101, 105–15, 120–32, 138, 143, 154, 155, 162–6, 175; see also *oratio*
Prickynge of Love 26, 33, 82, 87, 89, 91, 92, 140, 168, 171–7
Priscian 21, 22, 165, 165
probatio 134, 142; *see also* discernment
Prick of Conscience 25, 28, 39–49, 114, 168, 169
pride 15, 26, 30–4, 38, 49, 57, 71, 85–6, 91, 94, 117, 118, 133–40, 146–9
as *superbia* 15, 86, 164
Psalms 26, 52, 60, 68, 74, 121, 160, 163, 166, 170, 173–4
The Penitential Psalms 57, 59, 70, 71; *see also* Richard Maidstone
Pseudo-Kilwardby 22, 165
Purgation 9–11, 16, 17, 32, 53–6, 79, 84, 88, 116–17

Q
quadrivium 16, 18, 20

INDEX

R
recreatio 8, 18
regimen 7, 11, 16, 134, 162
Regimen sanitatis salernitanum 7
remedy 27, 33, 59–61, 86, 96, 104, 113, 124
Respice in Faciem Christi 81
Richard Misyn 56
Richard of St Victor
   De quatuor gradibus violentae caritatis 13, 113, 163, 174
   Benjamin Minor 33, 137, 163
Rigaldi, Odo 13
Rolle, Richard
   Ego Dormio 5, 56, 169
   Form of Living 19, 56, 169
   Incendium Amoris 56, 169, 173
   Oleum Effusum 56, 169
'root(s)e' 33, 38, 45, 59, 116, 124, 127, 149
rotten 46, 59
Ruben (drede personified) 33, 34; *see also* fear
rumination (*ruminatio*) 8, 133, 163

S
sacramental 19, 35, 39, 94
sadness 12, 14, 53
   as 'sorowe' 11, 20, 56, 71, 85, 96, 103, 156
   as *tristicia* 164, 175
Salerno 12
salvation (as spiritual health) 6, 12–15, 28–9, 88, 117, 151
sanatus 7, 85, 162
'Saule' 58, 112, 137
Scala Claustralium 176
Secretum Secretorum 7, 162
sickness 13–17, 26–8, 37, 51–4, 61, 66–9, 84–6, 95–8, 113, 119, 136–40, 144, 155
   caused by sin 27, 54, 95, 144
selfhood 4, 5, 88
   confessional self-awareness 51, 67, 68, 78, 96, 117, 148, 149
   relational self-awareness 30, 127
   self-hatred or 'holy hatrede' 94, 107, 139, 149
selfless 29, 108, 108, 115–17; *see also* meekness
signification 21, 22, 47
   per modum conceptus 21, 22
   per modum affectus 21–4, 121, 132
actus exercitus 23
actus significatus 23

sloth (spiritual torpor) 53, 54, 138, 140, 147
Speculum Vitae 25, 28, 35–40, 90, 115, 175
spes (hope) 164, 175; *see also* emotions
stimulus carnis 86–7, 91, 171
stomach 6, 8, 53, 54, 144
'surryp' 97
sweet 83, 97–9, 122, 124, 130, 131
syncategoremata 21, 165; *see also* interjection (part of speech)

T
taste 11, 44, 88, 98–102
Talking of the Love of God, A 26, 112, 121–32
therapy (etymology) 5
   as spiritual concept 2, 12, 16, 26
Timaeus 6, 22, 161
travel (effects of) 86–7, 135, 137, 172
Tretise of Ghostly Battle 92, 173
tribulation ('tribulacion') 52, 87–8, 91–5
trust ('triste') 33, 94; *see also* emotional complex
trivium 16, 18, 20
Troilus and Criseyde 51, 168
tumour 53, 85
   of pride 86, 91
   of conscience 9, 92
Twelve Profits of Tribulation 52, 87–8, 91, 168, 172–3

V
virtue (as opposite of vice) 13–20, 26–31, 37–8, 42–3, 55–8, 88, 90, 91, 119, 153
   and spiritual pathologies 144, 146, 147
   and discretion *see* discernment
'vndiscrecion' 142, 143
'vndiscreet' 134–7, 149

W
Walter Hilton 5, 32, 92, 134, 161
   Scale of Perfection 5, 34, 57, 91, 117, 137
   Eight Chapters on Perfection 141, 176, 177
   Of Angels Song 137, 140, 176, 177
   Epistle on the Mixed Life 142, 177
William of Auvergne 13, 16, 53–5, 169
   De Virtutibus 13
William de Montibus 16, 53, 164, 169
   Peniteas Cito 16, 53, 55, 169
William of St Thierry 13, 84
William Peraldus 30, 167
   Summae virtutum ac vitiorum 167

'wittes' (as aspects of psychology) 19, 34, 69, 70, 77, 101, 119, 137
  as 'wytte' 40, 45, 137
'woodnes' 134, 136, 137, 139
wrath 15, 31, 118; *see also* emotion

Y
'ydelnesse' (*accidia*) 140, 143; *see also* sloth
'ymaginacion' 34, 120, 135, 137; *see also* faculties, of the soul